The Toxicity of Methyl Mercury

The Johns Hopkins Series in Environmental Toxicology
Zoltan Annau, editor

also in this series:
Neurobehavioral Toxicology
edited by Zoltan Annau

Lead Toxicity: History and Environmental Impact
edited by Richard Lansdown and William Yule

Toxic Chemicals, Health, and the Environment
edited by Lester B. Lave and Arthur C. Upton

The Toxicity of Methyl Mercury

edited by
Christine U. Eccles and Zoltan Annau

The Johns Hopkins University Press
Baltimore and London

The Johns Hopkins University Press
701 West 40th Street
Baltimore, Maryland 21211
The Johns Hopkins Press Ltd., London

The paper used in this publication meets the minimum requirements of American
National Standard for Information Sciences—Permanence of Paper for Printed
Library Materials, ANSI Z39.48-1984.

Library of Congress Cataloging-in-Publication Data

The Toxicity of methyl mercury.

(The Johns Hopkins series of environmental toxicology)
Includes bibliographies and index.
1. Methylmercury—Toxicology. 2. Methylmercury—
Physiological effect. 3. Neurotoxic agents.
I. Eccles, Christine U., 1952–   . II. Annau,
Zoltan, 1936–   . III Series.
RA1231.M5T69 1987   615.9′25663   86-46278
ISBN 0-8018-3449-X (alk. paper)

Contents

List of Figures   vii

List of Tables   xi

Introduction   xiii

1. The Quantitative Measurement of Methyl Mercury
    Paul Mushak   1

2. Biological Target Sites of Mercurials
    Adil E. Shamoo   13

3. The Absorption, Distribution, and Excretion of Methyl Mercury
    Laszlo Magos   24

4. Dose-Response Relationships in Humans: Methyl Mercury Epidemics in Japan and Iraq
    David O. Marsh   45

5. The Experimental Neuropathology of Methyl Mercury
    Louis W. Chang   54

6. The Pathological Lesions of Methyl Mercury Intoxication in Monkeys
    N. Karle Mottet, Cheng-Mei Shaw, and Thomas M. Burbacher   73

7. Sensory Deficits Caused by Exposure to Methyl Mercury
    Zoltan Annau and Christine U. Eccles   104

8. Prenatal Exposure to Methyl Mercury
    Christine U. Eccles and Zoltan Annau   114

9. The Alteration of Protein Synthesis by Methyl Mercury
    David J. Thomas and Tore L. M. Syversen   131

10. The Neurochemical Effects of Methyl Mercury in the Brain
    Hannu Komulainen and Jouko Tuomisto   172

11. Neurophysiological Effects of Mercurials
    William D. Atchison   189

12. Tissue Culture: A Useful Model for Studying the Mechanism of Methyl Mercury Toxicity on Nerve Tissue
    Kedar N. Prasad   220

List of Contributors   253

Index   255

Figures

2.1. Side chain targets in heavy-metal binding   14

2.2. Mercury content in a blood-free brain homogenate   20

5.1. Electron histochemical method suggesting mercury's affinity for biological membranes   56

5.2. Proliferation of Bergmann's glial fiber projecting through the molecular layer from the Purkinje granule cell junction   60

5.3. Electron microscopy showing pyknotic and atrophic cerebellar granule cells in a rat intoxicated by methyl mercury   61

5.4. Dorsal root ganglion in a normal rat   62

5.5. Dorsal root ganglion in a rat intoxicated by mercury   62

5.6. Dorsal root ganglion in a rat treated with methyl mercury   63

5.7. Vacuolar change in a large dorsal root ganglion neuron in a rat intoxicated by methyl mercury   63

5.8. Large dorsal root ganglion neuron of a rat treated with methyl mercury, showing a part of the cytoplasm   64

5.9. Large area of a dorsal root neuron filled with fragments of endoplasmic reticulum in methyl mercury treated rat   64

5.10. Vacuolar degeneration of a large neuron in the dorsal root ganglion in a rat treated with methyl mercury   65

5.11. Accumulation of lysosomes and axoplasmic debris near the node of Ranvier in a methyl mercury treated rat   65

5.12. Protrusion of axoplasm at the node of Ranvier filled with axoplasmic debris, in methyl mercury treated rat   66

5.13. Breakdown of the myelin sheath in a dorsal root fiber, in methyl mercury treated rat   67

6.1. Kidney proximal convoluted cell containing inclusions similar to those described in the Paneth cells   79

6.2. Tip of a crypt of Lieberkühn   82

6.3. Portions of the Paneth cell cytoplasm   83

6.4. Graph of one of the Paneth cell lysosomes, showing a peak for mercury   84

6.5.   Liver and hepatocytes containing vacuoles that stain for lipid with oil red O stain   85

6.6.   Macaque myocardium   86

6.7.   Occipital cortex of a macaque with blood mercury level of above 2.5 ppm   88

6.8.   Cerebral cortex showing glial cells   89

6.9.   Abnormal morphology in spermatozoa of macaque with methyl mercury exposure   94

6.10.   Brain of an infant congenitally exposed to methyl mercury   96

11.1.   Time course of contraction inhibition with methyl mercury   191

11.2.   Effects of methyl mercury on EPP amplitude at the rat neuromuscular junction   194

11.3.   Effects of methyl mercury on EPP amplitude   195

11.4.   Effects of methyl mercury on neurotransmitter release at rat neuromuscular junction   197

11.5.   Effects of increasing $[Ca^{2+}]_o$ on MEPP frequency in the absence and presence of methyl mercury   201

11.6.   Time course of effects of methyl mercury on MEPP frequency   202

11.7.   End-plate depolarization produced by iontophoretic application of acetylcholine before and after methyl mercury   206

11.8.   Effects of methyl mercury on the resting membrane potential, and the potential responses induced by iontophoretic application of acetylcholine   207

11.9.   Absence of an effect of methyl mercury on dopamine-induced current in voltage-clamped neuroblastoma cell   208

11.10.   Current-voltage relationships for peak sodium current and steady-state potassium current before and during an application of methyl mercury chloride   209

11.11.   Effects of methyl mercury on components of voltage-dependent ionic current   210

11.12.   Effects of methyl mercury on the action potential   211

11.13.   Resting membrane potentials of muscle fibers after exposure to methyl mercury or $HgCl_2$ 211

12.1.   Sensitivity of NB and C-6 cells to CH_3HgCl 222

12.2.   Effect of PGE_1 on NB and C-6 cells   226

12.3.   Effect of R020-1724 on C-6 cells in presence of CH_3HgCl 228

12.4.   Effects of vitamin E on CH_3HgCl-induced toxicity   229

12.5.   Effect of vitamin C on CH_3HgCl growth inhibiting effect in NB
         cells   231

12.6.   Modification of glutamate effect on NB cells in culture by organic
         mercury   233

12.7.   Modification of glutamate effect on NB cells in culture by
         manganese chloride   234

12.8.   Effect of CH_3HgCl on protein phosphorylation in cytosol fraction of
         C-6 cells, as shown by results of polyacrylamide gel
         electrophoresis   239

12.9.   Effect of CH_3HgCl on protein phosphorylation in particulate
         fraction of C-6 cells   240

12.10.   Effect of CH_3HgCl on protein phosphorylation in crude nuclear
         fraction of C-6 cells   241

12.11.   Effect of CH_3HgCl on protein phosphorylation in cytosol fraction of
         NB cells   245

12.12.   Effect of CH_3HgCl on protein phosphorylation in particulate
         fraction of NB cells   246

12.13.   Effect of CH_3HgCl on protein phosphorylation in crude nuclear
         fraction of NB cells   247

Tables

1.1. Column packings for GLC analysis of methyl mercury   4

1.2. Detector systems for GLC analysis of methyl mercury   5

1.3. GLC analysis procedures for methyl mercury   6

3.1. Distribution of methyl mercury between red blood cells and plasma   27

3.2. Organ to blood mercury concentration ratios after methyl mercury treatment   29

3.3. Mercury in brain after nontoxic dose of methyl mercury   30

3.4. Biological half time of mercury after exposure to methyl mercury   34

4.1. Frequency of paresthesia according to estimated peak concentration of blood mercury   49

8.1. Neuropathology produced by developmental exposure to methyl mercury   120

8.2. Behavioral effects of developmental exposure to methyl mercury   121

10.1. Effect of methyl mercury on brain cholinergic neurotransmission   174

10.2. Effect of methyl mercury on brain dopaminergic neurotransmission   177

10.3. Effect of methyl mercury on brain noradrenergic neurotransmission   178

10.4. Effect of methyl mercury on brain serotonergic neurotransmission   180

10.5. Effect of methyl mercury on brain GABAergic and amino-acid related transmission   182

12.1. Modification by prostaglandins of CH_3HgCl effect in glioma cells in culture   227

12.2. Effect of glioma "factor(s)" on CH_3HgCl-induced growth inhibition in NB and glioma cells in culture   231

12.3. Modification by metals of glutamate effect on NB cells in culture   232

12.4. Binding of [^{3}H]-glutamic acid with 50,000 × g pellet of mouse neuroblastoma cells   235

12.5. Effect of methyl mercuric chloride on prostaglandin E$_1$ sensitive adenylate cyclases in glioma and neuroblastoma cells in culture   236

12.6. Effect of methyl mercuric chloride on changes in amounts of phosphorylation of cytosol proteins of glioma cells   242

12.7. Effect of methyl mercuric chloride on changes in amounts and phosphorylation of proteins of particulate fraction of glioma cells   243

12.8. Effect of methyl mercuric chloride on changes in amounts of phosphorylation of crude nuclear proteins of glioma cells   244

Introduction

Environmental exposure to organic mercury is a significant health problem, as the abundant clinical reports that followed the Japanese and Iraqi epidemics of methyl mercury poisoning demonstrated. Attention to mercury intensified after it was established that mercuric ion can be methylated biologically upon distribution in rivers, estuaries, and lakes. Once formed, mercuric ion is rapidly removed from the aquatic environment through bioaccumulation. Recognition of these processes is important when the continuing widespread industrial use of chiefly inorganic forms of mercury is considered. High levels of contamination by environmental mercury have been reported recently in the United States.

Reports from the literature on clinical and experimental studies demonstrate that neurological disturbances dominate the clinical features of methyl mercury poisoning. The chapters in this book review a wide range of effects of methyl mercury, with primary emphasis on its neurotoxicity. Much of this information is not covered in review form elsewhere. Material reviewed previously is included here because of its overall importance to the subject. Furthermore, a brief survey of the literature on methyl mercury reveals that, following a surge of clinical and experimental studies in the 1960s and 1970s, relatively little attention has been given to this organometal.

Selected reviews of topics related to the toxicity of methyl mercury, which have not been previously organized in a single volume, are included in this book. The information presented here is intended primarily to assist clinicians, researchers, and regulatory scientists who want to become familiar with a broad range of studies in clinical and experimental toxicity. Chapters 1, 2, and 3 describe fundamental information necessary for understanding the problems related to a quantitative analysis of organic and inorganic mercury in biological tissue (physicochemical properties of mercurials) and principles of absorption, distribution, and excretion in experimental animals. Chapter 4 reviews dose-response relationships observed in human epidemics in Japan and Iraq. Chapters 5 and 6 review experimental pathology observed after exposing rodents and primates to methyl mercury. Much of the primate work described is the result of recently completed studies not previously published. Chapter 7 addresses the consequences of prenatal exposure to methyl mercury, with a focus on the experimental literature. Chapters 8, 9, 10, and 11 deal with subjects that are related to possible mechanisms of toxicity and review the effects of exposure to methyl mercury on protein synthesis, neuro-chemistry, and neurophysiology. The use of tissue culture models as a means of answering mechanistic questions related to the toxicity of mercury is discussed in Chapter 12.

The Toxicity of Methyl Mercury

ONE

The Quantitative Measurement of Methyl Mercury

Paul Mushak

Until the 1960s, the measurement of mercury in various media invariably involved determining total element levels. Since then, the focus has shifted to measurement of specific chemical forms associated with discrete effects, for example, methyl mercury and associated neurotoxicity. Details of such speciation analysis, with particular reference to methyl mercury, are the subject of this chapter.

Over the years, several reviews have described methods for the analysis of methyl mercury in biological systems (Mushak 1973; Mushak 1977; Rodriguez-Vazquez 1978), and this discussion summarizes the earlier data and includes more recent reports of analytical methodology for this agent. In many cases, it is necessary to carry out combined analyses of methyl mercury as well as total or inorganic mercury analyses to interpret fully the agent's behavior in biological systems. Methods for these additional determinations are included in this section. Since speciation analysis requires sampling and sample manipulation procedures that are different from those used for total element measurement, we will deal with those steps separately.

Sampling and Sample Handling

Even under conditions of excessive exposure, levels of methyl mercury in biological systems are present at trace levels, and the usual precautions must be taken both to minimize loss of mercury from the sample and to avoid sample contamination. The risk of contamination of samples by methyl mercury is less than for the inorganic form.

Standard protocols for sampling steps in trace analysis work are now widely distributed in the literature (e.g., Stoeppler et al. 1979) and will not be detailed here. It is enough to say that every precaution should be taken (1) to employ mercury-free ware in sample collection, (2) to minimize the time lapse between sample collection and analysis, and (3) to preserve the amount of the specific form of the mercurial being analyzed, in this case methyl mercury, via either direct loss or artifactual transformation to the inorganic element.

While there is considerable controversy in the literature concerning the use of scalp hair as an "internal" indicator of exposure to inorganic metals because of the difficulty in distinguishing between internal deposition and external or surface contamination, we would not expect this difficulty to apply as readily to methyl mercury, where the risk of external contamination is comparatively low. The problem would be more severe with inorganic mercury and might affect studies in which levels of both methyl mercury and inorganic mercury in hair are being measured.

In analysis of soft tissues for mercury or other elements, it is often the practice to homogenize samples in which there is heterogeneity of the agent's distribution. This is usually done with an ordinary laboratory apparatus, but some laboratories have attempted to minimize contamination problems by alternative methods. In the method of Nichols and Hageman (1979), biological samples wrapped in layers of polyethylene are immersed in liquid nitrogen, and the frozen samples are pulverized.

As noted above, a major consideration with sample-handling for analysis of methyl mercury is the preservation of the amount of this form at the time of sampling. This includes both sample storage and sample manipulation just prior to analysis.

Suzuki and Yamamoto (1982) observed that levels of methyl mercury in stored hair samples are stable up to 11 years, indicating both stability toward outright loss from the matrix and stability of the carbon-metal bond. Various tissues from animals exposed to methyl mercury-203 were found by Kelman et al. (1977) to retain the mercury label over the 7-day interval studied and at temperatures of $8°$ C and $24°$ C. While this study indicates that, under these conditions, mercury itself is not lost from samples, one cannot conclude that there was no change in the amount of methyl mercury via demethylation, since retention was studied by total label radiometry. This author has observed (unpublished data) that levels of methyl mercury in experimental animal soft tissue decline at ambient temperature and at relatively short time periods. This is probably attributable both to bacterial action and to continuing transformation activity in the tissue.

Sample-processing steps prior to laboratory analysis will differ for methyl mercury, compared with analysis of total mercury, for example. Sample mineralization cannot be carried out in the analysis of methyl mercury because such a process will also demethylate the mercurial. Hence, one must strike a balance between sample treatment that is chemically mild enough to keep methyl mercury structurally intact, but vigorous enough to liberate the agent from tight binding to matrix components. The general approach has usually been partial matrix modification, through use of a mineral acid in tandem with other agents, such as metal ions. Both acid and added agents work in concert either to compete with methyl mercury for binding sites or to compete with binding sites for methyl mercury, while acid further functions to fragment or otherwise modify tissue components. This topic is discussed in more detail below.

The Measurement of Methyl Mercury in Biological Media

Virtually all known procedures for measuring methyl mercury in biological media have specifically involved the monomethyl form. In most cases, dimethyl mercury is either absent or too volatile to remain in samples during homogenizing or other sample preparation. With most procedures, which usually involve acid treatment of samples, any dimethyl mercury present would undergo dealkylation to monomethyl mercury. Since it is the monomethyl form that is of direct interest in human neurotoxicity, the greater focus on this form is appropriate.

Gas-Liquid Chromatography

In its various analytical manifestations, chromatography is a powerful tool for separation and subsequent specific measurement of a vast variety of chemical species, so it is not surprising that chromatographic methods have been widely exploited in analysis of methyl mercury.

General Considerations   Methyl mercury has the requisite properties—thermal stability and adequate volatility—for gas-liquid chromatography (GLC), the form of chromatography most commonly employed. Two major components of the GLC system are of particular importance in methyl mercury analysis: the column/column packing and the detection system.

While methyl mercury and its various covalent derivatives have sufficient thermal stability for GLC analysis, this property is strongly influenced by the material from which the column is fabricated. Because metal columns (e.g., stainless steel) can promote degradation of methyl mercury at elevated temperatures, glass columns are generally necessary, particularly for measurements at the trace level (Johansson et al. 1970). Similarly, direct, on-column injection is preferable to contact with the heated metal surface in an injection port.

A number of column packings have been employed in GLC measurement of methyl mercury (see Table 1.1). Solid supports have commonly been of the diatomaceous earth type and have been treated in various ways, for example, acid-washing and silanization, to minimize adsorptive loss of the mercurial. Such column retention is particularly troublesome at very low levels of methyl mercury. Even with quite inert supports, it is frequently necessary to treat or "dress" the column with samples of the mercurial to maintain adsorptive site saturation.

While silicone gums and oils as stationary phases have found some application in GLC procedures for methyl mercury, better performance in this case seems to reside with the polyester phases, for example, diethyleneglycol

Table 1.1 Column packings for GLC analysis of methyl mercury

Packing	Loading (%)	Performance	Reference
1. Silicones			
Mixture of OV-17/QF-1 on Chromosorb 101.	2.0, OV-17 2.0, QF-1	Working sensitivity for methyl mercury in fish, 0.05-0.1 ppm.	Bache and Lisk 1971
Mixture of OV-17/QF-1 on 80/100 Chromosorb-W-HP.	1.5, OV-17 2.0, QF-1	Measure of methyl mercury in blood, feces, fish, hair, soft tissue at relatively low temperatures (110°C) and high sensitivity (2 ppb).	Cappon and Smith 1977
2. Polyesters			
Diethyleneglycol succinate on Chromosorb S or Celite 545.	5.0–25.0	DEGS and other polyesters better than silicone and hydrocarbon oil phases; detection limit ca. 1.0 picogram.	Sumino 1968
Butane-1,4-diol succinate on 100/120 Chromosorb W, AW/DMCS.	2.0	Methyl mercury in fish and grain products; detection limit 20 picograms.	Newsome 1971
Poly (ethylene glycol) succinate on Chromosorb G, AW/DMCS.	2.0	PEGS column superior to other phases. Methyl mercury residue on fruits and vegetables.	Tatton and Wagstaffe 1969
3. Polyethyleneglycols			
Carbowax 20M on Chromosorb W, AW/DMCS, or Teflon 6.	10.0	Methyl mercury in fish, meats, eggs, other foodstuffs; working detection limit several ppb.	Westöö 1966, 1968
Carbowax 20M on Chromosorb G, 80/100, AW/DMCS.	2.5	Methyl mercury in fish; detection comparable to Westöö.	Analytical Methods Committee 1977
4. Chemically Bonded Packing			
Carbowax 400 (low K') on Proasil.	—	Soft tissues and urine; detection limit ca. 20 ppb.	Zarnegar and Mushak 1974

succinate (DEGS) and polyethyleneglycol succinate (PEGS), as well as certain of the polyethyleneglycol coatings (e.g., Carbowax 20M). Use of a packing in which the phase is chemically bonded to the support minimizes the necessity for column maintenance. For instance, Zarnegar and Mushak (1974) employed Durapak Carbowax 400 (low K') in analysis of methyl mercury over extended periods of time without any perceptible loss of system sensitivity attributable to analyte adsorption in the column.

A number of GLC detection systems have been employed in analysis of methyl mercury (see Table 1.2). The most common of these has been electron capture (EC) detection, employing assemblies fitted with either tritium or nickel-63 foils. This mode of detection offers excellent sensitivity down to picogram levels. Since the tritium EC system is much more sensitive than one having nickel-63, and operates at more moderate temperatures for optimal response, it has been more popular. On the other hand, it is more easily contaminated and may entail considerable maintenance time.

Detectors of the EC type have the drawback of nonspecificity for mercurials, and interferents such as halogenated compounds can cause difficulties. This intrinsic limitation has prompted the use of methyl mercury specific or mercury specific detection systems as an alternative.

Use of a mass spectrometer as a detector (GLC-MS) provides the most specific means of identification (e.g., Johansson et al. 1970), and the more recent technique of mass fragmentography, where one or more fragments are selectively analyzed under computer control, permits detection at levels even below that of the EC detector.

Given the considerable expense and required operator expertise involved in GLC-MS, such alternatives as atomic emission or atomic absorption spectroscopy appear to offer the best compromise between accessibility and specificity without loss in sensitivity.

Table 1.2   Detector systems for GLC analysis of methyl mercury

Detector Type	Advantages	Disadvantages	Reference
1. Electron capture detectors, generally ^{3}H foil.	Excellent sensitivity, easy to use.	Sensitive to all electron-capturing agents, ^{3}H foil easily contaminated.	Westöö 1966
2. GLC unit interfaced with mass spectrometer.	Highly specific for methyl mercury, excellent sensitivity.	High cost, high level of operator expertise.	Johansson et al. 1970
3. GLC unit interfaced with flameless atomic absorption system.	Specific for mercury in column effluents, relatively simple to operate and maintain, reasonable sensitivity.	Initial interfacing of GLC and AA units.	Longbottom, 1972; Dressman 1972; Gonzalez and Ross 1972; Bye and Paus 1979
4. GLC unit interfaced with argon plasma emission system.	Specific for mercury in effluents, excellent sensitivity.	Somewhat more complicated than AA detector in installation and operation.	Bache and Lisk 1971

The cold-vapor atomic absorption (AA) method widely employed for inorganic mercury measurement has been adapted for function as an element-specific detector (Longbottom 1972; Dressman 1972; Gonzales and Ross 1972; Bye and Paus 1979). In all cases, methyl mercury in the GLC effluent must first be decomposed, with mercury from decomposition being swept into the measurement cell of an atomic absorption spectrometer. Of these procedures, that of Bye and Paus (1979) appears most feasible for most laboratories. GLC effluent is passed through a pyrolysis tube maintained at a temperature high enough to "crack" the methyl mercury, the elemental mercury then being measured in a cuvette positioned in the light beam of the spectrometer unit. In the approach of Bache and Lisk (1971), mercury in GLC effluent is subsequently measured by emission spectroscopy in a microwave-generated helium plasma. All these approaches are sensitive enough to measure the levels of methyl mercury occurring in biological media, with the plasma emission technique being sensitive to the subpicogram range.

The above specific detection modes generally allow less processing and fewer purification steps than EC detectors do, although the cold vapor AA technique does require exclusion of other ultraviolet-absorbing material.

Bioanalytical Applications   Extensive use of gas-liquid chromatography for measurement of methyl mercury in biological media (Table 1.3) dates to the detailed work in the late 1960s by Westöö in Sweden (Westöö 1966, 1967, 1968). In outline, the Westöö method entails the treatment of homogenized

Table 1.3   GLC analysis procedures for methyl mercury

Media	Sample Treatment	Form Analyzed	Reference
Fish, meat, kidney, etc.	Homogenized samples + HCl, cysteine used for separation from GLC interferents.	Methyl mercuric chloride	Westöö 1966, 1967, 1968
Fish	HBr used instead of HCl, copper (II) ion instead of mercury (II), toluene instead of benzene.	Methyl mercuric bromide	Uthe et al. 1972
Cereal grains	A mixture (10:1) of benzene-formic acid used instead of benzene.	Methyl mercuric bromide	Newsome 1971
Hair	Initial alkaline digestion, then acidification as per Westöö method.	Methyl mercuric chloride	Giovanoli-Jakubczak et al. 1974
Blood, fish, soft tissues, etc.	Initial alkaline digestion, acidification in HBr, use of thiosulfate as mercurial partitioning agent.	Methyl mercuric bromide	Cappon and Smith 1977

(if necessary) samples of fish, meat, kidney, eggs, and so on, with a hydrohalic acid (usually hydrochloric acid) in tandem with other added agents, to liberate the mercurial from its binding with ligands in the matrix. Liberated mercurial is then partitioned into an organic solvent such as benzene. Since this first extract is heavily contaminated with chromatographic interferents, the mercurial is then repartitioned into an aqueous phase using a complexing agent such as cysteine. The original organic phase is discarded, and the relatively clean aqueous fraction containing the mercury is sequentially acidified to liberate methyl mercury. Finally, the organomercurial is reextracted into benzene or another solvent.

The level of acidification adequate to strip the mercurial from matrix binding but sufficiently moderate to preserve the carbon-metal bond in the Westöö approach appears to be 2N in hydrochloric acid. Agents such as mercuric chloride and molybdic acid function in various ways to further promote mobilization of the mercurial into the liquid medium. While cysteine is used in the Westöö method for complexation and subsequent cleanup, other reagents have been found to serve the purpose.

Over the years, various steps in the basic Westöö scheme have been modified with use of different acids, dissociation promotion agents, and extraction solvents, as well as repartitioning chelants for the methyl mercury (e.g., Newsome 1971; Uthe et al. 1972), hydrobromic in lieu of hydrochloric acid, copper (II) ion instead of mercury (II), toluene instead of benzene, and thiosulfate instead of cysteine as a complexing/extracting agent.

More involved modifications of the original scheme include that of Giovanoli-Jakubczak et al. (1974), in which samples such as hair are first subjected to alkaline digestion, which strongly promotes dissociation of the mercurial. Subsequently, Cappon and Smith (1977) applied and extended such a preliminary alkaline digestion step to blood, fish, soft tissue, feces, and grain.

The basic Westöö procedure has been the subject of several external method validation surveys in which various laboratories measured the methyl mercury content of specially prepared samples. In the survey described by Holden (1973), a group coefficient of variation of 20 percent was obtained in the measurement of the mercurial in fish samples. A more recent survey (Analytical Methods Committee 1977), in which 10 laboratories received a special lot of canned tuna at two levels of methyl mercury, provided coefficients of variation (calculated by this author) of 8.7 percent and 11.3 percent for low and high levels, respectively. In a third interlaboratory survey (Schafer et al. 1975), also involving canned tuna fish samples, the basic Westöö method yielded an interlaboratory coefficient of variation of 5.8 percent, while preliminary alkalinizing of samples (as homogenates) gave a corresponding figure of 7.8 percent.

Other Chromatographic Approaches

High-performance liquid chromatography (HPLC) has recently become a promising alternative to gas-liquid chromatography for a number of chemical agents of biological/toxicological interest. At present, however, only limited use of this type of chromatography has been applied to measurement of mercurials. While HPLC would appear to offer limited advantage in cases where just methyl mercury itself is to be determined, it probably has much more flexibility in multimercurial measurement, for example, methyl mercury plus inorganic mercury. On the other hand, most of the commonly employed detector systems for HPLC use offer limited promise in terms of the sensitivity required for trace or ultra-trace analysis of mercurials.

MacCrehan and Durst (1978) employed reverse-phase HPLC and differential pulse electrochemical detection to analyze simple mixtures of methyl, ethyl, and phenyl mercury, as well as certified samples of tuna fish or shark meat for methyl mercury content. Using a Spherosorb ODS column and ammonium acetate in methanol/water, the organomercurial mixture was separated within 14 minutes. Detection limits rival that of GLC-EC (e.g., 2 ppb for methyl mercury). A major drawback to this particular HPLC system has to do with the electrochemical reduction mode of detection. As with many organometals, reduction occurs at an electrical potential where oxygen interferes, requiring a totally inert system. The authors enclosed their apparatus in an inert atmosphere chamber.

Brinckman et al. (1977) described the use of an HPLC system interfaced to a graphite-furnace atomic absorption spectrometer with automated sampling. Mobile phases were either ammonium acetate in water or 2-mercaptoethanol in methanol using a Lichrosorb C_8 column in the isocratic mode. The problem here is one of sensitivity of detection, most mercurials (methyl, ethyl, propyl, and butyl) being measurable only at parts-per-million (ppm) range—considerable analyte dilution occurs because of the basic configuration of the system.

A somewhat better system is that of Fujita and Takabatake (1983), where a conventional HPLC assembly has been interfaced with cold-vapor atomic absorption spectrometry via a continuous-flow reducing vessel. Eluates are mixed with an oxidant in a mixing coil and passed into a reduction chamber, and the liberated elemental mercury is swept into the cell of a mercury analyzer. Sensitivity appears to be much better than direct analysis of eluates.

Combined Analysis of Methyl and Total/Inorganic Mercury

Inorganic mercury in biological systems has generally been measured (1) by sequential measurement of both total and methyl mercury, the difference being assigned to the inorganic fraction, or (2) by specific quantitation of inorganic mercury content.

Estimation of inorganic mercury by difference is probably most problematic in cases where different approaches are used for total versus methyl mercury. These disparate techniques may have quite differing characteristics in terms of accuracy, bias, specificity, and so on.

In the reports of Westöö (see above), total mercury was routinely determined by neutron activation, and methyl mercury by GLC-EC. More commonly, total mercury analysis involves atomic absorption spectrometry of wet-ashed samples. In one interlaboratory survey procedure (Analytical Methods Committee 1977), samples of fish were mineralized with a mixture of sulfuric and nitric acids and hydrogen peroxide. After decomposition of excess peroxide, there is sequential sample treatment with, first, hydroxylamine and then tin (II) chloride in an aeration vessel. The tin (II) ion generates elemental mercury vapor, which is swept into the measurement cell of an atomic absorption spectrometer. Mercury is measured at 253.7 nm. Methyl mercury is measured simultaneously by GLC. The reduction/aeration step of the total mercury procedure is that of Magos (1971), discussed below.

A number of reports describing analysis of inorganic and organic mercury by relatively similar methods have appeared, avoiding the problems referred to earlier. The most popular of these approaches is that of Magos (Magos 1971; Magos and Clarkson 1972)—the cold-vapor atomic absorption technique. Partially digested samples (with organic mercury kept intact structurally) in a closed aeration vessel are first treated with a solution of stannous chloride to form elemental mercury vapor from liberated inorganic mercury (II), followed by sweeping of the vapor into a gas cell mounted in either a mercury analyzer or a conventional atomic absorption spectrometer (AAS), with measurement of the signal at 253.7 nm. Subsequent use of a solution containing a mixture of stannous and cadmium chloride results in the reductive volatilization of all mercury present, organic and inorganic. The difference in these measurements is an estimation of organic mercury content. Since the discrete form of the organomercurial cannot be determined in this way, GLC can be used in tandem with the cold vapor AAS method (Giovanoli-Jakubczak et al. 1974) for determination of both forms—methyl mercury and inorganic mercury, for example. The Magos method has found application in the analysis of such media as hair, kidney, brain, liver, and tuna fish.

An alternative approach for measurement of methyl mercury and inorganic mercury involves use of GLC for both forms, via conversion of inorganic mercury to an organomercurial amenable to GLC measurement. In the studies of Mushak et al. (Mushak et al. 1973; Zarnegar and Mushak 1974), inorganic mercury in urine or soft tissue homogenates was converted to either phenyl or methyl mercury in one approach (Zarnegar and Mushak 1974), and to pentafluorophenyl mercury in an alternative route (Mushak et al. 1973), using various organometallic or other reagents. Use of the reagent methyl (pentacyanocobaltate) to form methyl mercury from the inorganic precursor entails sequential GLC analysis, if methyl mercury already present as such is also determined. With the reagent, total methyl mercury is measured. Difference between this value and the organomercurial level without use of reagent gives inorganic mercury content. Working detection limits in various media are of the order of 20–50 parts per billion. In the related approach of Cappon and Smith (1977), inorganic mercury is converted to methyl mercury via reaction with tetramethyl tin (IV).

Direct measurement of methyl mercury and inorganic mercury, without the need for derivatizing the inorganic form, would appear feasible with HPLC. In the Fujita and Takabatake (1983) study discussed earlier, inorganic mercury is readily separated from mixtures of organomercurials. However, sensitivity of detection with existing detection systems still appears to be a limitation of this approach.

References

Analytical Methods Committee (1977). Determination of mercury and methyl mercury in fish. *Analyst* 102:769–776.

Bache, C. A., and Lisk, D. J. (1971). Gas chromatographic determination of organic mercury compounds by emission spectrometry in a helium plasma. *Anal Chem* 43:950–952.

Brinckman, W. R.; Blair, W. R.; Jewett, K. L.; and Iverson, W. P. (1977). Application of a liquid chromatograph coupled to a flameless atomic absorption detector for speciation of trace organometallic compounds. *J Chromatogr Sci* 15:493–503.

Bye, R., and Paus, P. E. (1979). Determination of alkylmercury compounds in fish tissue with an atomic absorption spectrophotometer used as a specific gas chromatographic detector. *Anal Chim Acta* 107:169–175.

Cappon, C. J., and Smith, J. C. (1977). Gas-chromatographic determination of inorganic mercury and organomercurials in biological materials. *Anal Chem* 49:365–369.

Dressman, R. C. (1972). The conversion of phenyl mercuric salts to diphenyl mercury and phenyl mercuric chloride upon gas-chromatographic injection. *J Chromatogr Sci* 10:468–472.

Fujita, M., and Takabatake, E. (1983). Continuous flow reducing vessel in determination of mercuric compounds by liquid chromatography / cold vapor atomic absorption spectrometry. *Anal Chem* 55:454–457.

Giovanoli-Jakubczak, T.; Greenwood, M. R.; Smith, J. C.; and Clarkson, T. W. (1974). Determination of total and inorganic mercury in hair by flameless atomic absorption and of methyl mercury by gas chromatography. *Clin Chem* 20:222–229.

Gonzalez, J. G., and Ross, R. T. (1972). Interfacing of an atomic absorption spectrophotometer with a gas-liquid chromatograph for the determination of trace quantities of alkyl-mercury compounds in fish tissue. *Anal Lett* 5:683–694.

Holden, A. V. (1973). Mercury and organochlorine residue analysis of fish and aquatic mammals. *Pestic Sci* 4:399–408.

Johansson, B.; Ryhage, R.; and Westöö, J. (1970). Identification and determination of methyl mercury compounds in fish using combination gas chromatograph-mass spectrometer. *Acta Chem Scand* 24:2349–2354.

Kelman, B. J.; Bush, D. M.; Sasser, L. B.; and Jarboe, G. E. (1977). Respiration of mercury from rats and release of mercury from stored rat tissues treated with methyl mercury chloride. *Health Phys* 33:139–141.

Longbottom, J. E. (1972). Inexpensive mercury-specific gas chromatographic detector. *Anal Chem* 44:1111–1112.

MacCrehan, W. A., and Durst, R. A. (1978). Measurement of organomercury species in biological samples by liquid chromatography with differential pulse electrochemical detection. *Anal Chem* 50:2108–2112.

Magos, L. (1971). Selective atomic absorption determination of inorganic mercury and methyl mercury in undigested biological samples. *Analyst* 96:847–853.

Magos, L., and Clarkson, T. W. (1972). Atomic absorption determination of total inorganic and organic mercury in blood. *J Assoc Off Anal Chem* 55:966–971.

Mushak, P. (1973). Gas-liquid chromatography in the analysis of mercury (II) compound. *Environ Health Perspect* 2:55–60.

—— (1977). Advances in the analysis of toxic heavy elements having variable chemical forms. *J Anal Toxicol* 1:286–291.

Mushak, P.; Tibbetts, F. E. III; Zarnegar, P.; and Fisher, G. B. (1973). Perhalobenzene sulfinates as reagents in the determination of inorganic mercury in various media by gas-liquid chromatography. *J Chromatogr* 87:215–226.

Newsome, W. H. (1971). Determination of methyl mercury in fish and in cereal grain products. *J Agr Food Chem* 19:567–569.

Nichols, J. A., and Hageman, L. R. (1979). Non-contaminating, representative sampling by shattering of cold, brittle, biological tissues. *Anal Chem* 51:1591–1593.

Rodriguez-Vazquez, J. A. (1978). Gas-chromatographic determination of organomercury (II) compounds. *Tolanta* 25:299–310.

Schafer, M. L.; Rhea, U.; Peeler, J. T.; Hamilton, C. H.; and Campbell, J. E. (1975). Method for the estimation of methyl mercuric compounds in fish. *J Agr Food Chem* 23:1079–1083.

Stoeppler, M.; Valenta, P.; and Nurnberg, H. W. (1979). Application of independent methods and standard materials: An effective approach to reliable trace and ultra trace analysis of metals and metalloids in environmental and biological matrices. *Fresenius. 2. Annal Chem* 297:22–34.

Sumino, K. (1968). Analysis of organic mercury compounds by gas chromatography, I: Analytical and extraction methods for organic mercury compounds. *Kobe J Med Sci* 14:115–130.

Suzuki, J., and Yamamoto, R. (1982). Organic mercury levels in human hair with and without storage for eleven years. *Bull Environ Contam Toxicol* 28:186–188.

Tatton, J. O'G., and Wagstaffe, P. J. (1969). Identification and determination of organomercurial fungicide residues by thin-layer and gas chromatography. *J Chromatogr* 44:284–289.

Uthe, J. F.; Colomon, J.; and Guft, B. (1972). Rapid semimicromethod for the determination of methyl mercury in fish tissue. *J Assoc Off Anal Chem* 55:583–589.

Westöö, G. (1966). Determination of methyl-mercury compounds in foodstuffs, I. *Acta Chem Scand* 20:2131–2140.

———— (1967). Determination of methyl mercury compounds in foodstuffs, II: Determination of methyl mercury in fish, eggs, meat and liver. *Acta Chem Scand* 21:1790–1800.

———— (1968). Determination of methyl mercury salts in various kinds of biological media. *Acta Chem Scand* 22:2277–2280.

Zarnegar, P., and Mushak, P. (1974). Quantitative measurement of inorganic mercury and organomercurials in water and biological media by gas-liquid chromatography. *Anal Chim Acta* 69:389–401.

T W O

Biological Target Sites of Mercurials

Adil E. Shamoo

Heavy metals and their derivatives have many deleterious effects on health (Nordberg 1976; Clarkson et al. 1983; O'Neill and Holtzman 1984; U.S. EPA 1984*a*, 1984*b*, 1984*c*). The heavy metals that are of concern in environmental issues are cadmium (Cd^{2+}), lead (Pb^{3+}), mercury (Hg^{2+}), manganese (Mn^{2+}), and arsenic (As^{3+}). Cadmium, lead, and mercury have no known essential role in the biological metabolic pathways, and at certain concentrations they are toxic metals. However, manganese is an essential element at very low concentrations and toxic at higher levels. Arsenic, at low concentrations, is reported to be an essential element for some animal species, and yet toxic at higher levels. Each heavy metal may exist in a variety of forms, and each form can differ a great deal in its toxic action. Mercury, in addition to being a cation, can covalently bind to proteinaceous molecules by forming either R-S-Hg$^+$ or R-S-Hg-S-R. Other heavy metals act as deleterious divalent cations either by substitution for another divalent cation that is acting as a cofactor, or as a ligand.

Physical-Chemical Characteristics of Heavy Metals

In order to understand the toxic effects of a heavy metal such as mercury, one must understand the chemistry of heavy-metal molecules and how they interact with target molecules. Heavy metals usually react with sites that contain side chains with oxygen (O), sulfur (S), and nitrogen (N). The primary distinction among heavy metals that endows them with different properties is whether they are in an inorganic form or an organic form.

Inorganic Heavy Metals

Inorganic heavy metals form "coordinated" complexes—"ionic bonds"— with various chelating agents, peptides, proteins, and other compounds. The toxic effects of heavy metals vary, depending on the strength of the bonds formed with the target site, which depend primarily on ionization potential and charge-radius ratio (Williams 1984). It is worth noting that covalent and ionic bonds are just two extreme forms of the same bonding relationship. Heavy metals, because of their high affinity to negatively charged groups of proteins, may cause changes in protein conformation leading to inhibition of various enzymes. We can loosely classify heavy-metal actions into three categories: covalent, coordinate, and Ca^{2+} antagonist.

Covalent   Covalent linkage of heavy metals into a target site could have deleterious effects on peptides, proteins, and nucleotides because of the following reaction:

$$R\text{-}SH + Hg^{2+} \qquad R\text{-}S\text{-}Hg^+ + H^+$$
$$R\text{-}S\text{-}Hg^+ + R'\text{-}SH \qquad R\text{-}S\text{-}Hg\text{-}S\text{-}R' + H^+$$

where R and R′ could represent two different proteins or residues in the same protein.

Coordinated   Heavy metals form metal ligand complexes, where the ligand can be amino acids, peptides, nucleotides, or other compounds with a negative residual charge. An example of the sites that heavy metals can utilize to form a metal ligand complex is one or more of the side chains illustrated in Figure 2.1.

Ca^{2+} Antagonist   Heavy metals are cations, as is the calcium ion (Ca^{2+}). Heavy metals differ in size and charge from the calcium ion. They bind to calcium sites with differing strengths and can easily displace it. As we shall

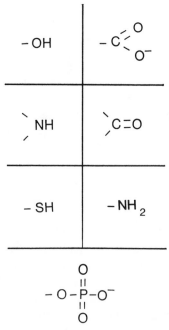

Figure 2.1.   Side chain targets in heavy-metal binding.

see, calcium sites could be specific structures, such as those needed for calcium carriers, channels, and pump proteins, or nonspecific structures, whereby they are merely negatively charged groups similar to some of those shown in Figure 2.1. The most likely structures of proteins involved in binding of heavy metals are the hydroxyl and carboxyl groups, or a mixture of the two. These specific structures are ideal for binding heavy metals, and they bind with even greater affinity than calcium. The nonspecific structures are merely one or two of the aforementioned structures that could provide negative ionic sites for calcium. Heavy metals can also bind at these sites and with greater strength than calcium, thereby displacing it. One can therefore rationalize how heavy metals can inhibit specific calcium transport systems and also interfere with structures that depend on divalent cation binding for their integrity, that is, membranes.

Organic Heavy Metals

Heavy metals form organometallic compounds by binding covalently to carbon molecules. Examples are tetramethyl lead and methyl mercury. These compounds differ considerably from their respective inorganic heavy metals: (1) They are bulkier; (2) they are considerably less soluble in aqueous solutions; and (3) neither competes with or binds to Ca^{2+} binding sites. If residual valency remains in the organic structure, it will react with sites that are accessible to the large-size organometal. An example of this is methyl mercury.

$$R\text{-SH} + CH_3Hg^+ \quad R\text{-S-Hg-}CH_3 + H^+$$

Interaction of Heavy Metals with Cell Components

If one could envision an "idealized cell," it would contain "all" relevant structures and functions. The "idealized cell" is an aggregate of all cellular components known to be in different cells. Cells from different organs or types simply have a different distribution and amount of these components. For example, at one extreme is the skeletal-muscle cell, which is rich in well-developed endoplasmic reticulum called sarcoplasmic reticulum. The skeletal muscle does not have the receptor and transmitter portion shown in the idealized cell. In cardiac muscle, however, the cell contains the receptor portion, but in two different sections of the cell membranes.

The "idealized cell" identifies potential targets for heavy-metal interaction. The "idealized cell" also has all the known regulatory mechanisms involved in calcium homeostasis, and thus targets of heavy-metal interaction (for details of calcium in a cardiac cell, see Shamoo and Ambudkar 1984). Briefly, it contains the following:

A.   Plasma membrane
1.   Channels. For Na^+, K^+, and Ca^{2+}; all involved in action potentials.
2.   Carriers. The Na^+:Ca^{2+} exchange carrier involved in Ca^{2+} regulation.
3.   Receptors. A variety of transmitters and hormone receptors are involved in the regulation of Na^+ and K^+ channels and cAMP (cyclic adenosine monophosphate) production. Regulation of cellular cAMP ultimately results in modulation of cellular Ca^{2+}.
4.   Transmitters. There are a variety of neurotransmitters, and calcium plays an integral role in their release.
5.   Pumps. There are several pumps, such as the Na^+:K^+-ATPase (adenosine triphosphatase) and Ca^{2+}-ATPase pumps involved in the active transport of Na^+, K^+, and Ca^{2+}, respectively, and therefore potential targets for heavy-metal interaction.
B.   Intracellular organelles
1.   Mitochondria. Mitochondria contain the following:
a.   ATP synthesis machinery of oxidative phosphorylation.
b.   A Ca^{2+} uniporter, responsible for Ca^{2+} influx. This system is driven via the membrane potential generated by the electron transport chain (ETC). In general, heavy metals are taken up by the same Ca^{2+} uniporter system, as well as by their leakage into mitochondria. Once inside, these metals are strongly bound.
c. Na^+:Ca^{2+} exchange carrier responsible for calcium efflux.
d.   Enzymes responsible for transmitter synthesis, i.e., acetylcholine (ACh).
2.   Endoplasmic reticulum. The endoplasmic reticulum contains the Ca^{2+}:Mg^{2+}-ATPase, a Ca^{2+} accumulating pump, and also channels necessary for calcium release.
3.   Lysosomal enzymes.
4.   Nucleus.
C.   Intracellular soluble proteins (e.g., enzymes, calmodulin). Any proteins containing sulfhydryl groups or depending on Ca^{2+} for their activity could be the target of heavy metals. A good example is calmodulin, a crucial and wide-range regulatory protein that depends on calcium-binding for its activity. Thus, heavy-metal interaction with calmodulin can disrupt, in part, all the regulatory functions that calmodulin exerts on multiple systems.

Mercury Compounds

Recently there has been a wide range of studies on the toxicity of mercury compounds. The early 1970s saw a rise in environmental concerns following accidental mercury compound intoxications that led to serious health effects accompanied by death or relatively permanent nervous system impairment in many instances (Bakir et al. 1973; Clarkson et al. 1983). Mercury compounds exist primarily in three oxidation states: Hg^{2+} (mercuric), Hg_2^{2+} (mercurous), and Hg^0 (metallic). The mercuric ion, in addition to forming salts, also forms organometallic compounds such as methyl mercury (CH_3Hg^+) and phenyl mercury. These organometallic compounds, especially methyl mercury, are very toxic because of their hydrophobic nature. The hydrophobic characteristics endow the compound with extremely easy transport across membrane barriers. This enables these compounds to attack quickly organ sites distal to the point of ingestion, such as the brain.

Inorganic Mercury

Inorganic mercury compounds, such as mercurous salts, are not very toxic because of their very low solubility. However, ingestion of 1 gram of mercuric chloride can lead to death in an adult human (Gleason et al. 1963). Inorganic mercury is highly nephrotoxic when the kidney is infused with the compound (Barnes et al. 1980). Children are more susceptible to damage by ingestion of inorganic compounds, such as calomel. The main symptom is painful extremities (acrodynia) or so-called "pink disease" (Cheek 1980), which is characterized by bluish-pink hands and feet, rosy cheeks, sweating, painful joints, irritability, and other nervous system abnormalities. Mercury vapor, however, produces erethism, tremor, and gingivitis (Goldwater 1964). As one can see, early detection of inorganic intoxication based on diffuse clinical symptoms is difficult. Buchet adopted an approach similar to the one he developed for cadmium, which required measuring protein levels in urine (Buchet et al. 1980). He found that large-molecular-weight proteins, such as albumin, increased in the urine following mercury intoxication, in contrast to small-molecular-weight proteins like β_2-microglobulin, which appear in the urine due to cadmium toxicity.

Inorganic mercury is a powerful inhibitor of Ca^{2+} transport processes as a result of two types of action exerted by the compound. The first is that Hg^{2+} can directly compete with Ca^{2+} like Mn^{2+}. The second action of Hg^{2+} is that it can covalently link to the sulfhydryl group of the proteins involved in the Ca^{2+} transport system. In the case of Mn^{2+}, the major metabolic route for manganese in the cell is through the transport of Mn^{2+} into mitochondria via the calcium carrier (Chappel et al. 1963; Chance and Mela 1966; Saris and Akerman 1980). In the cell, manganese is sequestered by mitochondria (Maynard and Cotzias 1955; Bygrave 1978). The specificity of divalent cation influx into mitochondria is $Ca^{2+} > Sr^{2+} > Mn^{2+} > Ba^{2+}$, but these ions do not transport Mg^{2+}. The use of manganese as a spectroscopic probe had made it possible to purify the calcium carrier, calciphorin (Jeng and Shamoo 1980*a*, 1980*b;* Shamoo and Ambudkar 1984; Ambudkar et al. 1984; Herrmann et al. 1984; Shamoo et al. 1984). Isolated calciphorin has been shown to transport calcium and manganese in numerous experimental procedures. However, manganese is not released from mitochondria in exchange for Na^+ ions, as is Ca^{2+} through the $Na^+ : Ca^{2+}$ exchange system (Gunter et al. 1978). Furthermore, both calcium and Mn^{2+} passively leak out of mitochondria, but not with the same mechanism (Gunter et al. 1983). Since calcium is a crucial divalent cation in a multitude of cellular functions, such as in receptor activity, secretion, synthesis, and so on, it is clear that increased cellular Mn^{2+}, to the extent of replacing calcium, could result in deleterious effects. It is worth noting that Mn^{2+} can be carried via the calcium carrier into mitochondria but does not substitute for calcium in most instances where calcium is needed. Depending on Mn^{2+} levels, Mn^{2+} could have sometimes harmful effects at low doses. For example, Mn^{2+} has been shown to stimulate Ca^{2+} uptake in a way that is similar to the action of Mg^{2+} on Ca^{2+} uptake into mitochondria (Hughes and Exton 1983). Also, Mn^{2+} was shown to prevent Ca^{2+}-induced inhibition of ATP synthesis in brain mitrochondria (Hillered et al. 1983).

As shown by Shamoo and MacLennan (1976), essential sulfhydryl groups are blocked in the skeletal-muscle sarcoplasmic reticulum Ca^{2+} transport system. The action of inorganic mercury on various enzymes through covalent linkage to sulfhydryl groups is similar to that of methyl mercury, but it does differ in that Hg^{2+} can react with two sulfhydryl groups in close proximity, as well as compete for calcium sites.

Organic Mercury

The first indication that methyl mercury may have deleterious effects on public health came from the epidemics of Minamata Bay and Niigata in Japan. These episodes came to be known as the "Minamata disease." During the period 1953–60, a total of 121 people were poisoned with methyl mercury. Some 46 people died. In a large study initiated in the 1960s in Sweden, it was found that increasing industrial and agricultural use of mercury resulted in an increased mercury concentration in fish from polluted waters. A second outbreak occurred in Japan in 1970 in Niigata, with 47 people poisoned and 6 deaths reported. Careful investigation revealed that the villagers were eating fish and that the bay water was contaminated with methyl mercury, as were the fish.

The upper limit set by government agencies for the amounts of methyl mercury permitted in fish and fish products used for consumption is usually in the range of 0.5–1.0 part per million (ppm) (U.S. EPA 1984*a*).

Mechanism of Toxicity

There is overwhelming evidence that patients poisoned with methyl mercury have mild to severe neuromuscular disorders. Several lines of investigation into the site and mechanism of such neuromuscular disorders have been initiated, and several possible drugs and treatment courses have also been undertaken. One of the earliest such studies was conducted directly on afflicted patients.

Neurophysiological Characterizations

The first direct evidence for the involvement of the cholinergic system was obtained by Von Burg and Landry (1976), who showed that methyl mercury treatment shifted the dose-response curve for muscle contraction induced by acetylcholine to the right.

Atchison et al. (1984) have recently shown that in rat diaphragms methyl mercury at 20 μM irreversibly and nearly completely blocked the end-plate potential (EPP) after 30 minutes. The data are consistent with the blocking action of methyl mercury on junctional transmission and voltage-evoked ACh release. It is also known that inorganic mercury inhibits voltage-evoked ACh release by inhibiting Ca^{2+} entry through the calcium channel (Nachshen 1983). However, methyl mercury did not inhibit the calcium channel, and thus its inhibition of voltage-evoked ACh release must be due to other factors.

Methyl mercury first increases the spontaneous release of ACh (Atchison et al. 1984), probably because of an increase in intracellular calcium; a later effect is complete cessation of the spontaneous ACh release (Atchison et al. 1984). This block in the spontaneous release of ACh by methyl mercury may well be attributable to the inhibitory action of methyl mercury on intracellular metabolic enzymes involved in maintenance of ATP levels.

Biochemical Characterizations

Biotransformation of Methyl Mercury   When methyl mercury is administered (intravenously) to rats, one finds about 3–6 percent of the total brain mercury present in the inorganic form. Figure 2.2 illustrates that injection of methyl mercury results in more inorganic mercury in the brain than if an equal amount of inorganic mercury is injected into rats. Thus, the time course of the inorganic mercury content into the brain is dependent on the compound administered. Earlier studies have shown that 4–7 percent of total methyl mercury in the brain tissue is detected as inorganic mercury (Syverson 1974). It is of interest to note that myelin and mitochondria accumulate more inorganic mercury than other subcellular fractions (Syverson 1974). (See Chapter 3, below.)

Interaction of Mercury Compounds with Receptors   Mercurial compounds such as Hg^{2+} and methyl mercury inhibit in an in vivo and in vitro experiment the nicotinic and muscarinic acetylcholine receptors (Von Burg et al. 1980; Abd-Elfattah and Shamoo 1981; Abdallah and Shamoo 1984). Fur-

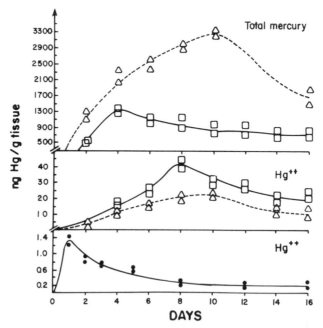

Figure 2.2. Mercury content in a blood-free brain homogenate in relation to time after a single injection of [203]Hg-labeled methyl mercuric chloride or mercuric chloride. Results from the 10 mg/kg CH_3HgCl (*closed triangles*), 5 mg/kg CH_3HgCl (*closed squares*), and 5 mg/kg $HgCl_2$ (*closed circles*). (From Syverson 1974)

thermore, *d*-penicillamine and dimercaptosuccinic acid (DMSA) reverse the mercurial inhibition to these receptors. The mechanism of inhibition appears to be the result of the covalent linkage of the mercurials to the essential sulfhydryl groups on the receptor.

Conclusion

Heavy metals, and mercurials in particular, are very toxic if they come in contact with appropriate target sites. The inhibitory effect of mercurials can be reversed with chelating agents. In the case of methyl mercury, a small percentage is transformed to inorganic mercury, and thus exerts its action both as a heavy metal and as an organic compound.

Acknowledgment

This work was supported in part by the U.S. Department of Energy (DE-AS0580EV 10329).

References

Abdallah, E. A. M., and Shamoo, A. E. (1984). Protective effect of dimercaptosuccinic acid on methylmercury and mercuric chloride inhibition of rat brain muscarinic acetylcholine receptors. *Pest Biochem Physiol* 21:385–393.

Abd-Elfattah, A. S., and Shamoo, A. E. (1981). Regeneration of a functionally active rat brain muscarinic receptor by *D*-penicillamine after inhibition with methylmercury and mercuric chloride. *Mol Pharmacol* 20:492–497.

Ambudkar, I. S.; Kima, P. E.; and Shamoo, A. E. (1984). Characterization of calciphorin, the low molecular weight calcium ionophore, from rat liver mitochondria. *Biochim Biophys Acta* 771:165–170.

Atchison, W. D.; Clark, A. W.; and Narahashi, T. (1984). Presynaptic effects of methylmercury at the mammalian neuromuscular junction. In *Cellular and Molecular Neurotoxicology,* edited by T. Narahashi, pp. 23–43. New York: Raven Press.

Bakir, F.; Damluji, S. F.; Amin-Zaki, L., Murtadha, M., Khalidi, A.; Al-Rawi, N. Y.; Tikriti, S.; Dhahir, H. I.; Clarkson, T. W.; Smith, J. C.; and Doherty, R. A. (1973). Methylmercury poisoning in Iraq. *Science* 181:230–291.

Barnes, J. L.; McDowell, E. M.; McNeil, J. S.; Flamenbaum, W.; and Trump, B. F. (1980). Studies on the pathophysiology of acute renal failure. *Virchows Archiv B Cell Pathol* 32:233–260.

Buchet, J. P.; Roels, H.; Bernard, A.; and Lauwerys, R. (1980). Assessment of renal function of workers exposed to inorganic lead, cadmium, and mercury vapor. *J Occup Med* 22:741–750.

Bygrave, F. L. (1978). Mitochondria and the control of intracellular calcium. *Biol Rev* 53:43–79.

Chance, B., and Mela, L. (1966). Calcium and manganese interactions in mitochondrial ion accumulation. *Biochemistry* 5:3220.

Chappel, J. B.; Cohn, M.; and Grenville, G. D. (1963). The accumulation of divalent ions by isolated mitochondria. In *Energy-Linked Functions of Mitochondria,* edited by B. Chance, pp. 219–235. New York: Academic Press.

Cheek, D. B. (1980). Acrodynia. In *Brennermann's Practice of Pediatrics,* edited by V. C. Kelley, vol. 1, rev. ed., chap. 17D. New York: Harper & Row.

Cheung, W. Y. (1984). Calmodulin: Its potential role in cell proliferation and heavy metal toxicity. *Fed Proc* 43:2995–2999.

Clarkson, T. W.; Weiss, B.; and Cox, C. (1983). Public health consequences of heavy metals in dump sites. *Environ Health Perspect* 48:113–127.

Gleason, M. N.; Gosselin, R. E.; and Hodge, H. C. (1963). *Clinical Toxicology of Commercial Products.* 2nd ed. Baltimore: Williams & Wilkins.

Goldwater, L. J. (1964). Occupational exposure to mercury: The Harben Lectures. *J R Inst Public Health* 27:279–301.

Gunter, T. E.; Chace, J. H.; Puskin, J. S.; and Gunter, K. K. (1983). Mechanism of sodium independent calcium efflux from rat liver mitochondria. *Biochemistry* 22:6341–6351.

Gunter, T. E.; Gunter, K. K.; Puskin, J. S.; and Russell, P. R. (1978). Efflux of Ca^{2+} and Mn^{2+} from rat liver mitochondria. *Biochemistry* 17:339–345.

Herrmann, T. R.; Jayaweera, R. A.; Ambudkar, I. S.; and Shamoo, A. E. (1984). Characterization of calciphorin by laser-excited europium luminescence. *Biochim Biophys Acta* 774:11–18.

Hillered, L.; Muchiri, P. M.; Nordenbrand, K.; and Ernster, L. (1983). Mn^{2+} prevents the Ca^{2+}-induced inhibition of ATP synthesis in brain mitochondria. *FEBS Lett* 154:247–250.

Hughes, B. P.; and Exton, J. H. (1983). Effect of micromolar concentrations of manganese ions on calcium-ion cycling in rat liver mitochondria. *Biochem J* 212:773–782.

Jeng, A. Y., and Shamoo, A. E. (1980a). Isolation of a Ca^{2+} carrier from calf heart inner mitochondrial membrane. *J Biol Chem* 255(14):6897–6903.

——— (1980b). The electrophoretic properties of a Ca^{2+} carrier isolated from calf heart inner mitochondrial membrane. *J Biol Chem* 255(14):6904–6912.

Maynard, L. S., and Cotzias, G. C. (1955). The partition of manganese among organs and intracellular organelles of the rat. *J Biol Chem* 214:489–495.

Nachshen, D. A. (1983). Selectivity of Ca^{2+} binding sites in synaptosomal Ca^{2+} channels: Inhibition of Ca^{2+} influx by multi-valent metal cations. *J Gen Physiol* 83:941–967.

Nordberg, G. F. (1976). *Effects and Dose-Response Relationships of Toxic Metals.* Amsterdam: Elsevier Press.

O'Neill, J. J., and Holtzman, D. (1984). Heavy metal toxicity and energy metabolism in the developing brain: Lead as the model. In *Cerebral Energy Metabolism and Metabolic Encephalopathy,* edited by D. W. McCandless, pp. 391–424. New York: Plenum Press.

Saris, N.-E., and Akerman, K. E. O. (1980). Uptake and release of bivalent cations in mitochondria. *Curr Top Bioenergetics* 10:103–179.

Shamoo, A. E., and Ambudkar, I. S. (1984). Regulations of calcium transport in cardiac cells. *Can J Physiol and Pharmacol* 62:9–22.

Shamoo, A. E.; Jayaweera, R. A.; and Ambudkar, I. S. (1984). Calciphorin-calcium carrier in artificial membranes. In *Proceedings of "Calcium and Phosphate Transport Across Biomembranes,"* Second International Workshop, Vienna, Austria, edited by F. Bronner and M. Peterlik. New York: Alan R. Liss.

Shamoo, A. E., and MacLennan, D. H. (1976). Separate effects of mercurial compounds on the ionophoric and hydrolytic functions of the $(Ca^{++} + Mg^{++})$-ATPase of sarcoplasmic reticulum. *J Memb Biol* 25:65–74.

Syverson, T. L. M. (1974). Biotransformation of Hg-203 labeled methylmercuric chloride in rat brain measured by specific determination of Hg^{2+}. *Acta Pharmacol Toxicol* 35:277–283.

U.S. Environmental Protection Agency (1984a). Health Issue Assessment. In *Mercury Health Effects Update.* Washington, D.C.: U.S. Government Printing Office.

——— (1984b). *Health Assessment Document for Manganese.* Washington, D.C.: U.S. Government Printing Office.

——— (1984c). *Health Assessment Document for Lead.* Washington, D.C.: U.S. Government Printing Office.

Von Burg, R., and Landry, T. (1976). Methylmercury and skeletal muscle receptor. *J Pharm Pharmacol* 28:548–551.

Von Burg, R.; Northington, F. K.; and Shamoo, A. (1980). Methylmercury inhibition of rat brain muscarinic receptors. *Toxicol Appl Pharmacol* 53:285–292.

Williams, R. J. P. (1984). Structural aspects of metal toxicity. In *Changing Metal Cycles and Human Health,* edited by J. O. Nriagn, pp. 251–263. Springer-Verlag: New York.

THREE

The Absorption, Distribution, and Excretion of Methyl Mercury

Laszlo Magos

In the mammalian organism, every form of mercury is converted to bivalent mercury, predominantly attached to sulfhydryl and chloride ligands. The conversion can be so fast that mercury clears from the body with the half time of mercuric mercury, or is so slow that in many organs the concentration of mercury declines with the half time of the original form. Thus, half times for the original forms of mercury (see Magos 1981) correlate only loosely with conversion rates. The faster the conversion, as in the oxidation of Hg^0 to Hg^{2+}, the more faithfully the conversion rate is reflected by the half time of the original form. When the conversion is slow, as in the decomposition of methyl mercury, then excretion influences the half time of the original form more than its conversion to Hg^{2+}. From the point of view of neurotoxicity, half times for the original forms of mercury are extremely important, because mercury accumulation in the nervous system depends on the ability of a given form of mercury to cross membranes and barriers before it is converted to Hg^{2+}.

The intercompartmental mobility of atomic mercury is so high that exposure to mercury vapor results in pronounced mercury accumulation in the brain (Berlin et al. 1966; Magos 1968), in spite of the extremely short (less than 1 min) half time (see Magos 1981). Though the half times of phenyl and methoxyethyl mercury are significantly longer (12 hrs), these organomercurials do not raise the brain concentration of mercury above levels observed after the parenteral injection of inorganic mercury salts (Friberg et al. 1957; Swensson and Ulfvarson 1968). One reason for their limited intercompartmental mobility may be that these organomercurials have—as phenyl mercury has—higher affinities for plasma proteins than methyl mercury (Fang and Fallin 1976) and consequently have less chance to associate with thiol carriers. In the case of methyl mercury, the increased chance of diffusable complex formation both with small molecular weight sulfhydryl compounds and chloride favors intercompartmental mobility (Magos 1981). The effects of these favorable conditions are accentuated by the lack of preferential renal accumulation, which leaves a large proportion of the dose available for extra renal distribution (Magos 1973), as well as by the slow decomposition and long half time of methyl mercury.

Absorption

The biological methylation of methyl mercury and its subsequent accumulation in the aquatic food chain assure that ingestion is the most common form of methyl mercury intake. Pulmonary and percutaneous absorptions are important only in occupational exposures. Compared with mass intoxications caused by ingestion of food containing high concentrations of methyl mercury (see Clarkson et al. 1976), occupational cases of methyl mercury intoxication are few (Kurland et al. 1960), and the relationship between exposure and uptake has not been established. The experimental interest in gastrointestinal absorption versus pulmonary and dermal absorption also has another, purely methodological reason. It is easier to quantitate absorption after methyl mercury is introduced into the gastrointestinal tract with food, drink, or by gastric gavage than to quantitate pulmonary or dermal absorption and extrapolate it to the conditions of human exposure.

Pulmonary Absorption

Methyl mercury can be inhaled in particulate form (dust or spray) or as vapor. Its chloride salt is more volatile than metallic mercury. At 20° C the atmosphere is saturated with 76 g/l Hg as methyl mercuric chloride and 13 g/l as mercury vapor. It is assumed that the pulmonary absorption of methyl mercuric chloride is the same as that of mercury vapor. This means that about 80 percent of inhaled methyl mercury is absorbed (Task Group 1973). This assumption is based on some similarities between methyl mercuric chloride and mercury vapor. Both are lipid-soluble, they have no charge, and the molecular weight of methyl mercuric chloride is only 25 percent larger than the atomic weight of mercury.

The vapor pressure of methyl mercury depends on the anionic part of the molecule. Thus the vapor pressure is decreased 370-fold when chloride is replaced by dicyandiamide (see Swensson and Ulfvarson 1963). Because of the higher affinity of methyl mercury for sulfhydryl than for chloride, absorbed methyl mercuric chloride is rapidly converted to a sulfhydryl complex. This conversion prevents passage through the alveolar membrane from blood to air. In contrast, dimethyl mercury must be decomposed before it can react with sulfhydryls, and therefore not all the absorbed dimethyl mercury is retained. Like mercury vapor (Magos 1968), some is exhaled after parenteral administration (Ostlund 1969).

Percutaneous Absorption

Methyl mercury can be absorbed through human skin, as indicated by the occurrence of severe methyl mercury intoxication in some patients treated topically with methyl mercury thioacetamide (Suzuki and Yoshino 1969).

Absorption has been quantitated in guinea pigs after the application of different amounts of methyl mercury dicyandiamide in 1 ml water/3.1 cm^2 of shaven abdominal skin. At low concentrations, percutaneous absorption increased with dose and reached a maximum at about 16 mg Hg/ml. At this concentration, 5.9 percent of the dose was absorbed in the first 5 hours, indicating a 55-hour absorption half time. At 24 mg Hg, half time increased to 200 hours, and did not change appreciably between 24 and 40 mg Hg. When the dose was increased to 48 mg Hg, absorption could not be detected at all (Friberg et al. 1961). At low concentrations, the saturation of sulfur-binding sites may accelerate, while at high concentrations the denaturation of proteins may inhibit absorption.

There is evidence that mercury attached to human skin can be partly removed by soaking the contaminated area in or rubbing it with d-penicillamine solution. This decontamination procedure was more effective against Hg^{2+} than against $MeHg^+$ (personal observation, unpublished), either because the monovalent MeHg binds more strongly to keratin, or because it penetrates deeper into the keratin layer. Whatever the mechanism, it does not affect percutaneous absorption because equimolar doses of $HgCl_2$ are absorbed by the skin at the same rate as methyl mercury dicyandiamide (Friberg et al. 1961).

Gastrointestinal Absorption

The distribution of $MeHg^+$ between halide and thiol ligands depends on pH and the relative concentration of these two ligands. Low pH and high chloride concentration in the stomach favor the formation of uncharged and lipid-soluble MeHgCl (Rabenstein and Evans 1978), which easily crosses the gastric wall. Thus, when methyl mercury acetate was injected into the ligated stomach of piglets, the blood concentration of mercury peaked after 15 minutes (Platonow 1968). Significantly more mercury disappeared from the whole stomach of piglets in the first 6 hours (87 percent) than from a 6-inch section of duodenum (44 percent) or jejunum (56 percent) (Platonow 1968). In rats, the order of absorption from ligated sections was duodenum > stomach = ileum > jejunum (Sasser et al. 1978). The disappearance of methyl mercury from the perfused intestinal section of jejunum and ileum was faster in rats when methyl mercuric chloride was added to the perfusate than when methyl mercuric cysteinate was used, though excess cysteine—at least after 30 minutes—accelerated absorption (Hirayama 1975). When the gastrointestinal tract is unligated, however, difference in absorption rate linked to the chemical form of methyl mercury is unimportant, because absorption takes place along the whole length of the gastrointestinal tract, allowing ample time for absorption. The experiments of Aberg et al. (1969) and Miettinen (1973) on human volunteers indicated that the gastrointestinal absorption of methyl mercury is the same whether this toxic chemical is ingested in its natural form in fish or as a methyl mercury salt. This conclusion was also confirmed by Turner et al. (1975). The absorption is approximately 95 percent in humans (Aberg et al. 1969; Miettinen 1973), in monkeys (Berlin et al. 1975), and in rats (Glockling et al. 1977).

Distribution

Differences exist in the concentration of methyl mercury in different organs and tissues, but these differences are not as significant as those observed after exposure to mercuric mercury. The reason is that, compared with Hg^{2+}, the distribution of methyl mercury is influenced less by compartmental barriers and more by concentration differences in nondiffusible binding sites. Moreover, the renal accumulation process, which assures that the kidneys contain most of the body burden of inorganic mercury, does not operate for methyl mercury.

Distribution in Blood

Human red blood cells, suspended in saline buffer, cleared 98 percent of the methyl mercury supplement from the bathing medium within 7 minutes, but after their resuspension in stroma-free hemolysate or serum bovine albumin, methyl mercury equilibrated between cellular and extracellular binding sites (White and Rothstein 1973). The equilibration between red blood cells and plasma shows species-dependent variation as shown in Table 3.1. Thus, the red blood cell to plasma (RBC : plasma) ratio is about 150 in the rat, but only 25 or less in other species. There is a good correlation between the ratio of glutathione (GSH) to hemoglobin-bound methyl mercury in the red blood cells, and the proportion of $MeHg^+$ released within 60 minutes into bovine albumin (Doi and Tagawa 1983). In the rat, 95 percent of methyl mercury is bound to hemoglobin, and only 2 percent to GSH, while in human and rabbit

Table 3.1   Distribution of methyl mercury between red blood cells (RBC) and plasma

Species	RBC : Plasma*	Reference
Man	21	Kershaw et al. 1980
Squirrel monkey	17	Berlin et al. 1975
Rhesus monkey	25	Task Group 1973
Pig	8	Task Group 1973
Dog	25	Task Group 1973
Guinea pig	25	Task Group 1973
Sheep	15	Kostyniak 1983
Rabbit	10	Berlin 1963
Rat	145	Vostal and Clarkson 1973
Mouse	7	Ostlund 1969

*Mean values.

red blood cells, 60 percent of methyl mercury is GSH-bound (Naganuma and Imura 1979). Thus, the most important factor in the distribution of MeHg$^+$ between red blood cells and plasma is the binding capacity of hemoglobin. It has been suggested that hemoglobin binds a higher proportion of intravascular methyl mercury in the rat than in other species, because rat hemoglobin has more sulfhydryl ligands (Naganuma and Imura 1979; Doi and Tagawa 1983). However, the number of sulfhydryl binding sites in hemoglobin may not be the sole factor responsible for the high RBC : plasma ratio. Trialkyl tins, another group of organometallic compounds, have a similarly higher RBC : plasma ratio in the rat than in other species, though trialkyl tin is bound to histidine and not to sulfhydryl residues of rat hemoglobin (Rose 1969; Brown et al. 1979; Aldridge et al. 1981).

Extravascular Distribution

After absorption, methyl mercury is distributed not only between red blood cells and plasma, but also between blood and extravascular tissues. Only a small percentage of total mercury is in inorganic form in all organs except the kidney. Thus, in rats treated daily with methyl mercury, the inorganic form was responsible for 4 percent of total mercury in blood, 3 percent in brain, and 6 percent in liver (Magos and Butler 1976). Kidneys, however, accumulate most of the inorganic mercury derived from the decomposition of the mercury-carbon bond. Both after a single dose (Norseth and Clarkson 1970) and in the course of prolonged daily exposure (Magos and Butler 1976), there is a time-dependent increase in the contribution of inorganic mercury. In the latter case, the proportion of inorganic mercury to total renal mercury increased from 12 percent after 4 doses to 46 percent after 24 doses, after which a steady state was achieved (Magos and Butler 1976).

A loose inverse correlation exists between red blood cell to plasma and organ to blood concentration ratios. Table 3.2 shows that organ to blood concentration ratios are lower by at least one order of magnitude in the rat, compared with other species. Table 3.2 also shows that the concentration of mercury is higher in the kidneys and liver than in other tissues, and that usually the renal concentration is highest. The variation in the concentration of mercury in brain, muscle, heart, and lung is small, and only in rats is the variation more than twofold. In the rat, but not in other species, the spleen has a higher concentration than the liver.

Though kidneys have higher mercury concentrations than other organs after treatment with methyl mercury, the accumulation of mercury in this organ is far less than after parenteral treatment with HgCl$_2$. Rats treated subcutaneously with methyl mercury had only about 4 percent of the dose in the kidney at 24 hours (Magos and Webb 1977), while after an equimolar dose of HgCl$_2$, 24 percent was present (Magos et al. 1974b). However,

Table 3.2 Organ to blood mercury concentration ratios after methyl mercury treatment

Species	Treatment*	Brain	Liver	Kidney	Spleen	Heart	Lung	Muscle	Reference
Squirrel monkey	M	3.80	11.00	5.80	—	—	—	—	Berlin et al. 1975
Macaque monkey	M	2.60	13.00	25.00	—	—	—	—	Evans et al. 1977
Pig	M	3.30	14.00	5.70	4.30	2.90	4.30	3.90	Platonow 1968
Guinea pig	S	1.70	5.00	16.00	1.40	1.70	1.70	2.50	Iverson et al. 1973
Guinea pig	M	1.20	5.00	12.00	—	—	—	—	Iverson et al. 1974
Rat	S	0.06	0.32	1.00	0.40	0.23	0.28	0.10	Fang 1980
Rat	M	0.06	0.29	0.91	0.43	0.20	0.20	0.27	Magos and Butler 1976
Mouse	S	1.30	3.30	23.00	—	—	—	—	Doi and Kobayashi 1982
Mouse	M	1.20	4.20	10.00	—	—	—	—	Suzuki et al. 1963

*M = multiple treatment; S = single treatment.

29

Table 3.3 Mercury in brain after nontoxic dose of methyl mercury

| Species | Time After Treatment | | Reference |
	3 days	7 days	
Macaque monkey	—	0.50*	Aaseth et al. 1976
Pig	0.63	0.56	Platonow 1968
Guinea pig	—	0.70	Iverson et al. 1973
Rat	0.32	0.34	Magos and Webb 1977
Mouse C5 7BL	0.40	0.33	Doi and Kobayashi 1982
Mouse BALB/c	0.32	0.28	Doi and Kobayashi 1982
Mouse ICR	0.22	0.16	Doi and Kobayashi 1982

Note: The values in the table express the brain mercury concentration relative to dose of mercury administered as follows:

$$\frac{\text{Concentration}}{\text{Dose}} = \frac{\text{ng Hg/g brain tissue}}{\text{ng Hg/g body weight}}$$

*6 days after treatment.

accumulation of inorganic mercury in this organ is only partially responsible for differences in various organ mercury concentrations.

The brain to blood concentration ratio is not constant because there is a delay in brain accumulation of methyl mercury (Magos et al. 1978*b*, 1980*b*). This ratio is more than one order of magnitude less in rats than in other species, though in relation to dose, brain concentrations show much less variation. Table 3.3 shows that after equimolar doses the brain concentration of mercury is about 60–100 percent higher in the guinea pig, pig, and macaque monkey than in the rat. In mice, the brain concentration of methyl mercury shows a strain-dependent variation and can be lower or higher than in rats (Doi and Kobayashi 1982). Differences in the degree of methyl mercury retention by red blood cells combined with different whole-body clearance rates (Doi and Tagawa 1983) may explain these variations in mice. In rats, methyl mercury accumulation in the brain is influenced by the sex of the animals. Both after a single injection and after prolonged treatment, the brain concentration of methyl mercury reached a higher level in female rats than in male rats, probably because female rats have a larger brain to body weight ratio than male rats (Magos et al. 1981).

There are no direct data on the brain to blood methyl mercury ratio in humans, but indirect evidence based on the retention of [203]Hg-labeled methyl mercury in the head (Aberg et al. 1969) and in blood (Miettinen 1973) indicates that the ratio may be about 6.0.

Mercury is not homogeneously distributed in the brain. In rats treated daily with methyl mercury, the concentration of mercury in the cerebral cortex was approximately the same as that in the cerebellum (Somjen et al.

1973; Magos et al. 1981). In another experiment, intoxicated rats had 50 percent higher concentration in the cerebellum than in the cerebrum, and the concentration in the spinal ganglia was twice as much as in the cerebellum (Jacobs et al. 1975). The difference between brain and spinal ganglia decreased with the length of exposure, but spinal ganglia always had twice the concentration of the ventral or dorsal roots or the sciatic nerve (Somjen et al. 1973). In the pig, the difference between the cerebrum and the cerebellum was negligible; the brain stem had a slightly higher mercury concentration, the spinal cord a slightly lower one (Platonow 1968). In the guinea pig, the concentration of mercury was lower in the cerebellum than in the whole cerebrum (Komszta-Szumska et al. 1983) or in the frontal or occipital lobe, calcarine area, hypothalamus, and caudate nucleus, the highest concentration being in the caudate nucleus (Iverson et al. 1974). In dog brain (Yoshino et al. 1966), the higher concentration was found in the calcarine area. In the cat, cerebellar concentration of mercury was about 50 percent higher than in the cerebral cortex and nearly 200 percent higher than in the spinal cord (Charbonneau et al. 1974). In macaque monkeys, the difference between the lowest and highest concentrations in the central nervous system was twofold (Evans et al. 1977). In the cerebrum, the highest concentration was found in the corpus callosum, and the lowest in the frontal pole, while in the cerebellum the highest concentration was in the dentate nucleus, and in the midbrain in the superior and inferior colliculi. In the whole brain, the highest concentration was located in the lateral geniculate nucleus (Shaw et al. 1975). After a single dose, the cerebrum—and after repeated doses the cerebellum—had higher mercury concentrations in the squirrel monkey (Hoskins and Hupp 1978). The occipital part of the cerebrum had a higher concentration than the frontal or temporal parts (Berlin et al. 1975).

In experimental animals, part of the body burden is in the pelt. In mice, 8 days after a single dose of methyl mercury 6 percent of the body burden (Kostyniak 1980) was in pelt, and in rats, after 10 daily doses of methyl mercury, 28 percent was in pelt, and after 40 doses 37 percent (Magos and Butler 1976). After a single dose, the mercury concentration in the fur does not follow changes in body burden. For example, after a single dose of methyl mercury in rats, mercury concentration in kidneys started to decline after 7 days, and in all other tissues or organs after 1–3 days, but concentration in fur increased during the whole 24-day observation period (Farris et al. 1977). Mercury concentration in fur or hair near the roots correlates with mercury concentration in blood. The concentration of mercury changed with distance from root in the wool of sheep killed 55 days after a single intravenous dose of methyl mercury. Sequential analysis of 0.5 cm segments revealed that, from the roots outward, the concentration increased and then suddenly declined at the segment that had been growing at the time of treatment. The distance from root to the location of maximum concentration corresponded to the 55-day period during which mercury concentration in blood had been measured. It was therefore possible to compare clearance from blood to wool and to calculate the corresponding wool to blood mercury concentration ratio. Mercury declined in hair and blood with the same half time, and the ratio of wool to blood mercury was 120 (Kostyniak 1983). A similar correlation exists for human hair and blood, with a ratio of 260 to 320 (Kershaw et al. 1980).

Methyl mercury is easily transported from maternal blood into the fetus. In pregnant rats treated with methyl mercury on day 9 to day 13 of gestation, the concentration in the fetus on day 18 to day 20 was the same as in the mother and remained unchanged from day 19 to day 20, in spite of a twofold increase in litter weight (Magos et al. 1980*a*). In the pig, as in the rat, fetal uptake but not fetal concentration increased with gestation time (Kelman et al. 1982). In the guinea pig after gestation day 40, in spite of increased fetal uptake, the fetal concentration of methyl mercury decreased with gestation time (Kelman et al. 1980). In mice the placental to maternal blood concentration ratio was independent of the treatment day in relation to gestation age, but the fetal to maternal blood concentration ratio increased (Olson and Massaro 1977).

The rat fetal brain contained twice as much methyl mercury per gram of tissue than the maternal brain (Null et al. 1973). Correction of brain mercury concentration to blood content did not change this ratio (Wannag 1976). The fetal brain in mice also had higher methyl mercury concentrations than the maternal brain, when exposure was below the level associated with fetal mortality (Satoh and Suzuki 1983).

The passage of methyl mercury through human placenta is also significant, as judged from cases of fetal methyl mercury poisonings (Marsh et al. 1977) or from the high mercury concentration found in the liver of the fetus of a pregnant woman who died during the methyl mercury epidemics in Iraq (Magos et al. 1976). The average mercury concentration in maternal blood collected from nine Japanese women at delivery was 22.9 ng/ml red blood cells and 30.8 ng/ml in the umbilical cord blood (Suzuki et al. 1971).

Biodegradation

The mechanism and site of methyl degradation, with the exception of bacterial degradation in the gut, has not been identified. Liver, kidney, and brain slices (Fang and Fallin 1974) or liver homogenate (Gage 1975) did not cleave the $Hg–CH_3$ bond, but decomposition proceeded fast in the buffered (pH 7.4) solution of ascorbate in the presence of Cu^{2+} and oxygen (Gage 1975), and at a very much slower rate, 0.4 percent per day, in 0.1 M cysteine (Norseth and Clarkson 1970).

Decomposition in vivo is probably not catalyzed by a single enzyme and occurs in most parts of the body, with the exception of fur (hair). Inorganic mercury concentrations observed after methyl mercury treatment show that the Hg–CH$_3$ bond is cleaved even in the brain, where in rats the peak concentration of Hg^{2+} was 30 times higher after injection of methyl mercury than after an equivalent dose of HgCl$_2$ (Syversen 1974). In rats treated daily with methyl mercury for 90 days, 3.2 percent of the total mercury in the brain was inorganic. In other tissues, relative inorganic mercury levels were 6.2 percent in liver, 4.1 percent in blood, and 8.6 percent in the pelt. The relative concentration of inorganic mercury in kidneys increased with time and leveled off at 45 percent after 7 weeks (Magos and Butler 1976). In guinea pigs, the contribution of inorganic mercury to total mercury also leveled off about the same time, and at a lower level with higher as compared with lower doses (Iverson and Hierlihy 1974). In squirrel monkeys, about 50 percent of the mercury was inorganic in the kidneys, 20 percent in the liver, and less than 5 percent in the brain (Berlin et al. 1975). The biodegradation of methyl mercury is much more pronounced in some other species. In mink fed on methyl mercury contaminated fish, the percentage of total mercury in inorganic form was as follows: 50 percent of mercury in the liver, 38 percent in the kidneys, 18 percent in the brain, and 8 percent in the spleen (Jernelov and Johansson 1976). Kidneys and the livers of seals contain more than 90 percent of total mercury in the inorganic form, and muscle contains about 70 percent inorganic mercury (Freeman and Horne 1973).

Bacterial degradation in the gut may contribute to the inorganic mercury concentration in some tissues. In rats dosed daily with methyl mercury, 70 percent of fecal mercury, which represented 0.5 percent of the body burden of total mercury, was in the inorganic form (Magos and Butler 1976). Assuming 5 percent absorption, the bacterial degradation converts each day 0.025 percent of the body burden to inorganic mercury. Though it is a small amount, it equals 50 percent of the inorganic mercury content of the liver. Before inorganic mercury formed in the gut can reach the splanchnic circulation, it must pass through the intestinal wall, where its elevated level may indicate the site of demethylation. Degradation probably takes place in the colon, because in mice about 20 percent of mercury was inorganic in the colon, compared with 4 percent in the small intestine (Norseth 1971).

Biological Half Time

The kinetics of methyl mercury varies from one species to another. Table 3.4 lists biological half times in a few mammalian species, but the variation is even larger when comparison is extended to aquatic organisms. Thus, in mollusks the biological half time is 700 days, and in eel and flounder it is about 1,000 days (Clarkson 1972). Biological half time characterizes the ability of a species or an individual to accumulate higher or lower body burdens from identical daily doses and higher or lower concentrations in whole body or individual tissues. The larger the proportion of the body

Table 3.4 Biological half time of mercury after exposure to methyl mercury

Species	Medium	Half Time in Days	Reference
Man	Whole body	72.0	Aberg et al. 1969
Man	Blood	52.0	Kershaw et al. 1980
Man	Blood	65.0*	Clarkson et al. 1981
Man	Hair	72.0*	Al-Shahristani and Shihab 1974
Squirrel monkey	Whole body	124.0	Berlin et al. 1975
Squirrel monkey	Blood	49.0	Berlin et al. 1975
Rhesus macaque	Blood	30.0	Finocchio et al. 1980
Macaque monkey	Blood	22.0	Evans et al. 1977
Sheep	Blood	14.0	Kostyniak 1983
Cat	Whole body	114.0	Hollins et al. 1975
Cat	Blood	39.0	Charbonneau et al. 1974
Rat	Whole body	35.0	Magos and Butler 1976
Rat	Blood	14.0	Magos and Butler 1976
Rat	Whole body	47.0	Magos et al. 1980b
Mouse CBA/J	Whole body	7.4	Kostyniak 1980
Mouse CFW	Whole body	3.0	Kostyniak 1980

*Half times obtained from clinical cases of intoxication.

burden excreted daily, the shorter the time in which daily excretion reaches the level of daily intake (steady state) or the time at which a fixed proportion of the body burden is excreted after the cessation of exposure. The biological half time is calculated from the elimination constant b:

$$T_{1/2} = \frac{\ln 2}{b} \tag{1}$$

and b from the following equation, which describes clearance from the whole body after the cessation of exposure:

$$b = \frac{\ln B_0 - \ln B_t}{t} \tag{2}$$

where B_0 = body burden at 0 time and B_t = body burden at t time, and t = time in days between the two measurements. With the help of the elimination constant, body burden can be predicted from a single measurement according to the following equation:

$$B_t = B_0 (e^{-bt}) \tag{3}$$

In equations 2 and 3, concentrations in blood or in any other tissue (but not in hair, fur, or wool) can be substituted for body burden, and therefore from C_0 and C_t the elimination constant can be calculated, or C_t can be predicted from b and C_0.

Table 3.4 shows that in experimental animals the biological half time of methyl mercury in the whole body is longer than in blood. The reason for this is that the whole body burden includes an amount that is already excreted from the body into the fur, and that the loss from this part is only by shedding. However, when the rate of fur (hair) growth is known, the distance from root can be used as a time scale. Biological half time given by the sequential analysis of fur (hair) is the same as the half time calculated from changes in blood concentrations.

When the elimination constant is known, body burden can be predicted for any time during the exposure period from the daily dose (or the average daily dose). The equation for this calculation is:

$$B_t = d/b \, (1 - e^{-bt}) \tag{4}$$

where d is the daily dose. When d is given as the total daily dose, B_t gives the total body burden; when d gives dose per body weight, B_t gives concentration in the whole body in the same unit. The same equation cannot be used without modification to predict C_t in a tissue. The modified equation includes accumulation factor f:

$$C_t = df/b \, (1 - e^{-bt}) \tag{5}$$

Depending on whether the concentration of methyl mercury in a tissue at steady state is higher or lower than in the whole body, the accumulation factor is either higher or lower than 1. A series of measured C_t values and doses can be used to calculate by approximation both f and b, which best fit equation 5 (see Magos and Butler 1976).

In most of the experiments, exposure is not long enough to reach the condition of steady state, that is, when time has no further influence on B_t because $B_t = B_{max}$. Body burden at steady state can be calculated from

$$B_{max} = d/b \tag{6}$$

All these calculations are based on the assumption that the elimination of methyl mercury approximates a simple exponential function, and that even when no distinction is made between methyl mercury and its decomposition product, the deviation from the simple exponential function does not cause a significant error. When data on the kinetics of mercury in rats treated for 13 weeks with methyl mercury (Magos and Butler 1976) were analyzed with a linear and a nonlinear model, which included the metabolic pathway, the more complicated model did not cause a consistent improvement in data fit (Fischer et al. 1983).

Compared with the imperfection of the linear model, a more significant error is caused by weight changes. Thus, after cessation of a treatment schedule that caused weight loss, the body concentration of methyl mercury at least temporarily increased. In the same experiment, exposure caused a larger weight loss in virgin rats than in pregnant rats, and therefore the elimination constant in the two groups was similar only for body burden, but not for the body concentration of methyl mercury (Magos et al. 1980*a*).

The elimination constant established for one group of animals may not be the same for another group of the same species. Variations in biological half times are caused only by variations in excretion, because methyl mercury is nearly completely absorbed from the gastrointestinal tract in all species. Thus, the significant variation in biological half times between different mouse strains is caused mainly by differences in their urinary excretion (Kostyniak 1980). Biological half times were significantly decreased in human patients (Greenwood et al. 1978), in rats (Magos et al. 1980*b*), and in mice (Greenwood et al. 1978) during lactation. The prevention of the reabsorption of methyl mercury excreted in bile shortened biological half time (Clarkson et al. 1973; Magos and Clarkson 1976), while the suppression of intestinal methyl mercury decomposition as observed in germ-free mice (Nakamura et al. 1977) or in antibiotic-treated rats (Rowland et al. 1980) prolonged the biological half time.

Dietary influences on biological half times are probably mediated through a change in the ability of intestinal flora to demethylate methyl mercury. The 10.9-day biological half time of mice fed a pelleted diet was reduced to 5.8 days by GIBCO 116 E.C. diet and increased to 19.2 days by milk diet (Landry et al. 1979). The difference in the ability of the cecal content to demethylate methyl mercury was demonstrated in vivo when the cecal contents of milk- and pellet-fed rats were incubated with methyl mercury (Rowland et al. 1983).

Excretion

Methyl mercury exposure in mammals increases the excretion of mercury in feces more than in urine. In the first 4 days after administration of a single oral dose of ^{203}Hg-labeled methyl mercury to human volunteers, 6 percent of the administered ^{203}Hg was excreted with feces and only a negligible quantity in urine. Although urinary excretion of ^{203}Hg progressively increased from the initial daily 0.01–0.02 percent to 0.1 percent 3 months later, urinary mercury even at that time accounted only for 20 percent of the total daily excretion (Miettinen 1973). In the first 2 weeks after dosing pigs eliminated only 1 percent of the dose in urine and 10–16 percent in feces (Platonow 1968; Gyrd-Hansen 1981). Rats eliminated 6 percent of the dose in urine and 22 percent in feces in the first 10–11 days after a single dose of approximately 1.0 mg/kg Hg as MeHg (Norseth and Clarkson 1971; Gabbard 1976). The fecal to urinary excretion ratio in rats was significantly higher when the dose was reduced by a factor of 10 (Swensson and Ulfvarson 1967), and lower after the sixth week of daily treatment with 0.84 mg/kg Hg as MeHgCl (Magos and Butler 1976). After a single dose, the fecal to urinary excretion ratio was lower in mice than in rats, and it increased with time within the limits of 1.2 and 2.0 (Magos and Clarkson 1976).

In rats, the proportion of inorganic mercury to methyl mercury increased with time both in kidneys and in urine over the course of a 3-month exposure period, but the relative contribution of inorganic mercury to total mercury always remained significantly less in urine than in kidneys. The contribution of inorganic mercury to total mercury fluctuated around 70 percent in feces and 6 percent in the liver during this exposure period (Magos and Butler 1976). The dependence of intestinal methyl mercury decomposition on bacterial flora may explain why in other experiments the relative concentration of inorganic mercury in feces was as low as 40–50 percent (Norseth and Clarkson 1970) or as high as 94 percent (Rowland et al. 1980). Enterohepatic circulation (Norseth and Clarkson 1971) and the intestinal degradation of methyl mercury result in more total mercury excretion and less inorganic mercury excretion in bile than in feces (Norseth and Clarkson 1971). When methyl mercury was trapped in the gut by administration of a polythiol resin, the biliary excretion of methyl mercury increased and the biological half time decreased (Clarkson et al. 1973; Magos and Clarkson 1976).

In rat bile, 4 percent of the total mercury was inorganic (Norseth and Clarkson 1971), and in mice this value was less than 2 percent in the first 2 days after a single dose and approximately 6 percent between 8 and 22 days (Norseth 1971). In the squirrel monkey, however, in which 20 percent of the liver mercury was in the inorganic form, 30–85 percent of the total biliary mercury was inorganic, and there was an inverse relationship between methyl mercury concentration in the blood and the relative concentration of inorganic mercury in the bile (Berlin et al. 1975). These large differences between rodents and monkeys indicate that the nonbacterial degradation of methyl mercury is a more important metabolic pathway in the squirrel monkey than in rodents and that bacterial degradation is more important in rodents. The formation of inorganic mercury in the liver of monkeys may have a depressing effect on the biliary excretion of methyl mercury. In rats, the biliary excretion of methyl mercury decreased by nearly 30 percent when they were given 0.65 mg/kg Hg as $HgCl_2$ 48 hours before the administration of methyl mercury (Cikrt et al. 1984).

Methyl mercury is excreted into bile as a glutathione complex (Refsvik and Norseth 1975). Its excretion depends not only on the availability of GSH, but also on the availability of ligandin, a transport protein (Magos et al. 1978a, 1979). The induction of ligandin by phenobarbitone thus increased the biliary excretion of methyl mercury (Magos et al. 1974a). Indocyanine green (a nonsubstrate ligand oligandin) decreased the biliary excretion of methyl mercury by competition for the transport protein (Magos et al. 1979). Thiol compounds that cannot be metabolized to GSH increased the biliary excretion of methyl mercury probably by increasing the availability of non-protein-bound methyl mercury. Thus *DL*-penicillamine and acetylpenicillamine were shown to cause a temporary increase in biliary excretion of methyl mercury (Norseth 1973; Refsvik 1983). Dimercaptosuccinic acid had no such effect (Magos et al. 1978), probably because it overwhelmingly promotes the urinary excretion of this organomercurial and therefore causes depletion of methyl mercury in blood and liver (Magos 1976).

An additional excretory route is present in humans but important only in furry animals. When hair or fur develops from the matrix cells of follicular invaginations, it takes up methyl mercury from blood. The significant differences between biological half time estimations based on blood and whole body (see Table 3.4) demonstrate the importance of this excretory route. Fur may withdraw more methyl mercury from the body than is lost by fecal excretion. In sheep treated with a single dose of methyl mercury only 11.5 percent of the dose was eliminated in feces in the first 8 days, while 18 percent was eliminated in wool (Kostyniak 1983).

The fourth important excretory route is restricted to the period of lactation. Experiments on mice (Greenwood et al. 1978) and rats (Magos et al. 1980*b*) showed a significantly accelerated elimination during lactation. These experiments validated the observation made on lactating female patients during the methyl mercury epidemics in Iraq. The rate of decline in the blood concentration of methyl mercury in these patients indicated that lactation decreased the average biological half time from 66 days to 45 days (Greenwood et al. 1978). However, a discrepancy existed between the extent of this change and the concentration of mercury in milk. The decrease in biological half time from 66 to 45 days requires excretion of an additional 0.5 percent of the body burden per day. Considering an above-average milk production of 1.0 liter per day and that 1 percent of the body burden is in 1 liter of blood (Miettinen 1973), the concentration of mercury in milk should have been 50 percent of the concentration in blood. However, in 43 paired samples the concentration of mercury in milk averaged 3 percent of the concentration in blood (Bakir et al. 1973). Thus it seems that, in addition to excretion in milk, lactation accelerated the elimination of methyl mercury by other routes, for example, decomposition and/or increased biliary excretion.

Conclusion

The kinetics of absorption, distribution, and excretion of methyl mercury is distinctly different from the kinetics of any other mercurials. Methyl mercury, like other organomercurials and unlike inorganic mercuric salts, is nearly completely absorbed from the gastrointestinal tract. It is more resistant to degradation than other organomercurials, and therefore its role as a precursor of inorganic mercury is not important. It does not accumulate in the kidneys to the same extent as mercuric mercury, but it does cross barriers more easily than any other mercurial, with the exception of metallic mercury. It does not cross the blood-brain barrier as fast as metallic mercury, but it accumulates in the nervous system after a single dose over a period of days, and not seconds, as metallic mercury does. Though the one compartmental model and elimination according to a single exponential function is only an approximation, for any practical purpose such a model describes its distribution, accumulation, and excretion quite satisfactorily.

References

Aaseth, J.; Wannag, A.; and Norseth, T. (1976). The effect of *N*-acetylated *DL*-penicillamine and *DL*-homocysteine thiolactone on mercury distribution in adult rats, rat foetuses, and macaca monkeys after exposure to methyl mercuric chloride. *Acta Pharmacol* 39:302–311.

Aberg, B.; Ekman, L.; Falk, R.; Greitz, U.; Persson, G.; and Snihs, J. O. (1969). Metabolism of methyl mercury (^{203}Hg) compounds in man. *Arch Environ Health* 19:478–484.

Aldridge, W. N.; Brown, A. W.; Brierley, A. W.; Verscholyle, R. D.; and Street, B. W. (1981). Brain damage due to trimethyltin compounds. *Lancet* 2:692–693.

Al-Shahristani, H., and Shihab, K. (1974). Variation of biological half-life of methyl mercury in man. *Environ Health* 28:242–244.

Bakir, F.; Damluji, S. F.; Amin-Zaki, L.; Murtadha, M.; Khalidi, A.; Al-Rawi, N. Y.; Tikriti, S.; Dhahir, H. I.; Clarkson, T. W.; Smith, J. C.; and Doherty, R. A. (1973). Methyl mercury poisoning in Iraq. *Science* 181:230–241.

Berlin, M. (1963). Renal uptake, excretions, and retention of mercury, II: A study in the rabbit during infusion of methyl- and phenylmercuric compounds. *Arch Environ Health* 6:626–633.

Berlin, M.; Carlson, J.; and Norseth, T. (1975). Dose-dependence of methyl mercury metabolism. *Arch Environ Health* 30:307–313.

Berlin, M.; Jerksell, L. G.; and Ubisch, H. (1966). Uptake and retention of mercury in the mouse brain. *Arch Environ Health* 12:33–42.

Brown, A. W.; Aldridge, W. N.; and Street, B. W. (1979). The behavioural and neuropathologic sequelae of intoxication by trimethyltin compounds in the rat. *Am J Pathol* 97:59–82.

Charbonneau, S. M.; Munro, I. C.; Nera, E. A.; Willes, R. F.; Kuiper-Goodman, T.; Iverson, F.; Moodie, C. A.; Stoltz, D. R.; Armstrong, F. A. J.; Uthe, J. F.; and Grice, H. C. (1974). Subacute toxicity of methyl mercury in the adult rat. *Toxicol Appl Pharmacol* 27:569–581.

Cikrt, M.; Magos, L.; and Snowden, R. (1984). The effect of interaction between subsequent doses of MeHgCl or $HgCl_2$ on the biliary excretion of mercury from each individual dose. *Toxicol Lett* 20:189–194.

Clarkson, T. W. (1972). Recent advances in the toxicology of mercury with emphasis on the alkylmercurials. *Crit Rev Toxicol* 1:203–234.

Clarkson, T. W.; Amin-Zaki, L.; and Al-Tikriti, S. (1976). An outbreak of methyl mercury poisoning due to consumption of contaminated grain. *Fed Proc* 35:2395–2399.

Clarkson, T. W.; Magos, L.; Cox, C.; Greenwood, M. R.; Amin-Zaki, L.; Majeed, M. A.; and Al-Damluji, S. F. (1981). Test of efficacy of antidotes for removal of methyl mercury in human poisoning during the Iraq outbreak. *J Pharmacol Exp Therap* 218:74–83.

Clarkson, T.W.; Nordberg, G.F.; and Sager, T. (1983). *Reproductive and Developmental Toxicity of Metals.* New York: Plenum Press.

Clarkson, T. W.; Small, H.; and Norseth, T. (1973). Excretion and absorption of methyl mercury after polythiol resin treatment. *Arch Environ Health* 26:173–176.

Doi, R., and Kobayashi, T. (1982). Organ distribution and biological half-time of methyl mercury in four strains of mice. *Jpn J Exp Med* 52:307–314.

Doi, R., and Tagawa, M. (1983). A study on the biochemical and biological behaviour of methyl mercury. *Toxicol Appl Pharmacol* 69:407–416.

Evans, H. L.; Garman, R. T.; and Weiss, B. (1977). Methyl mercury: Exposure duration and regional distribution as determinants of neurotoxicity in nonhuman primates. *Toxicol Appl Pharmacol* 41:15–33.

Fang, S. C. (1980). Comparative study of uptake and tissue distribution of methyl mercury in female rats by inhalation and oral routes of administration. *Bull Environ Contam Toxicol* 24:65–72.

Fang, S. C., and Fallin, E. (1974). Uptake and subcellular cleavage of organomercury compounds by rat liver and kidney. *Chem Biol Interact* 9:57–64.

——— (1976). The binding of mercurial compounds to serum proteins. *Bull Environ Contam Toxicol* 15:110–117.

Farris, F. F.; Poklis, A.; and Griesmann, G. E. (1977). Effect of dietary cysteine on toxicity, tissue distribution, and elimination of methyl mercury in the rat. *ERDA Symposium Series* 42:465–477.

Finocchio, D. V.; Luschei, E. S.; Mottet, N. K.; and Body, R. (1980). Effects of methyl mercury on the visual system of Rhesus Macaque (Macaca Mulatta), I: Pharmacokinetics of chronic methyl mercury related to changes in vision and behaviour. In *Neurotoxicity of the Visual System,* edited by W. H. Merigan and B. Weiss, pp. 113–122. New York: Raven Press.

Fischer, H. L.; Thomas, D. J.; Sumler, M.; and Mushak, P. (1983). A physiological model of methyl mercury retention, metabolism, and excretion. Lecture presented at the 1983 meeting of the Society of Toxicology, Las Vegas, 1983. Abstract in *Toxicologist* 3:138.

Freeman, H. C., and Horne, D. A. (1973). Mercury in Canadian seals. *Bull Environ Contam Toxicol* 10:172–180.

Friberg, L.; Odeblad, E.; and Forssman, S. (1957). Distribution of two mercury compounds in rabbits after a single subcutaneous injection. *Arch Indust Health* 16:163–168.

Friberg, L.; Skog, E.; and Wahlberg, J. E. (1961). Resorption of mercuric chloride and methyl mercury dicyandiamide in guinea pigs through normal skin and through skin pretreated with acetone, alkylaryl-sulphonate, and soap. *Acta Derm Venerol* 41:40–52.

Gabbard, B. (1976). Treatment of methyl mercury poisoning in the rat with sodium 2,3-dimercaptopropane-1-sulfonate: Influence of dose and mode of administration. *Toxicol Appl Pharmacol* 38:415–424.

Gage, J. C. (1975). Mechanism for the biodegradation of organic mercury compounds: The actions of ascorbate and of soluble proteins. *Toxicol Appl Pharmacol* 32:225–238.

Glockling, F.; Hosmane, N. S.; Mahale, V. B.; Swindall, J. J.; Magos, L.; and King, T. J. (1977). Mono-, bis-, and tris- (trimethylsilyl)methyl derivatives of mercury. *J Chem Res (M)* 1201–1256.

Greenwood, M. R.; Clarkson, T. W.; Doherty, R. A.; Gates, A. H.; Amin-Zaki, L.; Elhassani, S.; and Majeed, M. A. (1978). Blood clearance half times in lactating and non-lactating members of a population exposed to methyl mercury. *Environ Res* 16:48–54.

Gyrd-Hansen, N. (1981). Toxicokinetics of methyl mercury in pigs. *Arch Toxicol* 48:173–181.

Hirayama, K. (1975). Transport mechanism of methyl mercury: Intestinal absorption, biliary excretion, and distribution of methyl mercury. *Kumamoto Med J* 28:151–163.

Hollins, J. G.; Willes, R. F.; Bryce, F. R.; Charbonneau, S. M.; and Munro, I. C. (1975). The whole body retention and tissue distribution of (^{203}Hg) methyl mercury in adult cats. *Toxicol Appl Pharmacol* 33:438–449.

Hoskins, B. B., and Hupp, E. W. (1978). Methyl mercury effects in rat, hamster, and squirrel monkey. *Environ Res* 15:5–19.

Iverson, F.; Downie, R. H.; Paul, C.; and Trenholm, H. L. (1973). Methyl mercury: Acute toxicity, tissue distribution, and decay profiles in the guinea pig. *Toxicol Appl Pharmacol* 24:545–554.

Iverson, F.; Downie, R. H.; Trenholm, H. L.; and Paul, C. (1974). Accumulation and tissue distribution of mercury in the guinea pig during subacute administration of methyl mercury. *Toxicol Appl Pharmacol* 27:60–69.

Iverson, F., and Hierlihy, S. L. (1974). Biotransformation of methyl mercury in the guinea pig. *Bull Environ Contam Toxicol* 11:85–91.

Jacobs, J. M.; Cavanagh, J. B.; and Carmichael, N. (1975). The effect of chronic dosing with mercuric chloride on dorsal root and trigeminal ganglia of rats. *Neuropathol Appl Neurobiol* 3:321–337.

Jernelov, A., and Johansson, A. H. (1976). Methyl mercury degradation in mink. *Toxicology* 6:315–321.

Kelman, B. J.; Steinmetz, S.; Walter, B.; and Sasser, L. (1980). Absorption of methyl mercury by the guinea pig during mid to late gestation. *Teratol* 21:161–165.

Kelman, B. J.; Walter, B. K.; and Sasser, L. B. (1982). Fetal distribution of mercury following introduction of methyl mercury into porcine maternal circulation. *J Toxicol Environ Health* 10:191–200.

Kershaw, T. G.; Clarkson, T. W.; and Dhahir, P. H. (1980). Studies on the relationship between blood concentrations and dose of methyl mercury in man. *Arch Environ Health* 35:28–36.

Komszta-Szumska, E.; Czuba, M.; Reuhl, K. R.; and Miller, D. R. (1983). Demethylation and excretion of methyl mercury by the guinea pig. *Environ Res* 32:247–257.

Kostyniak, P. J. (1980). Differences in elimination rates of methyl mercury between two genetic variant strains of mice. *Toxicol Lett* 6:405–410.

―――― (1983). Pharmacokinetics of methyl mercury in sheep. *J Appl Toxicol* 3:35–38.

Kurland, L. T.; Faro, S. N.; and Siedler, H. (1960). Minamata disease. *World Neurol* 1:270–292.

Landry, T. D.; Doherty, R. A.; and Gates, A. H. (1979). Effects of three diets on mercury excretion after methyl mercury administration. *Bull Environ Contam Toxicol* 22:151–158.

Magos, L. (1968). Uptake of mercury by the brain. *Br J Indust Med* 25:315–318.

―――― (1973). Factors affecting the uptake and retention of mercury by kidneys in rats. In *Mercury, Mercurials, and Mercaptans,* edited by M. W. Miller and T. W. Clarkson, pp. 166–184. Springfield, Ill.: Charles C Thomas.

―――― (1976). The effects of dimercaptosuccinic acid on the excretion and distribution of mercury in rats and mice treated with mercuric chloride and methyl mercury chloride. *Br J Pharmacol* 56:479–484.

―――― (1981). Metabolic factors in the distribution and half time of mercury after exposure to different mercurials. In *Industrial and Environmental Xenobiotics,* edited by I. Gut, M. Cikrt, and G. L. Plaa, pp. 1–15. Berlin: Springer-Verlag.

Magos, L.; Bakir, F.; Clarkson, T. W.; Al-Jawad, A. M.; and Al-Soffi, M. H. (1976). Tissue levels of mercury in autopsy specimens of liver and kidneys. *Bull WHO* 53 (Suppl.):93–96.

Magos, L., and Butler, W. H. (1976). The kinetics of methyl mercury administered repeatedly to rats. *Arch Toxicol* 35:25–39.

Magos, L., and Clarkson, T. W. (1976). The effect of oral doses of a polythiol resin on the excretion of methyl mercury in mice treated with cysteine, *d*-penicillamine, or phenobarbitone. *Chem Biol Interact* 14:325–335.

Magos, L.; Clarkson, T. W.; and Allen, J. (1978a). The interrelationship between non-protein bound thiols and the biliary excretion of methylmercury. *Biochem Pharmacol* 27:2203–2208.

Magos, L.; Clarkson, T. W.; and Snowden, R. (1979). The effects of bromosulphthalein, indocyanine green, and bilirubin on the biliary excretion of methylmercury. *Chem Biol Interact* 26:317–320.

Magos, L.; MacGregor, J. T.; and Clarkson, T. W. (1974a). The effect of phenobarbital and sodium dehydrocholate on the biliary excretion of methyl mercury in the rat. *Toxicol Appl Pharmacol* 30:1–6.

Magos, L.; Peristianis, G. C.; Clarkson, T. W.; Brown, A.; Preston, S.; and Snowden, R. (1981). Comparative study of the sensitivity of male and female rats to methylmercury. *Arch Toxicol* 48:11–20.

Magos, L.; Peristianis, G. C.; Clarkson, T. W.; Snowden, R. T.; and Majeed, M. A. (1980a). Comparative study of the sensitivity of virgin and pregnant rats to methyl mercury. *Arch Toxicol* 43:283–291.

Magos, L.; Peristianis, G. C.; Clarkson, T. W.; and Snowden, R. T. (1980b). The effect of lactation on methyl mercury intoxication. *Arch Toxicol* 45:143–148.

Magos, L.; Peristianis, G. C.; and Snowden, R. T. (1978b). Postexposure preventive treatment of methyl mercury intoxication in rats with dimercaptosuccinic acid. *Toxicol Appl Pharmacol* 45:463–475.

Magos, L., and Webb, M. (1977). The effect of selenium on the brain uptake of methyl mercury. *Arch Toxicol* 38:201–207.

Magos, L.; Webb, M.; and Butler, H. (1974*b*). The effect of cadmium pretreatment on the nephrotoxic action and kidney uptake of mercury in male and female rats. *Br J Exp Pathol* 55:589–594.

Marsh, D. O.; Myers, G. J.; Clarkson, T. W.; Amin-Zaki, L.; and Tikriti, S. (1977). Fetal methylmercury poisoning: New data on clinical and toxicological aspects. *Trans Am Neurol Assoc* 102:1–3.

Miettinen, J. K. (1973). Absorption and elimination of dietary mercury (Hg^{2+}) and methylmercury in man. In *Mercury, Mercurials, and Mercaptans*, edited by M. W. Miller and T. W. Clarkson, pp. 233–240. Springfield, Ill.: Charles C Thomas.

Naganuma, A., and Imura, N. (1979). Methyl mercury binds to low molecular weight substance in rabbit and human erythrocytes. *Toxicol Appl Pharmacol* 47:613–616.

Nakamura, I.; Hisokawa, K.; Tamura, H.; and Miura, T. (1977). Reduced mercury excretion with feces in germ-free mice after oral administration of methyl mercury chloride. *Bull Environ Contam Toxicol* 17:528–533.

Norseth, T. (1971). Biotransformation of methyl mercuric salts in the mouse studied by specific determination of inorganic mercury. *Acta Pharmacol Toxicol* 29:375–384.

––––––– (1973). The effect of chelating agents on biliary excretion of methyl mercuric salts in the rat. *Acta Pharmacol Toxicol* 32:1–10.

Norseth, T., and Clarkson, T. W. (1970). Studies on the biotransformation of [203]Hg-labeled methyl mercury chloride in rats. *Arch Environ Health* 21:717–727.

––––––– (1971). Intestinal transport of [203]Hg-labeled methyl mercury chloride. *Arch Environ Health* 22:577–658.

Null, D. H.; Gartside, P. S.; and Wei, E. (1973). Methyl mercury accumulation in brains of pregnant, non-pregnant, and fetal rats. *Life Sci* 12(2):65–72.

Olson, F. C., and Massaro, E. J. (1977). Pharmacodynamics of methyl mercury in the murine maternal/embryo: Fetal unit. *Toxicol Appl Pharmacol* 39:263–273.

Ostlund, K. (1969). Studies on the metabolism of methyl mercury and dimethyl mercury in mice. *Acta Pharmacol Toxicol* 27(Suppl. 1):5–132.

Platonow, N. (1968). A study of the metabolic fate of methyl mercury acetate. *Occup Health Rev* 20:9–19.

Rabenstein, D. L., and Evans, C. A. (1978). The mobility of methyl mercury in biological systems. *Bioinorg Chem* 8:107–114.

Refsvik, T. (1983). The influence of some thiols on biliary excretion of methyl mercury. *Acta Pharmacol Toxicol* 52:22–29.

Refsvik, T., and Norseth, T. (1975). Methyl mercuric compounds in rat bile. *Acta Pharmacol Toxicol* 36:67–68.

Rose, M. S. (1969). Evidence for histidine in the triethyltin-binding site of rat haemoglobin. *Biochem* 111:129–137.

Rowland, I. R.; Davies, M. J.; and Evans, J. G. (1980). Tissue content of mercury in rats given methyl mercuric chloride orally: Influence of intestinal flora. *Arch Environ Health* 35:155–160.

Rowland, I. R.; Robinson, R. D.; Doherty, R.; and Landry, T. L. (1983). Are developmental changes in methyl mercury metabolism and excretion mediated by the intestinal microflora? In *Reproductive and Developmental Toxicity of Metals*, edited by Clarkson, T.W.; Nordberg, G.; and Sager, P.R., pp. 747–758. New York: Plenum Press.

Sasser, L. B.; Jarboe, G. E.; Walter, B. K.; and Kelman, B. J. (1978). Absorption of mercury from ligated segments of the rat gastrointestinal tract. *Proc Soc Exp Biol Med* 157:57–60.

Satoh, H., and Suzuki, T. (1983). Embryonic and fetal death after in utero methyl mercury exposure and resultant organ mercury concentrations in mice. *Indus Health* 21:19–24.

Shaw, C.-M.; Mottet, K.; Body, R. L.; and Luschei, E. S. (1975). Variability of neuropathologic lesions in experimental methylmercurial encephalopathy in primates. *Am J Pathol* 80:451–469.

Somjen, G. G.; Herman, S. P.; Klein, R.; Brubaker, W. H.; Brinder, J. K.; Goodrich, J. K.; Krigman, M. R.; and Haseman, J. K. (1973). The uptake of methyl mercury (^{203}Hg) in different tissues related to its neurotoxic effects. *J Pharmacol Exp Therap* 187:602–611.

Suzuki, T.; Miyama, T.; and Katsunuma, H. (1963). Comparative study of bodily distribution of mercury in mice after subcutaneous administration of methyl, ethyl, and *n*-propyl mercury acetate. *Jpn J Exp Med* 33:277–282.

────── (1971). Comparison of mercury contents in maternal blood, umbilical cord blood, and placental tissues. *Bull Environ Contam Toxicol* 5:502–508.

Suzuki, T., and Yoshino, Y. (1969). Effects of *d*-penicillamine on urinary excretion of mercury in two cases of methyl mercury poisoning. *Jpn J Indust Health* 11:487–488.

Swensson, A., and Ulfvarson, U. (1963). Toxicology of organic mercury compounds used as fungicides. *Occup Health Rev* 15(3):5–11.

────── (1967). Experiments with different antidotes in acute poisoning by different mercury compounds. *Int Arch Gewerbepathol Gewerbehyg 2.* 4:12–50.

────── (1968). Distribution and excretion of various mercury compounds after single injections in poultry. *Acta Pharmacol Toxicol* 26:259–272.

Syversen, T. L. (1974). Biotransformation of ^{203}Hg labeled methyl mercuric chloride in rat brain measured by specific determination of Hg^{2+}. *Acta Pharmacol Toxicol* 35:277–283.

Task Group on Metal Accumulation (1973). Accumulation of toxic metals with special reference to their absorption, excretion, and biological half-times. *Env Phys Biochem* 3:65–107.

Turner, M. D.; Smith, J. C.; Kilper, R. W.; Forbes, G. B.; and Clarkson, T. W. (1975). Absorption of natural methyl mercury (MeHg) from fish. *Clin Res* 23:225A.

Vostal, J. J., and Clarkson, T. W. (1973). Mercury as an environmental hazard. *J Occup Med* 15:649–656.

Wannag, A. (1976). The importance of organ blood mercury when comparing foetal and maternal rat organ distribution of mercury after methyl mercury exposure. *Acta Pharmacol Toxicol* 38:289–298.

White, J. F., and Rothstein, A. (1973). The interaction of methyl mercury with erythrocytes. *Toxicol Appl Pharmacol* 26:370–384.

Yoshino, Y.; Mozai, T.; and Nakao, K. (1966). Distribution of mercury in the brain and its subcellular units in experimental organic mercury poisonings. *J Neurochem* 13:397–406.

Dose-Response Relationships in Humans: Methyl Mercury Epidemics in Japan and Iraq

David O. Marsh

The dose-response for methyl mercury would ideally be the relationship between the dose of methyl mercury ingested to produce a certain brain concentration of methyl mercury, and the proportion of an exposed population that shows specific biological effects from this dose. Investigations of outbreaks of methyl mercury poisoning in human populations have of necessity been retrospective, with only limited data on dietary intake and rare opportunities for brain analyses. Under such circumstances, available body tissues such as hair and blood have been analyzed and used as indicators of dose. In steady-state situations, when intake equals elimination, hair and blood are good indicators; an average hair to blood ratio is about 250. After acute or subacute exposure, while the body burden is decreasing, the blood methyl mercury level is falling, and isolated blood analyses provide a limited indication of dose. In this case, segmental analysis of sufficiently long specimens of head hair may include the time of maximum exposure and provide a better index of dose. Head hair grows at an average rate of slightly over 1 cm per month, so segmental analysis of maternal hair may provide a good index of fetal exposure if the sample is long enough to cover the period of gestation.

Neurological Effects of Methyl Mercury

Postnatal

The first case reports on methyl mercury poisoning were by Edwards in 1885, and the first detailed account was by Hunter et al. in 1940, who reported on four men who had been exposed to methyl mercury in the manufacture of seed fungicides. Symptoms began 3–4 months after the onset of exposure and progressed after exposure had ceased. The most frequent initial symptom was paresthesia of the extremities, followed within a month by ataxia of gait, dysarthria, and impaired peripheral vision. The cardinal signs, confined to the nervous system, were constricted visual fields, ataxia, dysarthria, and sensory deficits (particularly impaired vibration), stereognosis, and two-point discrimination in the extremities.

The first mass outbreak of methyl mercury poisoning occurred in Minamata, Japan, and was caused by industrial pollution of the environment so that the effects were seen in the general population who ate contaminated fish. Between April and December 1956, 50 cases of the Hunter-Russell syndrome occurred in Minamata. Eventually the total number of recognized cases grew to 1,775 by late 1981 (Tokuomi et al. 1982), although many of these patients did not exhibit the full syndrome. This outbreak has been reviewed by Tsubaki and Irukayama (1977). The large number of cases allowed better definition of clinical effects. Again, the most common initial symptom was paresthesia of the extremities, sometimes accompanied by perioral paresthesia and followed by constricted visual fields, ataxia of limbs and gait, slow slurred speech that in severe cases progressed to anarthria, deafness to high tones, and sensory deficits. Vibration, joint position sensation, and two-point discrimination were impaired, as in the cases cited by Hunter et al. (1940), but in addition there was impairment of pain and touch sensation. This was commonly in glove and stocking distribution, but in some cases the deficit spread to the trunk. Less frequent signs included rigidity of the limbs with chorea or athetosis, mental impairment, emotional lability, depression, and excessive sweating. Deep tendon reflexes were more frequently increased than decreased. Plantar responses were extensor in a minority of cases. The most severely affected patients became comatose and died within a few months of the initial symptoms. By October 1960, 111 cases were recognized in the Minamata area, and by December 1965 some 37 percent of these had died.

The second Japanese outbreak of methyl mercury poisoning occurred in Niigata, and the first cases were recognized in 1965. Again, the source was consumption of fish with elevated concentrations of methyl mercury caused by industrial contamination of the Agano River. By the end of 1974, the total number of recognized cases was 520 (Tsubaki and Irukayama 1977).

During the winter of 1971–72, Iraq experienced the most extensive outbreak of methyl mercury poisoning. Methyl mercury treated wheat, intended for planting, was provided free to farmers throughout the country. They washed out the red dye, fed the grain to farm animals, and when they appeared unaffected, had it ground into flour, which was used for daily baking of bread. From December 1971 through March 1972, the total number of patients admitted to Iraqi hospitals and diagnosed as having methyl mercury poisoning was 6,500; some 459 of these patients died (Bakir et al. 1973). Many other cases were not admitted to hospitals. The clinical features were those reported from Japan, except for 6 patients with signs of optic atrophy (Rustam and Hamdi 1974) and improvement in many of the milder cases, especially among children (Amin-Zaki et al. 1974a), although blindness in children tended to persist (Amin-Zaki et al. 1978).

Prenatal

Harada (in Tsubaki and Irukayama 1977) reported 23 fetal cases in Minamata, born between 1955 and 1959 and diagnosed at ages 13 months to 9 years. Their mothers were asymptomatic during pregnancy, except that 5 experienced paresthesia. All these children had severe psychomotor retardation. None could crawl, stand, or say recognizable words until 3 years of age. Almost half remained unable to talk, and by 7 years of age, only 6 could walk without assistance. All were ataxic, and most had increased deep tendon reflexes, increased tone, involuntary movements, and incontinence. Cases with mild or moderate fetal effects were not identified in Minamata. The most important observation was that mothers with minor or no symptoms gave birth to severely affected infants. Despite clinical surveys, only one fetal case was identified in Niigata.

In 1974, Amin-Zaki et al. (1974*b*) reported 15 infant-mother pairs in Iraq who were exposed to methyl mercury during pregnancy. Several infants had severe psychomotor retardation similar to that observed by Harada, but others showed relatively mild effects. The same authors (Amin-Zaki et al. 1979) published a 5-year follow-up of 32 infants, including the above 15, and reported an increased mortality rate and emergence of clinical signs that were not apparent during the first few months of life.

Iraqi infant-mother pairs exposed during pregnancy to relatively low doses of methyl mercury were also studied (Marsh et al. 1980, 1981; Clarkson et al. 1981). Samples of maternal head hair were collected during 1972-74. Head hair grows at the rate of slightly over 1 cm per month, and the samples were long enough to cover gestation during the time the contaminated bread was consumed. Each sample of 50-100 strands of hair was analyzed in 1 cm segments by atomic absorption. The 84 mothers were questioned concerning the infants' early mental and physical development, and the infants were examined on several occasions. The peak maternal hair mercury concentrations during pregnancy were between 0.4 ppm (parts per million) and 640.0 ppm, indicating a wide range of fetal exposure. Observed effects on the children ranged from none to various degrees of psychomotor retardation ("cerebral palsy"). Maternal symptoms during pregnancy were mild and transient, with paresthesia as the most frequent symptom. The Iraq outbreak made it clear not only that there can be severe fetal effects, as reported in Minamata, but also that there can be less obvious effects, such as minor delay in achieving early developmental milestones. In both mild and severe cases, the mother may have no or merely mild and transient symptoms, indicating the much greater susceptibility of the developing fetal brain. Neuropathological studies (Choi et al. 1977; Takeuchi 1968) have indicated that the chief effects on the fetal brain are impaired migration of neurons to the cerebellar and cerebral cortices, together with deranged organization of the cerebral cortex. These features of impaired development and maturation of the fetal brain contrast with the areas of focal damage to the mature brain exposed in later life (Tsubaki and Irukayama 1977).

Dose-Response Relationship: Postnatal Exposure

Minamata

Most of the affected families ate fish from Minamata Bay every day. Berglund et al. (1971) estimated that the median concentration of total mercury in these fish was 11 mg/kg fresh weight, and that the maximum concentration in fish and shellfish was as high as 40 mg/kg. This contrasts with concentrations in most oceanic species of about 150 mg/kg fresh weight and higher levels in piscivorous species, such as tuna (350 mg/kg) and swordfish averaging about 1,150 mg/kg. Mercury in fish is predominantly in the methyl form. Consumption of fish with highly elevated mercury concentrations resulted in Minamata hair levels of approximately 700 μg/g at the time of onset of symptoms (Berglund et al. 1971). Blood mercury analyses were not made. The available data do not allow conclusions concerning dose-response relationship, except that daily intake of highly contaminated fish for several months or longer resulted in a severe outbreak of poisoning with a high mortality rate.

Niigata

Berglund et al. (1971) reported that blood mercury analyses were available for 17 patients, and hair mercury analyses for 36 patients. Dates of sampling and of onset of symptoms were uncertain in some cases. Analyses were performed by the colorimetric dithizone method, which was insensitive compared with later methods. The ratio of hair to blood mercury concentrations was 370, so the results of hair analysis may have greater validity. The number of cases was few, so Berglund et al. attempted to determine the blood or hair mercury concentration at the onset of symptoms, and hence the lowest blood or hair level associated with clinical effects. The lowest such hair concentration was stated to be 52 μg/g in June 1965 only 1–15 days after onset of symptoms and signs, which included sensory disorder, constricted visual fields, and ataxia. This was Niigata case 30. This hair sample was preserved and analyzed some years later by atomic absorption (Tsubaki et al. 1978). Tsubaki concluded that the hair mercury concentration at onset of symptoms was 96 μg/g and that the peak concentration was 200 μg/g. No other Niigata case had onset of symptoms associated with hair mercury concentration below 200 μg/g.

The many uncertainties in the data from Minamata and Niigata make it difficult to use them as the basis for the relationship between mercury concentration in hair or blood and clinical effects.

Iraq

Bakir et al. (1973) provided data relating blood levels to clinical effect (see Table 4.1). There were 40 controls with blood mercury concentrations from 0

Table 4.1 Frequency of paresthesia according to estimated peak concentration of blood mercury

Concentration of Mercury in Blood (ng/ml)		% (No.) with Paresthesia	No. of Cases
65 Days After Ingestion Ceased	At Estimated Peak		
0–100	0–200	9.5(2)	21
101–500	201–1,000	5.0(1)	19
501–1,000	1,001–2,000	42.0(8)	19
1,001–2,000	2,001–4,000	60.0(10)	17
2,001–3,000	4,001–6,000	80.0(20)	25
3,001–4,000	6,001–8,000	82.0(14)	17

Source: Based on data from Bakir et al. 1973.

to 500 ng/ml. Paresthesias were reported by three of the controls (7.5 percent). At higher blood mercury levels, the frequency of paresthesia, ataxia, visual signs, and death increased dramatically. The third line of the table indicates that there were 19 cases with blood mercury concentrations between 501 and 1,000 ng/ml, and increased frequency of paresthesia and other effects, compared with the control group. These blood mercury levels had been calculated from the primary data to give the estimated blood levels that would be expected 65 days after cessation of ingestion of methyl mercury. Given a clearance half time of about 65 days, these blood levels can be doubled to provide approximate peak mercury levels. This suggests that the lowest peak blood mercury concentration associated with symptoms or signs of methyl mercury poisoning in this group of 118 people was between 1,001 and 2,000 ng/ml, which corresponds to about 250–500 μg/g mercury in hair.

The 1976 World Health Organization report on mercury (WHO 1976) used the same data from Bakir et al. (1973) to estimate the minimum blood mercury concentration at which paresthesia became detectable. The mean blood mercury concentrations for each cohort were plotted on a logarithmic scale against the frequency of paresthesia. This approach attempted to determine the blood mercury concentration at which paresthesia caused by methyl mercury was detectable above the background frequency of paresthesia among the controls. Supposing a clearance half time of 65 days, the threshold blood mercury concentration for paresthesia was concluded to be 480 ng/ml. This calculation depends on the background frequency of paresthesia in the general population.

Paresthesia is a subjective sensation of tingling and numbness, such as one may experience on compression of circulation to an extremity. It can be an isolated symptom without neurological signs on examination, or it can be accompanied by signs of a lesion in a peripheral nerve or the central nervous system. Hyperventilation can cause paresthesia over the extremities and around the mouth. Common organic causes include alcoholism, diabetic neuropathy, and vitamin deficiency. Ayd (1961, p. 26) reported paresthesia in 60 percent of a group of depressed individuals, Turner et al.* (1981) elicited a history of paresthesia in 49.5 percent of 93 Peruvians in an agricultural village with low blood and hair mercury concentration, and in reporting the possibility of methyl mercury poisoning among Canadian Indians, Harada et al. (1976) said that 38 percent of a control group had sensory disturbances. Evans (1976) reported that 1 person in 4 or 5 experiences referred itching or prickling sensations, for example, scratching the skin produces prickling or itching sensations elsewhere. Aquagenic pruritis is said to be common, occurring in perhaps 16 percent of individuals after bathing (Greaves 1981), and does not depend on the temperature of the water. This is to be distinguished from itching skin weals that may develop under stress, after exposure to warm water, or on sweating after exertion. Thus paresthesia may be caused by a variety of factors, and several reports indicate a higher frequency than the 7.5 percent among controls in the Iraq study (Bakir et al. 1973). However, given this background frequency of paresthesia and a clearance half time of 65 days, the lowest peak blood mercury concentration for the earliest symptom, paresthesia, in 125 Iraq adults was between 1,001 and 2,000 ng/ml or, according to the calculations of the WHO report (1976), was 480 ng/ml. The latter would be equivalent to 120 μg/g mercury in hair, but the precise effect level in adults has assumed less importance, since there is evidence that the fetal brain is damaged at lower levels of exposure.

Dose-Response Relationship: Prenatal Exposure

Japan

In Minamata, samples of maternal head hair were obtained and analyzed too long after childbirth to reflect fetal exposure. Only one fetal case was identified in Niigata, and that was a boy whose mother had a peak hair mercury concentration during pregnancy reported to be over 200 μg/g (Tsubaki and Irukayama 1977). Little can be concluded from these observations, except that frequent maternal consumption of fish with highly elevated methyl mercury concentrations resulted in severe psychomotor retardation in their infants, although the mothers had only mild and transient symptoms.

Iraq

Amin-Zaki et al. (1974b) reported 15 infant-mother pairs. Six mothers had features of methyl mercury poisoning, and 6 infants had definite neurological abnormalities, including weakness, hyperreflexia, and abnormal tone. Four infants were blind, deaf, and mentally retarded. Only one mother of an affected infant was asymptomatic. The lowest blood mercury concentration in an abnormal infant was 564 ng/ml, and the 4 infants with the highest blood levels (1,053–4,220 ng/ml) all had severe neurological deficits. The infants were more severely affected than their mothers. The same authors (Amin-Zaki et al. 1979) reported a 5-year follow-up of 30 infants, including the above 15, and compared their progress with a control group. Mortality was 28 percent compared with 6 percent in controls. Surviving infants who had initially been identified as abnormal showed no improvement. Half the infants who had initially appeared normal suffered psychomotor retardation, and just over half demonstrated hyperreflexia and abnormal plantar reflexes. The mean of maximum maternal hair mercury concentrations for infants who died was 359 μg/g, compared with 160 μg/g for those who survived. These were the first reports of relatively mild fetal effect from exposure to methyl mercury, and they suggested that the severity of effect was related to the degree of exposure.

Marsh et al. (1980, 1981) studied 83 Iraq infant-mother pairs. Maternal symptoms and infant symptoms and signs increased in frequency according to the degree of exposure as reflected in the hair mercury levels. Severe neurological effects, clinically indistinguishable from cerebral palsy or psychomotor retardation caused by hypoxia, were noted in several infants whose mothers' peak hair mercury concentration was 165–320 μg/g. No infant effects were identified in those with maternal hair mercury levels below 18 μg/g. These data were evaluated further by Clarkson et al. (1981), with similar conclusions that for fetal exposure the clinical effect level is represented by a maternal hair mercury concentration of about 20 μg/g when the hair sample is a cluster of strands. Analysis of single strands may provide a somewhat higher peak concentration.

Thus, the Iraq outbreak of methyl mercury intoxication has provided relationships for dose-response (dose determined by hair analysis, response determined by clinical effects) for adult and fetal exposure. The average hair to blood ratio for methyl mercury is approximately 250, so that a mild fetal effect occurring at a hair concentration of 20 μg/g would correspond to 80 ng Hg/ml in blood (equal to 80 parts per billion or 8 μg/100 ml). According to data reviewed by the WHO task group (WHO 1976), this blood level might be achieved by a long-term daily intake of 1.2 μg/kg mercury as methyl mercury.

The dose-response conclusions derived from a limited amount of Iraq data were for ingestion of a methyl mercury fungicide applied to seed grain. Our usual consumption of methyl mercury is from seafood, which might not be toxicologically equivalent because selenium may counteract methyl mercury toxicity (Ganther 1980; Skerfving 1978). This issue awaits resolution by studies of populations eating large amounts of fish.

References

Amin-Zaki, L.; El-Hassani, S.; Majeed, M. A.; Clarkson, T. W.; Doherty, R. A.; and Greenwood, M. (1974*a*). Studies of infants postnatally exposed to methylmercury. *J Pediatr* 1974, 85:81–84.

Amin-Zaki, L.; El-Hassani, S.; Majeed, M. A.; et al. (1974*b*). Intrauterine methylmercury poisoning in Iraq. *Pediatrics* 54:587–95.

Amin-Zaki, L.; Majeed, M. A.; Clarkson, T. W.; et al. (1978). Methylmercury poisoning in Iraq children: Clinical observations over two years. *Br Med J* 11:613–616.

Amin-Zaki, L.; Majeed, M. A.; El-Hassani, S.; Clarkson, T. W.; Greenwood, M.; and Doherty, R. A. (1979). Prenatal methylmercury poisoning: Clinical observations over five years. *Am J Dis Child* 133:172–177.

Ayd, F. J. (1961). *Recognizing the Depressed Patient.* New York: Grune and Stratton.

Bakir, F.; Damluji, S. F.; Amin-Zaki, L.; Murtadha, M.; Khalidi, A.; Al-Rawi, N. Y.; Tikriti, S.; Dhahir, H. I.; Clarkson, T. W.; Smith, J. C.; and Doherty, R. A. (1973). Methylmercury poisoning in Iraq. *Science* 181:230–241.

Berglund, F.; Merlin, M.; Birke, G.; et al. (1971). Methylmercury in fish. *Nord Hyg Tidskr,* Suppl. 4.

Choi, B. H.; Lapham, L. W.; Amin-Zaki, L.; and Saleem, T. (1977). Abnormal neuronal migration in human fetal brain. *Am J Pathol* 86(2):417.

Clarkson, T. W.; Cox, C.; Marsh, D. O.; et al. (1981). Dose-response relationships for adults and prenatal exposure to methylmercury. In *Measurement of Risks,* edited by G. G. Berg and H. D. Maillie, pp. 111–129. New York: Plenum.

Edwards, G. N. (1885). Two cases of poisoning by mercuric methide. *St Bart's Hosp Rep* 1:141–150.

Evans, P. R. (1976). Referred itch. *Br Med J* 2:839–841.

Ganther, H. E. (1980). Interactions of vitamin E and selenium with mercury and silver. *Ann NY Acad Sc* 355:212–226.

Greaves, M. W.; Black, A. K.; Eady, R. A. J.; and Coults, A. (1981). Aquagenic pruritis. *Br Med J* 282:2008–2010.

Harada, M.; Fujino, T.; Akagi, T.; and Nishigaki, S. (1976). Epidemiological and clinical study and historical background of mercury pollution on Indian reservations in Northwestern Ontario, Canada. *Bull Inst Constit Med Kumamoto Univ* 26(34):169–184.

Hunter, D.; Bomford, R. R.; and Russell, D. R. (1940). Poisoning by methylmercury compounds. *Q J Med* 9:193–213.

Marsh, D. O.; Myers, G. J.; Clarkson, T. W.; et al. (1980). Fetal methylmercury poisoning: Clinical and toxicological data on 29 cases. *Ann Neurol* 7:348–353.

———— (1981). Dose-response relationship for human fetal exposure to methylmercury. *J Clin Toxicol* 18(11):1311–1318.

Rustam, H., and Hamdi, T. (1974). Methylmercury poisoning in Iraq. *Brain* 97:499–510.

Skerfving, S. (1978). Interactions between selenium and methylmercury. *Environ Health Perspect* 25:57–65.

Takeuchi, T. (1968). Pathology of Minamata disease. In *Minamata Disease,* edited by M. Kutsuma, pp. 141–228. Tokyo: Kumamoto University Press.

Tokuomi, H.; Uchino, M.; Imamura, S.; Yamanaga, H.; Nakanishi, R.; and Ideta, T. (1982). Minamata disease (organic mercury poisoning): Neuroradiologic and electrophysiologic studies. *Neurology* 32:1369–1375.

Tsubaki, T.; Hirota, K.; Shirakawa, K.; Kondo, K.; and Sato, T. (1978). Clinical, epidemiological, and toxicological studies on methylmercury. In *Proceedings of the First International Congress on Toxicology,* edited by G. L. Plaa and W. A. Duncan, pp. 339–357. New York: Academic Press.

Tsubaki, T., and Irukayama, K. (1977). *Minamata Disease.* New York: Elsevier.

Turner, M. D.; Marsh, D. O.; Rubio, C. E.; et al. (1981). Methylmercury in populations eating large quantities of marine fish. *Archiv Environ Health* 35(6):367–378.

World Health Organization (1976). *Environment Health Criteria 1: Mercury.* Geneva: World Health Organization.

FIVE

The Experimental Neuropathology of Methyl Mercury

Louis W. Chang

Methyl mercury is a highly toxic compound. Although it has long been recognized as a potential health hazard to industrial workers (Hunter et al. 1940; Hunter and Russell 1954), it was not until the massive outbreak in Minamata Bay, Japan, during the 1950s that scientists first recognized the potential of the organomercurial as an environmental toxicant (Kurland et al. 1960; Takeuchi 1968). Methyl mercury poisoning has since been termed "Minamata disease."

Toxic exposure to methyl mercury results primarily in neurological damage, characterized chiefly by ataxia, sensory disturbances, and changes in mental state. The pathology of Minamata disease in the adult has been well reviewed by Takeuchi (1968). This chapter will focus only on the neuropathological aspects of the effect of methyl mercury on experimental animals.

Effects on the Blood-Brain Barrier

The blood-brain barrier is a complex of multiple systems regulating the exchange of metabolic material between the brain and the blood (Broman 1967; Broman and Steinwall 1967; Steinwall 1961). Like many other chemical compounds, mercury was found to induce dysfunction of the blood-brain barrier (Steinwall and Olsson 1969; Chang and Hartmann 1972*d*). Steinwall and co-workers (Steinwall and Klatzo 1966; Steinwall and Snyder 1969) showed that an impairment of the blood-brain barrier occurred very rapidly following administration of a mercury compound. By means of light and electron microscopy, Chang and co-workers (Ware et al. 1974) also demonstrated that even a minute amount of mercury was capable of impairing the blood-brain system within hours, leading to an extravasation of normally barred plasma solutes.

Passow et al. (1961) indicated that mercury ions probably caused damage to the membrane structure by forming cross-linkages with the protein moiety of the cell membrane, resulting in impairment of the membrane functions as well as in the increase of its permeability ("leaky membrane" phenomenon). The increased permeability and dysfunction of the blood-brain barrier after mercury intoxication may reflect the damage of endothelial and glial membranes by the mercury ions, leading to leakage of the plasma solutes into the nervous parenchyma.

Distribution of Mercury

Distribution in the Nervous System

The distribution of mercury in the central nervous system has been studied by various investigators. By means of autoradiographic technique, Berlin and Ullberg (1963) demonstrated that when methyl mercury was given, accumulation occurred gradually over a period of a few days, and that the distribution in the brain was quite different from the distribution seen after injection of inorganic mercury. Unlike the heterogeneous distribution, as in the case of inorganic mercury, the distribution of methyl mercuric salt was more uniform. The areas that showed maximum concentration of mercury were the hippocampus and the cerebellar gray. In dogs, however, Yoshino et al. (1966) demonstrated that the calcarine cortex and the cerebellum initially showed higher mercury content than any other parts of the brain after administration of methyl mercury—but the distribution became relatively uniform 1 week after a single injection (Nordberg 1976). In pigs, the pattern of mercury distribution in the central nervous system was found to be: occipital cortex > cerebellum > brain stem > medulla oblongata > spinal cord > peripheral nerves (Platonow 1968). As a result of continuous administration of radioactive labeled methyl mercuric hydroxide, the spinal dorsal root ganglia of rats contained the highest concentration of mercury, followed closely by the cerebral cortex and the cerebellum, then by the subcortical part of the forebrain (Somjen et al. 1973). These distributions correlated well with pathological lesion distribution.

Cellular and Subcellular Distribution and Localization

Early study on the subcellular distribution of mercury in the rat nervous system was performed by means of biochemical fractionation and found that nearly all the mercury was in the protein fraction, whereas the lipid and nucleic acid fractions had low concentrations (Yoshino et al. 1966). Ultracentrifugation showed that mercury was largely distributed between the mitochondria, microsomal fractions, and supernatant fractions, while the nuclear fraction contained only very small amounts of mercury (Yoshino et al. 1966).

By means of an electron-microscopic histochemical method (metal-sulfide coupling), Chang and Hartmann (1972c) were able to demonstrate visually the actual localization of the mercury within the intact nervous tissues and cells. After intoxication with methyl mercuric chloride (CH_3HgCl) the general distribution of mercury among the nerve cells examined was found to be: dorsal root ganglion neurons > neurons of the calcarine cortex > Purkinje cells of the cerebellum > anterior horn motoneurons > granule cells of the cerebellum. As for the nerve fibers, the general distribution of mercury was: dorsal root fibers > sciatic nerves > ventral root fibers.

Intracellularly, mercury was found bound to most of the membranous structures, such as the mitochondria, the endoplasmic reticulum, the Golgi complex, and the nuclear envelope (Figure 5.1). In the nerve fibers, mercury was predominantly localized on the myelin sheaths and on the mitochondria. However, increasing amounts of mercury were detected in the general matrix of the cytoplasm and axoplasm as the intoxication progressed. Only a minute amount of mercury was found within the nuclei.

This observation was in good agreement with those obtained by biochemical analysis, which indicated that the subcellular distribution of mercury, in general, was: mitochondrial fraction > microsomal fraction > supernatant fraction > nuclear fraction (Massey and Fang 1968). As the intoxication progressed, there was a gradual increase in the mercury content in the supernatant fraction (Yoshino et al. 1966; Norseth 1967; Massey and Fang 1968). It has been indicated that the biological membranes are generally rich in sulfhydryl (-SH) groups (Passow et al. 1961; Clarkson 1972). This may explain the preferential binding of mercury to the membranous structures.

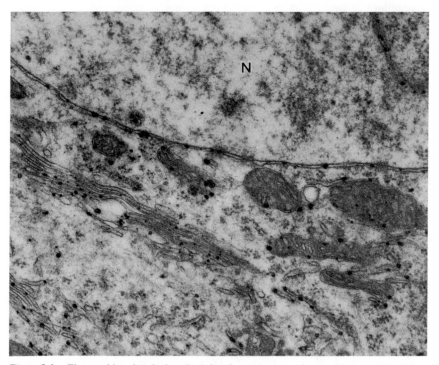

Figure 5.1. Electron histochemical method showing mercury as electron-dense particles binding to the nuclear envelope, mitochondria, Golgi complex, and endoplasmic reticulum, suggesting that mercury has a special affinity towards biological membranes. (N = nucleus.) (From Chang and Hartmann 1972*c*)

Biochemical and Metabolic Changes

Effects of Mercurials on Protein Synthesis

Yoshino et al. (1966) reported a comprehensive study on the biochemical changes in the rat nervous system following methyl mercury intoxication. It was found that incorporation of amino acid into the nervous system of mercury-intoxicated rats was markedly inhibited (a reduction of 43 percent) even before the development of any observable neurological symptoms or biochemical changes. Yoshino and his co-workers proposed that, since the disturbance in protein metabolism was the only alteration prior to all other biochemical changes, the selective inhibition of protein synthesis might have a bearing on the poisoning by alkyl mercury compounds.

Except for two reports in the literature (Brubaker et al. 1973; Richardson and Murphy 1974) claiming that there was a stimulatory effect on the synthesis of nucleic acids and protein in the brains of rats treated with methyl mercuric salts, findings in most laboratories (Cavanagh and Chen 1971a; Farris and Smith 1975; Verity et al. 1977; Syversen 1977; Omata et al. 1978; Chang 1983) confirmed and supported Yoshino's observation that incorporation of amino acids into the brain tissues was drastically reduced following mercury intoxication. It was postulated that the reduction of amino acids, and probably other metabolites, into the nervous system was a consequence of the impairment of the blood-brain barrier.

Changes in Enzymatic Activities

Yoshino et al. (1966) also reported the effects of methyl mercury on several sulfhydryl enzymes such as magnesium-activated adenosinetriphosphatase (ATPase), fructose-diphosphate aldolase, and succinic dehydrogenase. It was found that, except for succinic dehydrogenase, which showed a decrease in activity after the onset of neurological symptoms, there was no change in any of the enzymatic activities in the asymptomatic animals. In view of this, Yoshino postulated that the development of neurological symptoms and lesions was not a consequence of an inhibition of enzymatic functions or reduction in oxygen consumption in the nervous system, but rather that the reverse could be true.

Because of the central importance of the glycolytic pathway in energy production in the brain, enzymatic change in this pathway after mercury administration was extensively investigated. Using rodents as the animal models, Patterson and Usher (1971) and Salvaterra et al. (1973) reported a change in the glycolytic enzymatic activities after methyl mercury intoxication.

Patterson and Usher (1971) concluded that since there was an inhibition of such enzymes as phosphoglycerate mutase, enolase, pyruvate kinase, and pyruvate dehydrogenase toward the end of the glycolytic chain, there would be a drop in the level of adenosinetriphosphate (ATP). They further suggested that in the low-dose situation (0.05 mg Hg/kg) there might be an allosteric inhibition of glycogen phosphorylase, as indicated by a reduction in G-1-P and an unchanged GP shuttle activity. It was postulated that there might also be a decreased ATP usage, since there is an increase in ATP level at this dosage.

Salvaterra et al. (1973) also demonstrated dose-related and time-dependent changes in the levels of mouse brain phosphocreatine, adenosine nucleotides, α-glycerophosphate, and glycolytic intermediates. Based on their results, the authors postulated that the apparent inhibition may result in an allosteric suppression of glycolysis (Lowry et al. 1964; Rolleston and News-Holme 1967; Takagaki 1968).

Bull and Lutkenhoff (1975) studied the changes in the metabolic responses of rat brain tissue to stimulation, in vitro, produced by in vivo administration of methyl mercuric chloride. It was observed that methyl mercury enhanced the reductive response of NAD(P) (nicotinamide adenine dinucleotide (phosphate)) by electrical stimulation at low doses and inhibited it at high doses. The reductive response of the NAD(P) to addition to potassium was also enhanced by low doses of methyl mercury. While inhibition of this response was not apparent at high doses of mercury in these findings, the authors concluded that methyl mercury produced rather complex changes in the metabolic responses of the brain, suggesting that the coordination of energy metabolism to functional activity (i.e., metabolic control) had been impaired. Such alterations in intermediary metabolism of brain occurred at doses of methyl mercury far below those producing overt toxicity in rats.

Verity et al. (1975) reported an interesting finding in the synaptosomal preparations from rats that were intoxicated with methyl mercury. Synaptosomes isolated from the cerebrum and cerebellum following administration of methyl mercury revealed a significant decline in glutamate- and succinate-supported respiration during the phase of early neurotoxicity. A similar preparation from the cerebellum also revealed respiration defects during the latent period. These studies suggested that the primary site of organic mercurial action may not be the protein synthetic machinery per se, but may be associated with other processes coupled with the formation or regulation of protein synthetic apparatus. The perturbation of brain mitochondrial respiration in vivo and in vitro (Verity et al. 1975) may result in inhibition of synaptosomal protein synthesis (Verity et al. 1977).

Electrophysiological investigation of the characteristics of ganglionic block by methyl mercury revealed that at low concentrations there was a small increase in the amplitude of the compound action potential, whereas an inhibitory effect was observed with higher concentrations. The inhibitory effect was found to be temperature-dependent and was not reversible by washing (Alkadhi and Taha 1982). These authors said that this blocking effect of methyl mercury was exerted principally on the presynaptic nerve terminals and could be due to inhibition of acetylcholine release by interference with the function of calcium at the terminals.

By means of suspension cultures of HeLa cells, Frenkel and Harrington (1983) studied the effects of methyl mercury on mitochondrial synthesis of DNA and RNA compared with its effects on nuclear synthesis. It was found that in intact cells the compound inhibited both DNA and RNA synthesis in mitochondria at doses that were virtually identical to those that inhibited nuclear synthesis. DNA and RNA synthesis in isolated mitochondria was also found to be inhibited. Thus, the impact of methyl mercury on mitochondrial integrity and function was more than simply enzymatic disruption alone.

Sager et al. (1983) examined the effects of methyl mercury on cytoplasmic microtubules in cultured cells and on the in vitro polymerization of microtubules. It was found that methyl mercury caused disruption of cellular microtubules in a concentration- and time-dependent manner. In vitro polymerization was also directly inhibited by methyl mercury. Since microtubules (neurotubules) have an important function in the nervous system (both developmental and adult), the disruption of microtubule integrity may contribute significantly to the dysfunction of the nerve cells under the influence of methyl mercury.

The Neuropathology of Experimental Methyl Mercury Poisoning

Many experimental models have been used to study the neurotoxic effects of methyl mercury. Despite the large variations in experimental conditions and models tested, the basic neurotoxicity of methyl mercury is still comparable with that observed in human cases. It must be pointed out, however, that although the general pathological patterns induced in different species are similar, topographical differences in the location of lesions have still been noted (Chang 1977).

In methyl mercury poisoning, there is histologically a characteristic atrophy of the granule cell layer. Since the disappearance of granule cells takes place at first under the Purkinje cell layer, it was referred to as a centripetal type of cerebellar cortical atrophy (Morikawa 1961). Extensive loss of granule cells occurred, particularly at the depth of the sulci, with increased time of intoxication. As in human cases of methyl mercury poisoning, proliferation of the Bergmann's glial fibers can also be demonstrated (Figure 5.2). Such proliferation of Bergmann's glia is most prominent at the sites of granule cell loss, that is, most extensively at the depth of the sulci.

An increased extracellular space is also observed (Miyakawa and Deshimaru 1969). Most degenerating granule cells appear to be very electron-dense, having a coagulated appearance (Figure 5.3). As observed by Brown

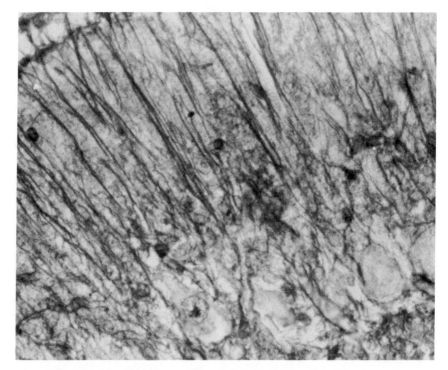

Figure 5.2. Proliferation of Bergmann's glial fiber projecting through the molecular layer from the Purkinje granule cell junction, one of the characteristic pathological findings in the cerebellum intoxicated by methyl mercury. (From Chang 1980)

and Yoshida (1965), degranulation of the rough endoplasmic reticulum is found in the nerve cells. Degeneration of the Purkinje neurons could also be observed in overtly affected animals (Chang and Hartmann 1972a). The necrotic Purkinje cells also have a coagulated appearance, with no recognizable cytoplasmic details. Nevertheless, Purkinje neurons are much more resistant to the mercury toxicity.

The sensory neurons of the dorsal root ganglia are found to be extremely sensitive to the toxicity of mercury (Chang and Hartmann 1972a, 1972b), resulting in extensive neuronal loss (Figures 5.4 and 5.5) in the ganglia. Such observation is confirmed by Herman et al. (1973) and Jacobs et al. (1977).

In methyl mercury intoxication, the early pathological change, in light microscopy, appears to be the formation of hyalinoid inclusion material within the neuronal cytoplasm (Figure 5.6). This hyalinoid material may eventually occupy the whole neuronal cytoplasm, and leads to intracellular

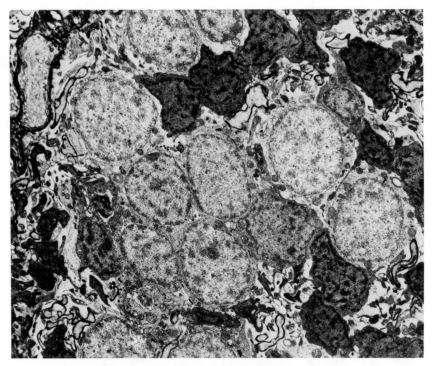

Figure 5.3. Electron microscopy showing pyknotic and atrophic cerebellar granule cells (increased in electron density) in a rat intoxicated by methyl mercury. (From Chang et al. 1977)

vacuolation of the neuron (Figure 5.7). With electron microscopy, it can be demonstrated that the earliest morphological change in these nerve cells consists of an increase in neuronal lysosomes and the disintegration of the rough endoplasmic reticulum (Figures 5.8 and 5.9), followed by focal cytoplasmic degradation and neuronal vacuolation (Figure 5.10). Such morphological findings are in good agreement with the biochemical data that indicate a significant reduction of RNA (Chang et al. 1972, 1973), a breakdown of polysomal structure (Sugano et al. 1975), and a reduction in RNA and protein synthesis (Yoshino et al. 1966; Cavanagh and Chen 1971*b;* Chang et al. 1972*a, 1972b*) in nerve cells after methyl mercury poisoning.

Degenerative changes of the nerve fibers have also been extensively investigated (Miyakawa et al. 1970, 1971; Cavanagh and Chen 1971*a;* Chang and Hartmann 1972*b;* Herman et al. 1973; Yip and Chang 1981). It was found that the sensory fibers are more sensitive and vulnerable to mercury intoxication than the motor fibers.

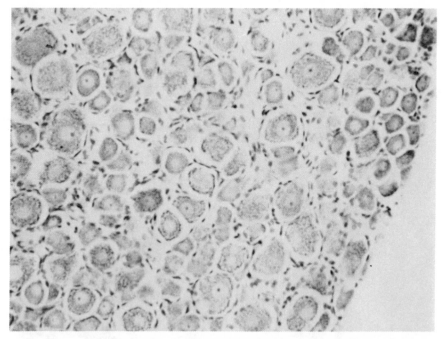

Figure 5.4. Dorsal root ganglion in a normal rat. The normal ganglion contains large numbers of neurons with prominent nuclei and Nissl substance. (From Chang et al. 1972)

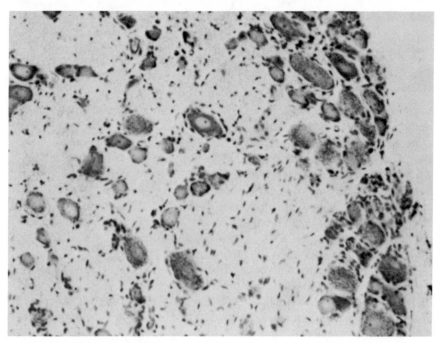

Figure 5.5. Dorsal root ganglion in a rat intoxicated by mercury. Significant loss of neurons was observed. (From Chang et al. 1972)

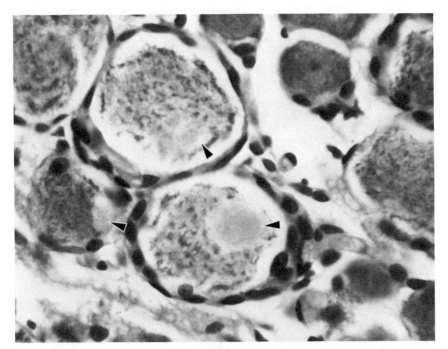

Figure 5.6. Dorsal root ganglion in a rat treated with methyl mercury. Large ganglion neurons showing cytoplasmic hyalinoid inclusions (arrow). (From Chang and Hartmann 1972*a*)

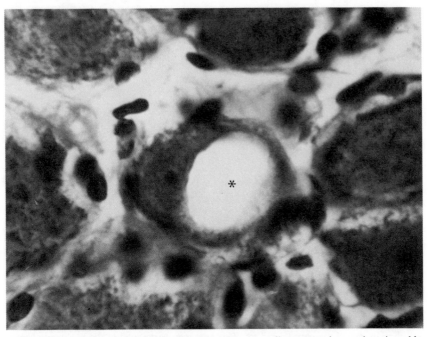

Figure 5.7. Vacuolar change (*) in a large dorsal root ganglion neuron in a rat intoxicated by methyl mercury. (From Chang and Hartmann 1972*a*)

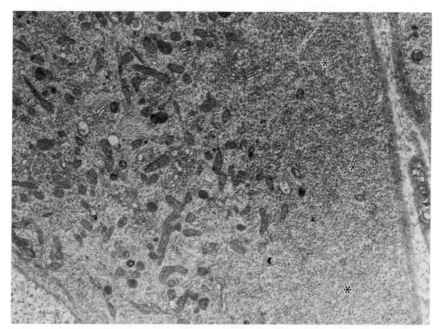

Figure 5.8. Large dorsal root ganglion neuron of a rat treated with methyl mercury, showing a large area (*) of the cytoplasm devoid of any well-organized Nissl substance. (From Chang 1983)

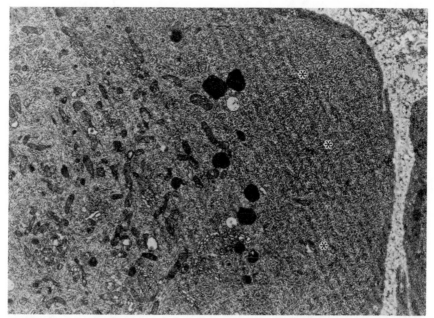

Figure 5.9. Large area (*) of a dorsal root neuron filled with fragments of endoplasmic reticulum in methyl mercury treated rat. This area may correspond to the hyalinoid changes observed via light microscopy. (From Chang 1979)

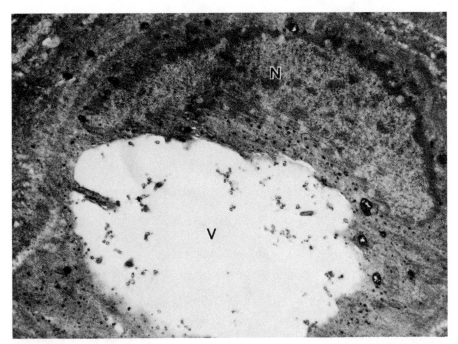

Figure 5.10. Vacuolar degeneration of a large neuron in the dorsal root ganglion in a rat treated with methyl mercury. (N = nucleus; V = cytoplasmic vacuole.) (From Chang and Hartmann 1972a)

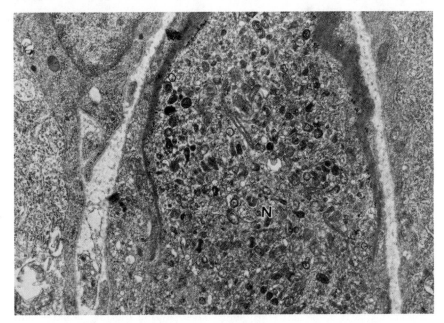

Figure 5.11. Accumulation of lysosomes and axoplasmic debris near the node of Ranvier (N) in methyl mercury treated rat. (From Chang 1980)

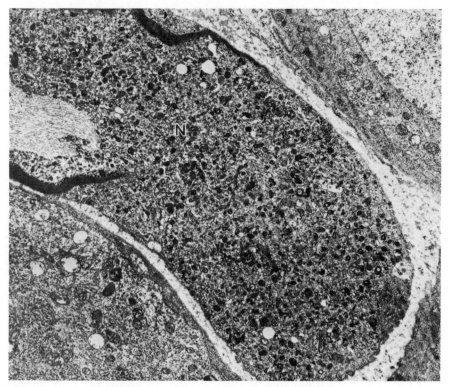

Figure 5.12.   Protrusion of axoplasm at the node of Ranvier (N) filled with axoplasmic debris, in methyl mercury treated rat.

After methyl mercury poisoning, the myelin sheaths of many nerve fibers appear to have lost their lamination and acquired a smudged appearance. The earliest lesion seems to begin at the node of Ranvier, where a large accumulation of lysosomes and cellular debris can be found (Figures 5.11 and 5.12). Many Schwann cells appear to be hyperfunctional after mercury poisoning. Layerings of myelin forming concentric figures or membranous structures are frequently observed in many nerve fibers (Chang and Hartmann 1972*b*). Degenerative changes of myelin sheaths were also observed (Figure 5.13). Similar concentric myelin structures have also been observed in INH (isonicotinic hydrazide) intoxication (Schroder 1971) or as onion-bulb structures in other forms of neuropathies (Dyck 1969; Webster et al. 1967; Ohta 1970), which may simply reflect a hyperreactive response of the supporting elements (Schwann cells). The Schwann cells are also found to play an important role as phagocytes (Chang and Hartmann 1972*b*) during the degenerative and regenerative phase of the nerve fibers after mercury intoxication. Similar

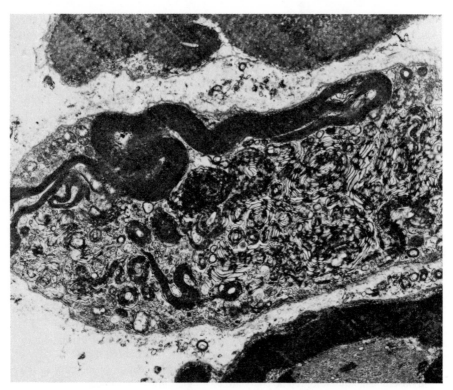

Figure 5.13.   Breakdown of the myelin sheath in a dorsal root fiber, in methyl mercury treated rat.

observations were reported by Miyakawa et al. (1971). Recent investigation also verified that the dorsal root fibers were even more vulnerable to methyl mercury than the dorsal root ganglion neurons (Yip and Chang 1981)

Conclusion

There is little debate that methyl mercury compounds are highly neurotoxic and pose an environmental hazard. Nerve cells and fibers, particularly those in the dorsal root ganglia and cerebellum, are extremely sensitive to the toxicity of methyl mercury. Both histochemical studies and biochemical studies indicated the high affinity of methyl mercury toward biological membrane systems and its ability to disrupt various vital functions (e.g., blood-brain barrier regulation, protein synthesis, glycolytic metabolism, mitochondrial function) of the cells.

It must be emphasized that methyl mercury is also a potent toxicant in the fetus, especially the developing nervous system. Such information has been covered in several recent reviews (Reuhl and Chang 1979; Chang et al. 1980; Chang and Annau 1984) and is not addressed here. Furthermore, despite its potent toxic impact on the nervous system, methyl mercury is a "systemic" toxicant, affecting other organ systems, such as kidney (Ware et al. 1975) and liver (Desnoyers and Chang 1975*a*, 1975*b;* Ware et al. 1974).

When examining the overall toxicity of methyl mercury, one must also bear in mind that various elements in the diet, such as selenium and vitamin E, will significantly modify the pathological impact of this toxic metal (Chang et al. 1977, 1978; Chang and Suber 1982; Yip and Chang 1982; Chang 1983; Gilbert et al. 1983).

Acknowledgment

Portions of the present review have been previously presented in various articles by the same author. The author wishes to thank Mrs. Laurie McDonald for her excellent assistance in the preparation of this manuscript.

References

Alkadhi, K. A., and Taha, M. N. (1982). Antagonism by calcium of the inhibitory effect of methylmercury on sympathetic ganglia. *Arch Toxicol* 51:175–181.

Berlin, M., and Ullberg, S. (1963). Accumulation and retention of mercury in the mouse. I: An autoradiographic study after a single intravenous injection of mercuric chloride. II: An autoradiographic comparison of phenylmercuric acetate with inorganic mercury. III: An autoradiographic comparison of methyl mercuric dicyandiamide with inorganic mercury. *Arch Environ Health* 6:589–616.

Broman, T. (1967). On basic aspects of the blood-brain barrier. In *Pathology of the Nervous System,* vol. 1, edited by J. Minckler, chap. 33. New York: Blakiston.

Broman, T., and Steinwall, O. (1967). Blood-brain barrier. In *Pathology of the Nervous System,* vol. 1, edited by J. Minckler, chap. 32. New York: Blakiston.

Brown, W. J., and Yoshida, N. (1965). Organic mercurial encephalopathy: An experimental electron microscopy study. *Adv Neurol Sci* (Tokyo) 9:34–42.

Brubaker, P. E.; Klein, R.; Herman, S. P.; Lucier, G. W.; Alexander, L. T.; and Long, M. D. (1973). DNA, RNA, and protein synthesis in brain, liver, and kidneys of asymptomatic methylmercury treated rats. *Exp Mol Pathol* 18:263–280.

Bull, R. J., and Lutkenhoff, S. D. (1975). Changes in the metabolic responses of brain tissue to stimulation, in vitro, produced by in vivo administration of methylmercury. *Neuropharmacol* 14:351–359.

Cavanagh, J. B., and Chen, F. C. K. (1971*a*). The effects of methyl mercury dicyandiamide on the peripheral nerves and spinal cord of rats. *Acta Neuropathol* (Berl) 19:208–215.

——— (1971*b*). Amino acid incorporation in protein during the "silent phase" before organo-mercury and ρ-bromophenyl-acetylurea neuropathy in the rat. *Acta Neuropathol* (Berl) 19:216–224.

Chang, L. W. (1977). Neurotoxic effects of mercury: A review. *Environ Res* 14:329–373.

—— (1979). Pathological effects of mercury poisoning. In *Biogeochemistry of Mercury,* edited by J. O. Nriagu. New York: Elsevier.

—— (1980). Mercury. In *Experimental and Clinical Neurotoxicology,* edited by P. S. Spencer and H. H. Schaumberg. Baltimore: Williams & Wilkins.

—— (1983). Protective effects of selenium against methylmercury neurotoxicity: A morphological and biochemical study. *Exp Pathol* 23:143–156.

Chang, L. W., and Annau, Z. (1984). Developmental neuropathology and behavioral teratology of methylmercury. In *Neurobehavioral Teratology,* edited by J. Yanai, pp. 405–432. Amsterdam: Elsevier.

Chang, L. W.; Desnoyers, P. A.; and Hartmann, H. A. (1972). Quantitative cyto-chemical studies of RNA in experimental mercury poisoning, I: Changes in RNA content. *J Neuropathol Exp Neurol* 31:389–501.

—— (1973). Quantitative cytochemical studies of RNA in experimental mercury poisoning, II: Changes in the base composition and ratios. *Acta Neuropathol* 23:77–83.

Chang, L. W.; Dudley, A. W., Jr.; Dudley, M. A.; Ganther, H. E.; and Sunde, M. L. (1977). Modification of the neurotoxic effects of methylmercury by sele-nium. In *Neurotoxicology,* edited by L. Roizin, H. Shiraki, and N. Grcevic, pp. 275–285. New York: Raven Press.

Chang, L. W.; Gilbert, M. M.; and Sprecher, J. A. (1978). Modification of the neurotoxic effects of methylmercury by vitamin E. *Environ Res* 17:356–366.

Chang, L. W., and Hartmann, H. A. (1972*a*). Ultrastructural studies of the nervous system after mercury intoxication, I: Pathological changes in the nerve cell bodies. *Acta Neuropathol* 20:122–138.

—— (1972*b*). Ultrastructural studies of the nervous system after mercury intoxica-tion, II: Pathological changes in the nerve fibers. *Acta Neuropathol* 20:316–334.

—— (1972*c*). Electron microscopic histochemical study on the localization and distribution of mercury in the nervous system after mercury intoxication. *Exp Neurol* 35:122–137.

—— (1972*d*). Blood-brain barrier dysfunction in experimental mercury intoxica-tion. *Acta Neuropathol* 21:179–184

Chang, L. W.; Pounds, J. G.; Reuhl, K. R.; and Wade, P. R. (1980). Prenatal and neonatal toxicity and pathology of heavy metals. In *Advances in Pharmacology and Chemotherapy,* vol. 17, edited by A. Goldin, F. Hawking, I. J. Kopin, and R. J. Schnitzer, pp. 195–231. New York: Academic Press.

Chang, L. W., and Suber, R. (1982). Protective effect of selenium on methylmercury toxicity: A possible mechanism. *Bull Environ Contam Toxicol* 29:285–289.

Clarkson, T. W. (1972). The pharmacology of mercury compounds. *Ann Rev Phar-macol* 12:375–406.

Desnoyers, P. A., and Chang, L. W. (1975*a*). Ultrastructural changes in the hepato-cytes following acute methylmercury intoxication. *Environ Res* 9:224–239.

—— (1975*b*). Ultrastructural changes of the liver after chronic exposure to methyl-mercury. *Environ Res* 10:175–189.

Dyck, P. J. (1969). Experimental hypertrophic neuropathy: Pathogenesis of onion-bulb formations produced by repeat tourniquet applications. *Arch Neurol* (Chi-cago) 21:73–75.

Farris, F. F., and Smith, J. C. (1975). In vivo incorporation of ^{14}C-leucine into brain protein of methylmercury treated rats. *Bull Environ Contam Toxicol* 13:451–455.

Frenkel, G. D., and Harrington, L. (1983). Inhibition of mitochondrial nucleic acid synthesis by methyl mercury. *Biochem Pharmacol* 32(8):1454–1456.

Gilbert, M. M.; Sprecher, J.; Chang, L. W.; and Meisner, L. F. (1983). Protective effect of vitamin E on genotoxicity of methylmercury. *J Toxicol Environ Health* 12:767–773.

Herman, S. P.; Klein, R.; Talley, F. A.; and Krigman, M. R. (1973). An ultrastructural study of methylmercury-induced primary sensory neuropathy in rats. *Lab Invest* 28:104–118.

Hunter, D.; Bomford, R. R.; and Russell, D. S. (1940). Poisoning by methylmercury compounds. *Q J Med* 33:193–213.

Hunter, D., and Russell, D. S. (1954). Focal cerebral and cerebellar atrophy in a human subject due to organic mercury compounds. *J Neurol Neurosurg Psychiat* 17:235–241.

Jacobs, J. M.; Carmichael, N.; and Cavanagh, J. B. (1977). Ultrastructural changes in the nervous system of rabbits poisoned with methylmercury. *Toxicol Appl Pharmacol* 39:249–261.

Kurland, L. T.; Faro, S. N.; and Siedler, H. (1960). Minamata disease: The outbreak of a neurological disorder in Minamata, Japan, and its relationship to the ingestion of seafood contaminated by mercuric compounds. *World Neurol* 1:370–395.

Lowry, D. H.; Passonneau, J. V.; Hasselberger, F. X.; and Schultz, D. W. (1964). Effects of ischemia on known substances and co-factors of the glycolytic pathway in the brain. *J Biol Chem* 239:18–30.

Massey, T. H., and Fang, S. C. (1968). A comparative study of the subcellular binding of phenylmercuric acetate and mercuric acetate in rat liver and kidney slices. *Toxicol Appl Pharmacol* 12:7–14.

Miyakawa, T., and Deshimaru, M. (1969). Electron microscopic study of experimentally induced poisoning due to organic mercury compound. *Acta Neuropathol* (Berl) 14:126–136.

Miyakawa, T.; Deshimaru, M.; Sumiyoshi, S.; Tersoka, A.; and Tatetsu, S. (1971). Experimental organic mercury poisoning: Regeneration of peripheral nerves. *Acta Neuropathol* 17:6–13.

Miyakawa, T.; Deshimaru, M.; Sumiyoshi, S.; Tersoka, A.; Udo, N.; Hattori, E.; and Tatetsu, S. (1970). Experimental organic mercury poisoning: Pathological changes in peripheral nerves. *Acta Neuropathol* (Berl) 15:45–55.

Morikawa, N. (1961). Pathological studies on organic mercury poisoning. *Kumamoto Med J* 14:71–86.

Nordberg, G. (1976). *Effects and Dose-Response Relationships of Toxic Metals.* New York: Elsevier.

Norseth, T. (1967). The intracellular distribution of mercury in rat liver after methoxyethyl mercury intoxication. *Biochem Pharmacol* 16:1645–1654.

Ohta, M. (1970). Ultrastructure of sural nerve in a case of arsenical neuropathy. *Acta Neuropathol* (Berl) 16:233–242.

Omata, S.; Sakimura, I.; Tsubaki, H.; and Sugano, H. (1978). In vivo effects of methylmercury on protein synthesis in brain and liver of the rat. *Toxicol Appl Pharmacol* 44:367–378.

Passow, H.; Rothstein, A.; and Clarkson, J. W. (1961). The general pharmacology of the heavy metals. *Pharmacol Rev* 13:185–224.

Patterson, R. A., and Usher, D. R. (1971). Acute toxicity of methylmercury on glycolytic intermediates and adenine nucleotides of rat brain. *Life Sci* 10:121–128.

Platonow, N. (1968). Les effets compares des agents chelateurs sur la distribution du mercure organique chez les porcelets. *Can Vet J* 9:142–148.

Reuhl, K. R., and Chang, L. W. (1979). Effects of methylmercury on the development of the nervous system: A review. *Neurotoxicology* 1:21–55.

Richardson, R. J., and Murphy, S. D. (1974). Neurotoxicity produced by intracranial administration of methyl mercury in rats. *Toxicol Appl Pharmacol* 29:289–300.

Rolleston, F. S., and News-Holme, E. A. (1967). Control of glycolysis in cerebral slices. *J Neurochem* 104:524–533.

Sager, P. R.; Doherty, R. A.; and Olmsted, J. B. (1983). Interaction of methylmercury with microtubules in cultured cells and in vitro. *Exp Cell Res* 146:127–137.

Salvaterra, P.; Lown, B.; Morganti, J.; and Massaro, E. J. (1973). Alterations in neurochemical and behavioral parameters in the mouse induced by low doses of methyl mercury. *Acta Pharmacol Toxicol* 33:177–190.

Schroder, J. M. (1971). Zur Pathogenese der Isoniazid-Neuropathie, I: Eine feinstruckturelle differenzierung gegenuber der Qallerschen degeneration. *Acta Neuropathol* (Berl) 16:301–323.

Somjen, G. G.; Herman, S. P.; Klein, R.; Brubaker, P. E.; Briner, W. H.; Goodrich, J. K.; Krigman, M. R.; and Maseman, J. K. (1973). The uptake of methylmercury (^{203}Hg) in different tissues related to its neurotoxic effects. *J Pharmacol Exp Ther* 187:602–611.

Steinwall, O. (1961). Transport mechanisms in certain blood-brain barrier phenomena: A hypothesis. *Acta Psychiat Neurol Scand* (Suppl. 150) 36:314–318.

Steinwall, O., and Klatzo, I. (1966). Selective vulnerability of the blood-brain barrier in chemically induced lesions. *J Neuropathol Exp Neurol* 25:542–559.

Steinwall, O., and Olsson, Y. (1969). Impairment of the blood-brain barrier in mercury poisoning. *Acta Neurol Scand* 45:351–361.

Steinwall, O., and Snyder, H. (1969). Brain uptake of C^{14}-cyclo-leucine after damage to blood-brain barrier by mercuric ions. *Acta Neurol Scand* 45:369–375.

Sugano, H.; Omata, S.; and Tsubaki, H. (1975). Methylmercury inhibition of protein synthesis in brain tissue, I: Effects of methylmercury and heavy metals on cell-free protein synthesis in rat brain and liver. In *Studies on the Health Effects of Alkylmercury in Japan*, pp. 129–136. Tokyo: Environmental Agency.

Syversen, T. L. M. (1977). Effects of methylmercury on in vivo protein synthesis in isolated cerebral and cerebellar neurons. *Neuropathol Appl Neurobiol* 3:225–236.

Takagaki, G. (1968). Control of aerobic glycolysis and pyruvate kinase activity in cerebral cortex slices. *J Neurochem* 15:903–916.

Takeuchi, T. (1968). Pathology of Minamata disease. In *Minamata Disease*, edited by M. Kutsuma, pp. 141–228. Tokyo: University of Kumamoto.

Verity, M. A.; Brown W. J.; and Cheung, M. (1975). Organic mercurial encephalopathy: In vivo and in vitro effects of methyl mercury on synaptosomal respiration. *J Neurochem* 25:759–766.

Verity, M. A.; Brown, W. J.; Cheung, M.; and Czer, G. (1977). Methyl mercury inhibition of synaptosome and brain slice protein synthesis: In vivo and in vitro studies. *J Neurochem* 29:673–679.

Ware, R. A.; Burkholder, P. M.; and Chang, L. W. (1975). Ultrastructural changes in renal proximal tubules after chronic organic and inorganic mercury intoxication. *Environ Res* 10:121–140.

Ware, R. A.; Chang, L. W.; and Burkholder, P. M. (1974). An ultrastructural study on the blood-brain barrier dysfunction following mercury intoxication. *Acta Neuropathol* (Berl) 30:211–224.

Webster, H. de F.; Schroder, J. M.; Asbury, A. K.; and Adams, R. D. (1967). The role of Schwann cells in the formation of "onion-bulbs" found in chronic neuropathies. *J Neuropathol Exp Neurol* 26:276–299.

Yip, R. K., and Chang, L. W. (1981). Vulnerability of dorsal root neurons and fibers toward methylmercury toxicity: A morphological evaluation. *Environ Res* 26:152–167.

—— (1982). Protective effects of vitamin E on methylmercury toxicity in the dorsal root ganglia. *Environ Res* 28:84–95.

Yoshino, Y.; Mozai, T.; and Nakao, K. (1966). Distribution of mercury in the brain and its subcellular units in experimental organic mercury poisoning. *J Neurochem* 13:397–406.

S I X

The Pathological Lesions of Methyl Mercury Intoxication in Monkeys

N. Karle Mottet, Cheng-Mei Shaw, and Thomas M. Burbacher

The different chemical forms of mercury to which an individual is exposed alter the target organ of principal injury. Thus, the pathological lesions will vary, depending on the chemical form. For example, inhalation of metallic mercury vapor causes severe toxic injury of the lung alveoli and blood vessels, which in turn results in pulmonary edema. This pathological sequence with the lung as the target organ is often the result of occupational exposures or misadventure (Moutinho et al. 1981; Natelson et al. 1971). Histopathologically, this edema is indistinguishable from pulmonary edema resulting from a myriad of other causes. Bichloride of mercury ($HgCl_2$) is readily absorbed through the gastrointestinal tract, but less efficiently than methyl mercury. The kidneys are the main target organ for bichloride of mercury. The Hg^{2+} ion is rapidly concentrated in the kidneys and liver. If the concentration is sufficient, it will cause necrosis of the epithelial cells and the lining of the kidney proximal tubules and may produce renal failure. Although the kidneys contain a high concentration of mercury regardless of the chemical form absorbed, they are the primary target organs for the mercuric form. In acute inorganic mercury poisoning (e.g., with mercuric chloride), it produces extensive damage to the proximal convoluted tubules, resulting in acute renal failure. At autopsy the kidneys are generally enlarged and pale, with a swollen cortex, and dark, congested pyramids. When death ensues during the first week of this type of exposure, the nephron lumen becomes filled with eosinophilic granular cytoplasmic debris, and casts will be seen in the lower portions of the nephron. Prior to the availability of artificial dialysis, the patient usually died in this stage of acute renal failure. With dialysis, however, the patient frequently survives, and the nephrons may regenerate. By 2–3 weeks after exposure, the tubules will have returned to normal. Remarkably, the basement membranes are not damaged in the process.

Absorbed methyl mercury is carried throughout the body mainly within erythrocytes, whereas much of inorganic mercury, such as bichloride of mercury, is transported by the plasma proteins. Thus, the inorganic mercury concentrates more quickly in the liver and kidneys and will achieve rapidly higher concentrations at those sites (Kershaw et al. 1980). Mercury compounds are eliminated from the body in the urine and feces (Clarkson 1971; Clarkson et al. 1980). However, some is also excreted in the bile, sweat, saliva, hair, and milk. Different chemical forms of mercury also have differ-

73

ent predominant routes of elimination (National Academy of Sciences 1978; Piotrowski and Inskip 1981). Metallic and mercuric mercury have the urinary excretion as their main route, whereas methyl mercury is excreted mostly in the feces.

Although poisoning with inorganic mercurials has been known since ancient times (Al-Damluji 1976), only relatively recently has there been greater attention paid to the organic mercury compounds (Amin-Zaki et al. 1974; Clarkson 1971; Clarkson et al. 1980; Turner et al. 1980). Methyl mercury readily passes through physiological barriers such as the blood-brain barrier, blood-testes barrier, and placenta, in contrast to the inorganic forms. Thus, methyl mercury is much more likely to target the nervous system, the testes, and the developing embryo/fetus. This chapter focuses on the spectrum of pathological changes of methyl mercury exposure.

The principal target organ for methyl mercury is the brain. It causes less dramatic lesions in the liver and kidneys, but it is more likely to produce major pathological changes in the nervous system of the adult, the fetus, and the reproductive tract. The modern era of the study of methyl mercury pathology began with the clinical and pathological reports of Hunter, Bomford, and Russell (1940) and Hunter and Russell (1954). These reports described the clinical features of methyl mercury exposure of four workers treating seed grain with methyl mercury and the autopsy findings in one of them 14 years later. To demonstrate that methyl mercury was the cause of the findings, they exposed rats to methyl mercury and investigated the pathological changes in one rhesus monkey. This report was followed by major outbreaks of mercury poisoning in humans in Iraq in 1950 and 1952 (Al-Damluji 1976), in Minamata, Japan, in 1956 (Kutsuma 1968; Tsubaki and Irukayama 1977), and in Iraq again in 1971 (Bakir et al. 1973; Jolili and Abbasi 1961). Although more than 8,500 human hospitalized cases for methyl mercury intoxication have occurred (with more than 500 deaths in these major epidemics), descriptions of the macroscopic, microscopic, and ultrastructural pathology are exceedingly sparse. Except for the central nervous system, the lesions are relatively subtle. The neuropathological changes have been well described. The reports (Kutsuma 1968; Tsubaki and Irukayama 1977) on Minamata disease deal with general pathology in only one paragraph, and the poisonings in Iraq resulted in only one brief report (Al-Saleem 1976) on four adult and four infant autopsies. However, a few case reports (see Mottet and Body 1974) have described some pathological findings and recorded the assay of organ mercury burden (Pazderova et al. 1974).

There is an increasing need for pathologists and toxicologists to recognize the differing morphological effects of mercury compounds under different conditions of exposure, particularly as in relation to methyl mercury. The major outbreaks referred to above represent hospitalized patients having high-dose exposure (often intermittent); there is virtually no reference to cases with subclinical levels of exposure. With the increasing risk of continuous low-level exposures attributable to the increasing level of methyl mercury in food as a result of acid rain, the pathological changes at low-level exposure become increasingly important. Identification of the pathology of low-level exposure is difficult in humans. In this chapter, nonhuman primates are shown to be relatively good models for the dose-pathological response to methyl mercury. The pathological findings reported here pertain to human and nonhuman primates. Dose-response relationships are deduced entirely from macaque monkeys. Laboratory rodent experiments will be mentioned and specifically identified.

During the past 15 years we have done 89 necropsies on macaque monkeys of known methyl mercury exposure and vehicle-exposed controls. Because pathological lesions reported here are from cases of known exposure, dose and duration, clinical signs, blood mercury levels, blood tests, liver and kidney function tests, serum electrolytes, and hemograms, which have been correlated with structural and functional changes, our investigations far exceed the human autopsy investigations in number and detail. Remarkably few investigations of methyl mercury toxicity have been done on nonhuman primates, and most of those were relatively high-dose exposures producing severe toxic signs and lesions. In addition to the report of Hunter, Bomford, and Russell (1940) mentioned above, Ikeda et al. (1973), Willes et al. (1978), Rice and Gilbert (1982), and Reynolds and Pitkin (1975) studied a total of 45 macaque monkeys in their investigations. The groups in Lund, Sweden (Berlin et al. 1975*a*, 1975*b*), and Rochester, New York (Garman et al. 1975), Joiner and Hupp (1978), and Vitulli (1974) used a total of 50 squirrel monkeys for their investigations. The following is a summary of the pathology as seen in the human and nonhuman primates.

The most extensive pathological studies of deaths due to methyl mercury poisoning are the reports of Takeuchi in Japan on the Minamata disease episode (Takeuchi and Eto 1977). In the 7 years following the exposure, 23 autopsy cases that had acute, subacute, or chronic exposure to methyl mercury were reported. Takeuchi's reports deal extensively with the nervous system lesions and also include some cases of congenital exposure to methyl mercury.

The Relationship of Blood Mercury to Lesions Observed

The background "normal" mercury burden in human organs and tissues is well established. We have reported (Mottet and Body 1974) the baseline organ and tissue levels of mercury (total) in 113 autopsies of human deaths of general hospital admissions ranging in age from 26 weeks of gestation to 88 years. More than 70 percent of all assays, irrespective of organ or age, had a burden of less than 0.25 μg/g of wet weight. Less than 10 percent had more than 0.75 $\mu g/g$. The kidney was the organ with the most variable burden, 29 percent of the assays being above 0.75 $\mu g/g$. The burden in fetal organs was more uniform than those in postnatal life. Multivariate statistical analysis indicated that urban-dwellers have a somewhat greater mercury burden than rural-dwellers. Our data did not reveal a statistically significant increase with age, suggesting that past environmental exposure levels did not exceed the capacity of the body to eliminate mercury. There was no correlation of mercury burden with the cause of death.

Our extensive studies with the macaque primate show a relatively close relationship between the blood level of mercury and the appearance of lesions (Finocchio et al. 1980; Luschei et al. 1977). This type of correlation was not possible with the human exposures, because in nearly all instances the extent of the exposure to mercury was determined retrospectively by indirect means, such as estimates of the amount of fish or loaves of bread eaten. Also, in Iraq, the exposure was for a short period at relatively high levels (Bakir et al. 1973; Magos et al. 1976). However, one must use caution in directly transposing the macaque whole-blood levels and lesions to the human, because the primate does not exactly correspond to the human. Our monkeys are healthy, normal, and well fed, and of course do not have the confounding personal habits of humans, such as smoking, alcohol consumption, or medications, which would tend to enhance the toxicity of methyl mercury. Also protecting the macaque is the fact that the hair of this very hirsute animal represents a sump for some of the mercury ingested, which may serve to diminish the blood level versus the dose received. More significant, there may be differences in the blood-brain barrier between the species, which would protect the macaque brain from higher blood levels of mercury. Furthermore, the human initial subjective symptom is paresthesia, which occurs at considerably lower blood levels than objective signs of mercury toxicity, such as ataxia, neurasthenia, visual and hearing loss, or spasticity and tremor, and so on. Working with monkeys, we can discern only signs and not symptoms. Finally, the biological half-time of methyl mercury in blood is less in the monkeys than in the humans (26 days vs. 60–70 days).

The occurrence of clinical signs of mercury intoxication in the macaque are remarkably consistent at a blood level of 2.8 parts per million (ppm) and above. Below this level, clinical lab tests are completely normal. Tests for liver function, renal function, electrolytes, and a hemogram are within the normal range. Above this level, particularly in the acute high-dose animals, abnormalities in liver-function tests and renal-function tests will occur. Ordinarily, gross macroscopic pathological lesions are not discernible below this level, but at levels above 3.0 one may see pallor of the liver and kidneys, diffuse edema and focal softening of the brain (particularly in the visual cortex), increased reproductive failure, and abnormal development. The absence of dramatic gross lesions, except in the most high-level acute poisoning, may account for the paucity of descriptions of the more subtle pathological findings. Microscopic lesions are seen in nonhuman primates with blood levels above 1 ppm. Lesions in the liver, kidney, and brain are consistently seen, and silent lesions in the brain at blood mercury levels between 1 and 2 ppm are seen in the absence of clinical signs of neurotoxicity. Ultrastructural changes in the liver, kidney, and intestine are seen at blood levels above 1 ppm.

Some significant negative findings are worth noting. There was no evidence of a particular intercurrent disease process associated with long-term mercury exposure. A recent report from Japan (Tamashiro et al. 1984) on autopsy and death findings on patients who had died many years after the Minamata exposure does not reveal an unusual spectrum of causes of death. Some reports raised the possibility of islet cell lesions in the pancreas, but diabetes has not been reported as associated with mercury intoxication, and the atherosclerosis associated therewith has not been predominant in the deaths. Similarly, anemia and bone marrow suppression have been suggested, but evidence for this is lacking both in the human and nonhuman primate. In the macaque, at blood levels below 2.5 ppm, the organs appear completely normal on macroscopic examination. The gastrointestinal ulcerations sometimes reported with bichloride of mercury ingestion were not found following methyl mercury exposure of the macaque, although some have been reported in humans. The colon lacks ulceration or other lesions, in spite of the high mercury content of the colonic wall. This high content of mercury in the colonic wall occurs even after administration of oral mercury has ceased, and it suggests that the mucosa may be a route of elimination of mercury from the body. Breast milk is a route of excretion of mercury in primates in high concentrations, but histological examination of the macaque breast tissue does not show the presence of specific lesions. The adverse effect on reproduction by methyl mercury (described later) is not reflected in gross or microscopic anatomical lesions in the reproductive organs. Finally, there are no residual lesions after high-level exposure, except in the central nervous system. The lesions in the liver, kidney, and intestines present at higher-level exposures are completely reversible, and the organs return to a normal appearance after exposure to mercury ceases (Chen et al. 1983).

Organ Pathology of Methyl Mercury

Kidney

In 1928, Goldblatt reviewed 38 cases of acute mercurial intoxication with bichloride of mercury, which caused 5 deaths. There were no definite signs of nervous system involvement, nor was there any pathology demonstrable to the skin, bone, joints, or muscles in this group of cases. The deaths appeared to be related to the severity of the renal injury. Macroscopically, no gross changes are seen, except that blood levels are above 3 ppm when slight pallor and swelling occurs. However, the microscopic changes seen in the kidneys at blood levels of 2.5 ppm and above are those of toxic acute tubular necrosis with swelling, and cellular necrosis with acidophilia of the proximal convoluted tubular cells (Verity and Brown 1970). With acute high doses this can be very extensive, with necrosis of the tubular epithelium ensuing. The basement membrane is not altered, but casts may accumulate in the lower segment of the nephron. The glomeruli are remarkably normal at high-level exposure, and there is no change in the interstitium. With chronic low-dose exposure to inorganic salts of mercury, elemental mercury, and mercury vapor, an immunologically induced membranous glomerulopathy may occur (Goyer 1985). At blood methyl mercury levels above 2 ppm ultrastructurally, one can see lysosomal lesions in cells of the convoluted tubules comparable to those seen in the Paneth cells. At these lower levels of exposure, the degeneration of necrosis is seen infrequently. In some regions, one can see the lysosomal inclusions being extruded from the tubular cells (Madsen and Christensen 1978). These changes in the kidneys were first identified by Fowler (1972).

As noted above, the kidneys are a major site of methyl mercury accumulation in the body. In the kidney, methyl mercury is metabolized to inorganic mercury. Long-term exposure (producing blood levels of 2.8 ppm and above in the macaque) to methyl mercury produces renal lesions similar to those described for inorganic mercury. Macroscopically, the kidneys are swollen and pale. Microscopically, toxic acute tubular necrosis involving principally the *pars recta* of the proximal convoluted tubular epithelium is seen. In later recovery phases from the injury, areas of regenerating epithelium are intermixed. The tubular basement membrane is remarkably intact, and the structure of the glomeruli and the distal tubular segments are not altered. Casts of cellular debris may be seen in the distal portions of the nephrons. These changes are entirely nonspecific. Large acidophilic inclusions are often seen in the cytoplasm before they become necrotic. Calcification of the necrotic debris is seen frequently. When clinical toxicity signs are evident, serum urea nitrogen and creatinine are usually elevated with this high-level exposure.

When the blood level of mercury is below 2.8 ppm with long-term exposure, the macroscopic appearance of the kidneys is often not altered, but scattered microscopic lesions may be seen in the absence of elevated blood urea nitrogen or creatinine. These lesions are similar to the above, but they are widely scattered and limited to a few nephrons. In the macaque, we have observed ultrastructural changes (lysosomal inclusions in tubular epithelial cells) similar to those described by Fowler in rats and to the inclusions we observed in the Paneth cells of the intestine. The lysosomes appear to be extruded from the cells, and portions of the cells are extruded (Figure 6.1). Ultrastructural studies on renal proximal tubules in mercury-intoxicated rats

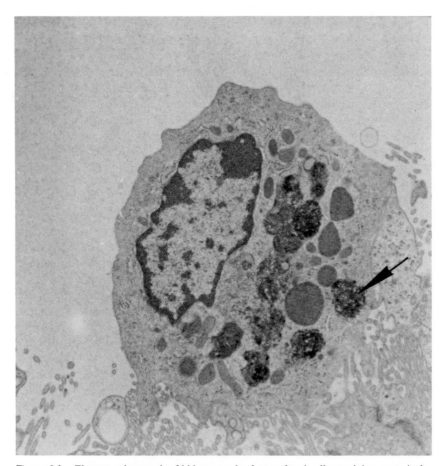

Figure 6.1. Electron micrograph of kidney proximal convoluted cell containing many inclusions similar to those described in the Paneth cells.

have provided evidence for structural-functional changes (Fowler et al. 1974; Gritzka and Trump 1968; Ware et al. 1975) and for the similarity of the Hg^{2+} lesions to the CH_3Hg^+ lesions.

Gastrointestinal Tract

In contrast to methyl mercury, which is almost 100 percent absorbed through the gastrointestinal epithelium, elemental mercury (Hg^0) is very poorly absorbed from the gastrointestinal tract. Soluble mercuric salts, but not the insoluble mercurous salts, are toxic to the gastrointestinal mucosa, leading to acute ulceration with inflammation and hemorrhage (Aaronson and Spiro

1973). Large bowel lesions may occur several weeks after ingestion. These lesions are associated with high-dose exposure (above 2 mg/kg) and may be fatal. Lower doses of inorganic mercury seldom cause ulcerations, but they may be associated with gingivitis and stomatitis. In contrast, methyl mercury is much less likely to produce gastrointestinal ulcerations. In our macaque experiments involving daily oral administration of doses up to 2 mg/kg, no gastrointestinal ulcerations or mucosal changes were seen. Within the small intestine, one could see some swollen and degenerating Paneth cells at the tips of the crypts of Lieberkuhn (Mottet and Body 1976). Takeuchi and Eto have reported islet beta cell lesions and atrophy of the taste buds (in Tsubaki and Irukayma 1977).

Light and electron microscopic observations on samples of duodenum and ileum following perfusion and immersion fixation in a glutaraldehyde para-formaldehyde fixative revealed numerous uniquely structured inclusions in the Paneth cells of the chronic low-dose macaques. Some necrotic Paneth cells were seen, especially in the most chronic and higher-dosed animals (Mottet and Body 1976). Acute high-dose treatment produced some inclusions in the Paneth cells similar to those of the chronic low-dose group, but degenerative and necrotic cells were more frequently seen. These alterations were not seen in other intestinal epithelial cells. Paneth cells were selectively injured. The severity of the change was generally dose-related. The cellular changes described below occurred sparsely in monkeys whose intestinal mercury burdens were in the range of 1 to 5 μg/g wet weight of intestinal wall. When the intestinal-wall burden was increased by one order of magnitude, the changes were seen much more frequently. High-dose acute exposure resulted in many necrotic cells. Although differences between the acute high dose and the chronic low dose were recognized, we were unable to recognize differences attributable to the variations of duration of exposure in the chronic low-dose group. The lesions of three groups will be described together, with their differences pointed out when appropriate. Cellular changes in the duodenal and ileal specimens were comparable and will also be described together. Comparable changes were not seen in the undifferentiated mucous goblet or in the enterochromaffin cells.

Virtually all the Paneth cells on light microscopy were somewhat enlarged, with a slightly basophilic reticular or frothy appearance to the cytoplasm. The Paneth cells occur with normal frequency. Degenerative and necrotic Paneth cells are frequently seen in the experimental groups. These latter cells are characterized by a pyknotic dense nucleus with virtually no discernible internal structure. Occasionally one can see a similar cell desquamated within the lumen of a crypt. Degeneration and necrosis seemed more frequent in the crypts of those cases where the intestinal burden was in excess of 10 μg/g.

Changes in Paneth cell organelles, as revealed by electron microscopy, were prominent in the cases of chronic exposure. Mitochondria were generally unremarkable. They were relatively large with numerous transverse cristae and frequent dense bodies. There was no increase in the distance between the unit membranes. Numerous profiles of smooth endoplasmic reticulum are seen in the Golgi region. Some form small vesicles. An elaborate Golgi apparatus caps the lumenal aspect of the nucleus. Transitional forms of small smooth vesicles and larger ones containing electron-dense secretory material are seen on the luminal aspect of the Golgi body. Numerous large membrane-bounded secretory granules fill the cytoplasm on the luminal aspect (Figure 6.2).

Within this region between the nucleus and the luminal aspect of the cells there are many characteristic inclusions. Very occasionally they may be seen lateral to or basal to the nucleus. The smallest inclusions are seen in the cytosol as an electron-dense concavo-convex structure. Whether they are altered smooth endoplasmic reticulum membranes or separate structures arising in the cytosol was not definitively discernible, though the former seemed more likely. Larger inclusions were relatively numerous and often attained a size equal to secretory granules. A complete spectrum of inclusions from the smallest to very large have similar morphological features. The single unit membrane boundary encloses clusters of coils, loops, and hoops of the electron-dense structures described above (and see Figure 6.3). The background matrix appears granular, and occasionally parallel membrane arrays (myelin figures) are also included. Some of the inclusions appear in continuity with lysosomal-like structures and secretory granules. The lysosomal structures were acid phosphatase positive. Some of the inclusions were also seen in large cytoplasmic vacuoles. Exocytosis of the inclusions was not observed.

Acute high doses of methyl mercury produced a somewhat different pattern of change in the Paneth cells (Mottet and Body 1976). As with the chronic low-dose animals, acute high-dose animals selectively produced degeneration in the Paneth cells. The inclusions described above were present though less prominent. Many more Paneth cells were in advanced stages of necrosis. The necrotic cells contained relatively few secretory granules. The most prominent change was the vesiculation of the rough endoplasmic reticulum throughout all regions of the cells. The vesiculation was moderate in the cells that were less severely altered and more prominent in those that had nuclear changes as well. Matrical swelling and some irregularity was seen in the mitochondria. This contrasts with the fine structural changes in mitochondria observed in acute inorganic mercury ($HgCl_2$) lesions in the kidney. Focal increases in the smooth endoplasmic reticulum were seen at the periphery of the Golgi region. Nuclear pyknosis with irregular clumping and margination of chromatin were seen in the more severely altered cells. Cell membranes, cell junctions, basal lamina, and intercellular space were unaltered. Autora-

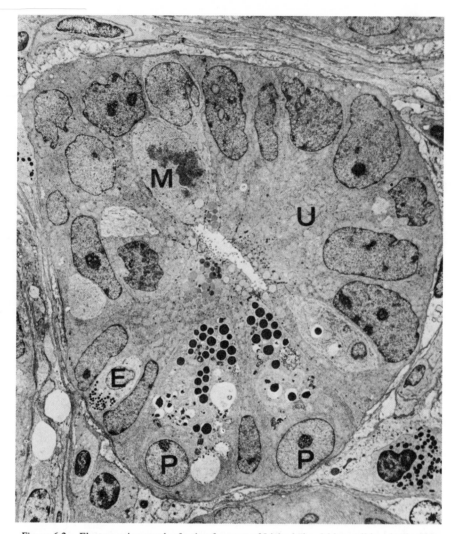

Figure 6.2. Electron micrograph of a tip of a crypt of Lieberkühn. M is a cell in mitosis. U is one of several undifferentiated or early differentiating mucous cells. E is an enterochromaffin cell. P is two Paneth cells. All the crypt cells are unremarkable, except the Paneth cells that contain lysosomes with granular material in the region between the nucleus and the secretory granules.

diographic studies have indicated that uptake of $^{203}HgCl_2$ by rat Paneth cells exceeded that of other cells of the small intestine. This finding suggested that Paneth cells may be a route of elimination of methyl mercury from the body. An alternate explanation would be that Paneth cells are much longer-lived than other intestinal mucosal epithelial cells and therefore have a greater opportunity to accumulate methyl mercury.

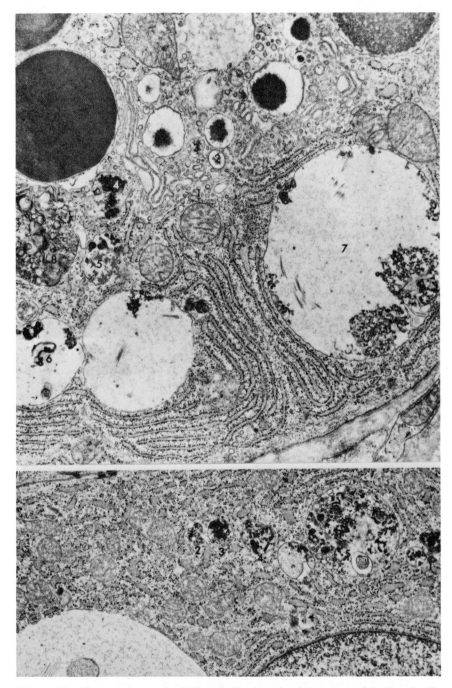

Figure 6.3. Electron micrographs, high magnification, showing portions of the Paneth cell cytoplasms. Numbers 1–8 indicate progressively larger lysosomal inclusions ranging from a small electron-dense portion of smooth endoplasmic reticulum to large lysosomes.

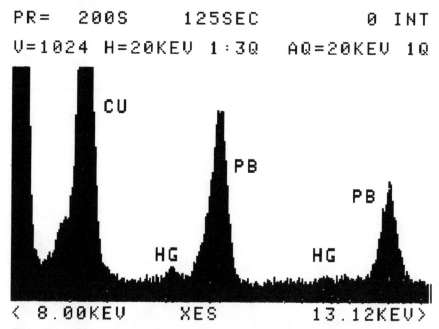

PR= 200S   125SEC   0 INT

V=1024 H=20KEV 1:3Q   AQ=20KEV 1Q

CU

PB

PB

HG

HG

< 8.00KEV   XES   13.12KEV>

Figure 6.4. Electron microprobe graph of one of the Paneth cell lysosomes, showing a peak for mercury (Hg). The copper (Cu) and lead (Pb) peaks are the result of sample preparation.

Some of the above-described lysosomal structures in mercury-dosed Paneth cells contain mercury as determined by x-ray microanalysis (Crooker et al. 1984). Electron-dense inclusions are present in the lysosomes in a variety of configurations, but when small granules are probed without interference from other inclusions, mercury-characteristic x-rays are detected (Figure 6.4). No mercury was detected in other organelles of Paneth cells or other intestinal epithelial cell types. Paneth cells from monkeys following blood clearance of mercury are free of the inclusions. The presence of mercury in lysosomes may be indicative of intracellular sequestration of a toxic mercury compound. Exocytosis of these bodies was not observed. Paneth cells may preferentially eliminate toxic mercury burdens by cell necrosis and desquamation.

Colon

The observation made on our macaque monkeys that the colon wall is among the tissues high in mercury burden with a level near the range of kidneys and liver is noteworthy. However, colonic ulcerations or changes in mucosal structure were not seen.

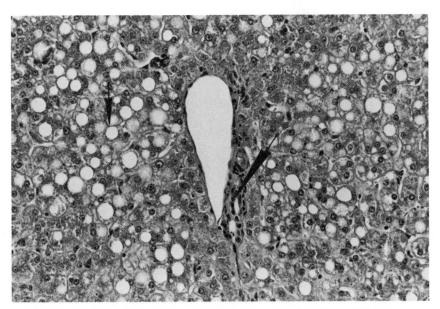

Figure 6.5. Photomicrograph of liver (× 400) showing a portal triad (*arrow*) surrounded by hepatocytes containing vacuoles that stain for lipid with oil red O stain. The central area of the lobules was free from this change. The blood mercury level was between 2.5 and 3.0 ppm for 10 weeks before sacrifice.

Liver

Macroscopic and microscopic lesions in the liver occur at dose levels comparable to those for kidney lesions (Desnoyers and Chang 1975). Macroscopically, the liver may appear swollen and pale at blood levels above 2.8 ppm in the monkey. Microscopically within the liver, however, the first change to appear is hepato-cellular swelling, particularly in the periphery of the lobules with fatty accumulation. At higher exposure levels, these changes become progressively more severe, and some liver cell necrosis may also be found. Abnormalities of the liver-function tests did not occur until general toxicity was observed. The liver lesions observed did not have characteristics that would differentiate them from fatty change due to a variety of toxic substances (see Figure 6.5).

I have been unable to find studies on the liver ultrastructural effects of methyl mercury in humans. Chronic exposure to 10 mg/kg MeHg in rats (Desnoyers and Chang 1975; Fowler and Woods 1977) reveals the dilatation of rough endoplasmic reticulum, mitochondrial swelling and liposomes, and peribiliary accumulation of lysosomes. Later, cytosegresomes containing degenerated organelles were seen. Our observations on primate liver at 2.8 ppm blood mercury and above are comparable to those seen in rats.

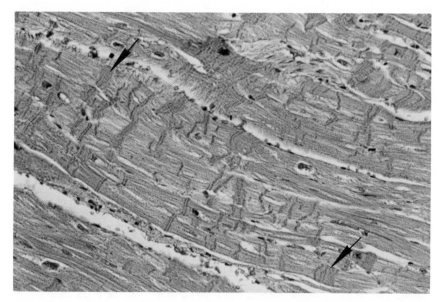

Figure 6.6.   Photomicrograph of macaque myocardium (× 500). Arrows point to two of many bands associated with myofibrillar degeneration. A blood mercury level at approximately 2.5–4.0 ppm was recorded for the final 41 days of life.

Heart

Previously I reported (Mottet 1974) the presence of myofibrillar degeneration and individual cell necrosis in the myocardium and a decreased force of contraction in vitro (Su and Chen 1979) in myocardium exposed to mercury. Although these changes have not been described in the human autopsies, we continue to find them in the macaque autopsies (see Figure 6.6). Recent reports from this department (Cowan et al. 1983; Reichenbach 1985) indicate that these lesions may be found in a small percentage of normal monkeys. Thus, the question of whether their presence is increased by methyl mercury remains unresolved. We rarely see the changes in our controls, but we have not quantitated the comparison.

Brain

Acute high-dose exposure to methyl mercury is severely neurotoxic. Much of the human neuropathology was originally defined by Hunter, Bomford, and Russell (1940) and later by Takeuchi and co-workers (1977). The widespread encephalopathy was associated with the characteristic symptoms and signs of methyl mercury brain injury to produce the clinical syndrome. In contrast, gastrointestinal and renal signs and symptoms predominate in inorganic divalent mercury exposure. The human neuropathological lesions are described elsewhere in this book. The clinical findings are paresthesia, ataxia, neurasthenia, vision and hearing loss, spasticity and tremor, and finally coma and death. Except for the brief reports of Al-Saleem (1976) and Choi et al. (1978), scant pathological studies on the brain have been reported from Iraq. The following is a description of our macaque monkey findings and their comparison to the human findings. Both human and nonhuman primate findings in the brain are remarkably similar, except for those in the cerebellum. The neuropathological observations revealed the cortex of the cerebrum to be selectively involved with focal neuronal degeneration followed by neuronal death and reactive gliosis and associated with relatively mild phagocytosis (Shaw et al. 1975). These changes are most prominent in the cerebral cortex along deeper fissures, such as in the calcarine and central cortex and insula. These destructive changes are associated with cerebral edema in the acute stage (Shaw et al. 1975).

Acute High-Dose Exposure   A single dose of 3 mg/kg body weight of methyl mercury produced no abnormalities, either clinically or pathologically, in macaque monkeys after 1 week. The blood mercury level was 0.7 μg/ml at 1 week. Another group receiving 2 mg/kg body weight daily for 16 days produced a blood mercury level of 10 μg/ml on day 17 when sacrificed. Apathy, clumsiness, tremor, and lethargy signs developed relatively abruptly 15 days after the onset of the experiment. The symptom—paresthesia—is not detectable in the monkeys. It is this symptom that occurs at much lower dose levels than the signs in humans.

Histopathologically, the major destructive lesions involved the deep nuclei of the cerebrum and cerebellum. The large neurons in these regions were markedly diminished in number, and the glia cells and capillaries had proliferated. Occasional mild perivascular lymphocytic cuffings were present (Figure 6.7). The remaining large neurons showed various types of degenerative changes, including central chromatolysis, Spielmeyer's "homogenizing" degeneration or Nissl's "chronic degenerative" changes, shrinkage (with pyknotic nuclei), and condensed cytoplasm, and frequently were surrounded by a cluster of neuroglia. Glial nodules without fragments of neuronal bodies in the center were also present. These changes were most marked in the dentate nucleus of the cerebellum and lateral geniculate nucleus; moderate in the thalamus (predominantly in the lateral nuclei), basis pontis, cranial nerve nuclei in the tegmentum pontis, and inferior colliculi; and mild in the claustrum, putamen, globus pallidus, and medial nuclei of the thalamus (Shaw et al. 1975). Neuronal loss was not striking in these regions, but active neuronophagia and glia nodules were numerous. Similar changes were also seen in the large neurons of the claustrum, putamen, globus pallidus, and medial parts of the thalamus. In the cerebral cortex, occasional neurons, including

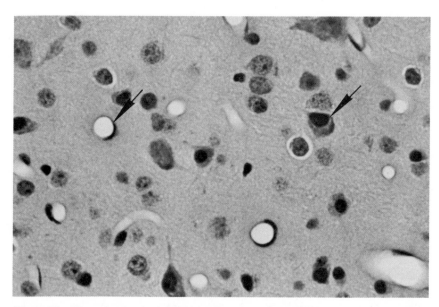

Figure 6.7. Photomicrograph of occipital cortex of a macaque that had a blood mercury level above 2.5 ppm for 3 months prior to sacrifice. Clinical signs of mercury encephalopathy were present throughout much of this period. Right arrow points to one of several degenerating neurons. Left arrow points to a lipid-filled phagocyte ($\times$ 200).

the calcarine and insular cortex, were involved, but neurons in the cerebellar cortex were practically uninvolved. With myelin stains, the white matter was diffusely pale. Stained myelin sheaths were sparse, fenestrated, and fragmented, but no focal necrosis or phagocytosis was evident (Figure 6.8). Proliferation of astrocytes and their fibers was diffuse and moderate throughout the white matter.

Continuous Low-Dose Exposure   A group of adult monkeys were given low doses of methyl mercury orally in apple juice for prolonged periods (Shaw et al. 1975). The doses ranged from 0.1 to 0.6 mg/day, and the total duration of the experiment ranged from 6.8 to 12.0 months.

The histopathological lesions in the monkeys that showed clinical signs differed only in severity and extent from the above, but their histological characteristics and anatomical localizations were remarkably similar. The main focus of destructive lesions was in the cerebral cortex, with a strong tendency to involve the cortex lining deep sulci. The midportion of the cortex lining the sulci was the center of the destructive lesions, which became less apparent as the cortex extended either to the depth of the sulcus or to the surface of the cerebral hemisphere. The calcarine, insular, and opercular

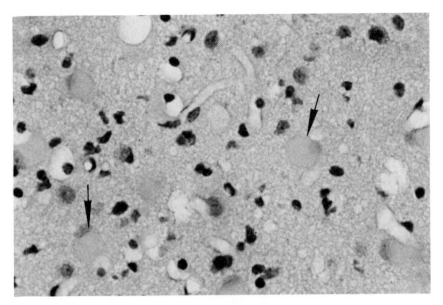

Figure 6.8. Photomicrograph (× 100) of the cerebral cortex. Arrows point to two of many glial cells. Gliosis is a prominent feature of the later stages of mercury injury.

cortices line the two deepest fissures—the calcarine and Sylvian. These cortices were most severely involved in all monkeys. Cortices lining the sagittal fissure were spared. The lesion extended centrifugally from the Sylvian fissure to the frontal, temporal, and parietal lobes, but still followed the general rule of involving the cortex in the depths of the sulci. Similar but less extensive spread was seen in the medial occipital lobes, where the lesion extended anteriorly along the calcarine fissure. The frontal and occipital poles were spared.

The type of histological lesions in these chronic animals had minor differences from those characteristic of acute mercurial encephalopathy. There was a tendency for the destruction to favor the small granular neurons, such as those located in layers II and IV of the calcarine cortex. In most instances, however, the lesions were too far advanced to show such selectivity. The most striking lesions, usually found in the calcarine and insular cortices, consisted of a spongy degeneration of the middle layers of the cortex, where marked diffuse neuronal loss and marked glial proliferation were evident. Most of the small vacuoles appeared empty, but some contained a nucleus in the center. Frozen sections stained with oil red O revealed no neutral lipids in these vacuoles. Hypertrophic astrocytes were abundant in all cortical layers, but most striking in the molecular layer. The transition between the involved and uninvolved cortex was gradual. At the areas of transition and in the thalamus and putamen, shrinkage and pyknosis of large neurons and perineural glial nodules, such as seen in the acute encephalopathy, were observed. Also in these areas, tiny vacuoles around the nuclei of small granular neurons in the middle layers of the cortex were found. If this finding represents an early lesion, then it implies that the small granular neurons are destroyed first. At any rate, lesions with different severity of destruction were present in the same specimen, and the different severities probably indicate different durations of the lesions.

The brains of monkeys with chronic poisoning show a fourfold to sevenfold increase of mercury above the highest level of the asymptomatic animals, ranging from 4 to 18 μg/g tissue, with the lowest level in the cerebellar hemisphere and the lower brain stem (Shaw et al. 1980). The concentration of mercury is slightly higher in the deep cerebral nuclei and the higher brain stem, but these areas do not show the greatest destructive lesions.

The brains of monkeys with acute poisoning show a ten- to twentyfold increase of mercury above the asymptomatic animals, with a similar tendency to show higher concentrations in the deep cerebral nuclei, high brain stem, colliculi, and dentate nucleus—the sites with the major destructive lesions.

Various types of histological changes in the nervous system have been described in both humans and experimental animals with organic mercury poisoning, but most investigators have agreed that these variations probably represent different stages in the sequence of the same pathological process. Thus, degenerative changes of neurons and neuroglia, phagocytosis of neurons, perivascular accumulation of inflammatory cells, and vascular and glial proliferation, as described in the two monkeys of our acute experiment, are typical findings of the early stage and are followed by a marked reduction in number of neurons, pseudolaminar spongy degeneration of the cerebral cortex, marked gliosis, and loss of myelin and axons, representing the late stage of the same process that was seen in our monkeys with chronic mercury poisoning.

Review of documented pathological data in the literature shows that there is a strong tendency for selective involvement of small granular neurons, especially of those in the granular cell layer of the cerebellum and calcarine cortex of the cerebrum. The putamen is probably the structure next most frequently involved. This tendency is especially true in humans. Different types of organic mercury compounds may also induce different types of lesions in the central nervous system, especially with regard to the site of the lesions. Ventral horn cells and pyramidal tracts in the spinal cord were involved in a case of phenyl mercury acetate poisoning and lesions in the white matter, such as the corpus callosum, anterior commissure, and subcortical white matter, in addition to the cerebellum and cerebral cortex in a case of ethyl mercuric chloride exposure.

Cerebellar lesions have not been reported in squirrel monkeys (Garman et al. 1975) or in a rhesus monkey (Hunter et al. 1940). In our experiments with macaque monkeys, varying the dose of methyl mercury and the duration of the mercury intake produced both acute and chronic mercurial intoxication but no lesions of granular cells or Purkinje cells. When cerebellar lesions were finally obtained by hyperacute and large-dose intoxication, they were in the dentate nucleus, not in the cerebellar cortex. Furthermore, large neurons, not the granular neurons of the koniocortex and cerebellum, were primarily involved in the hyperacute encephalopathy.

In addition to the species-specific variability of regional susceptibility of the brain in organic mercury poisoning shown by previous investigators and in the present report, we also observed an interesting phenomenon of a dualistic regional susceptibility in macaque monkeys produced by the different rate and mode of exposure to methyl mercury.

The regional susceptibility to a noxious agent is qualitative in nature and usually constant in mature animals of the same species. Alteration of the dose and the rate of administration of the agent can produce lesions that are quantitatively different in terms of their severity and extent, but it should not change the localization of the lesions. Different susceptible regions can be observed among animals of the same species only when they are in different stages of ontogenic development.

Cerebral cortical atrophy could be found if the animals were kept alive for a prolonged period after destruction of the gray matter and subsequent gliosis had begun. Observations on primate brains by our group (Shaw et al. 1975, 1979, 1980), by Berlin et al. (1975a, 1975b), and by Willes et al. (1978) are consistent with the above and provide a time, dose, and tissue-burden relationship. Shaw observed (Shaw et al. 1980) that in autopsies done more than a year after the cessation of exposure, cerebral atherosclerosis occurred in 4 out of 27 animals in the leptomeningeal arteries overlying the sites of parenchymal degeneration. Previous investigators have described the presence of cerebrovascular lesions in human cases of organic mercurial intoxication (Takeuchi and Eto 1977). These lesions were often seen years after exposure and after the cessation of acute intoxication symptoms. Whether the human cerebrovascular changes were coincidental or causally related to the mercury intoxication remained moot. We have studied the parenchymal and cerebrovascular lesions in 27 macaques in six groups ranging in methyl mercury exposure from none to acute high-dose and chronic low-dose exposure for more than a year (Shaw et al. 1979). Cerebrovascular lesions were found in 4 macaques. The lesions occurred in leptomeningeal arteries and arterioles in association with parenchymal degeneration. The lesions were morphologically similar to those seen in humans and associated with hypertension— principally intimal thickening, smooth-muscle-cell degeneration, and adventitial fibrosis.

Sacrifice of macaque monkeys with blood levels above 2 ppm but without signs of mercury poisoning revealed in a few instances the presence of the neurological lesion in the cerebral cortex, showing that "silent damage" occurs at lower blood levels when clinical signs of toxicity are not present. Whether "silent damage" occurs at blood mercury levels below 2 ppm remains moot.

A system of grading the severity of chronic methyl mercury encephalopathy has been developed by Shaw (unpublished) based on his extensive study of the macaque. Grade I lesions represent small focal cortical degenerations in the depths of a few sulci, such as the calcarine, Sylvian, superior, temporal, or central sulci. Grade II lesions have cortical degenerations in the depths of most sulci, whereas grade III lesions have diffuse cortical degeneration, which occurs both at the depths of sulci and at the crests of gyri. Grade IV lesions are characterized by diffuse cortical degeneration in the depths of sulci and at the crest of gyri degeneration of the basal ganglia. No lesions have been seen in the hippocampus, brain stem, and cerebellum in chronic methyl mercury intoxication in the macaque. Cortical atrophy and arteriosclerosis probably reflect the duration, but not the severity, of the degenerative processes.

Reproductive Effects of Methyl Mercury

Outcome of Pregnancy

Studies of the human epidemics of methyl mercury poisoning in Japan (see Takeuchi and Eto 1977; Tsubaki and Irukayama 1977) and in Iraq (Amin-Zaki et al. 1974; Bakir et al. 1973) have not reported effects of methyl mercury on the outcome of pregnancy. Perhaps the nature of these population exposures and the ill-defined population at risk precluded the possibility of defining the rate of pregnancy, abortion rate, and so on. A surprise finding in our primate studies was that methyl mercury decreased the pregnancy rate and increased the abortion rate at maternal blood levels above 1 ppm (Burbacher et al. 1984). Our findings have been recently reported (Mottet et al. 1985). Below the maternal 1 ppm blood mercury level, we have not detected adverse effects on pregnancy outcome, but in this group we have only six offspring. At 1.1–1.5 ppm, we had 2 adverse outcomes in 7 females (1 miscarriage and 1 nonconception). At 1.6–2.0 ppm there were 9 adverse outcomes with 13 females (3 stillbirths, 2 miscarriages, and 4 nonconceptions). At 2.1 ppm and above, we had no viable offspring in 3 females (1 abortion and 2 nonconceptions). Because in our experimental situation we are able to select fertile females of known pregnancy history, control their environment extensively, control the mating, and observe the occurrence of miscarriages, delivery, and offspring, these findings are significant. This effect of methyl mercury appears to be principally on the ovarian and uterine component of pregnancy. To date, our studies on the hormones and pituitary morphology are negative, except in the highest exposure group (unpublished). Further, our autopsies subsequently revealed that the female reproductive tracts were anatomically normal and were characteristic of fertile young females. One had a slightly bicornuate uterus, but that was judged to be of no functional significance.

Spermatogenesis

There appears to be only one report in the literature (Popescu 1978) suggesting decreased spermatogenesis in humans due to alkyl mercury exposure. In laboratory rodents it has been shown that methyl mercury breaches the blood-testes barrier and is present in the seminiferous epithelial cell region of the seminiferous tubules. Dr. Mohamed, in my laboratory, has conducted studies on the effect of methyl mercury on macaque sperm in vitro. A decrease in sperm motility was shown as decreased swimming speed quantitated by a new laser light scattering method (Mohamed et al. 1986). Using the laser light scattering technique, further information on dose-effect relationships of methyl mercury on sperm motility was obtained. The technique provides a quantitative evaluation of sperm swimming speed. Semen samples were collected from normal male *Macaca fascicularis* monkeys by anal electroejaculation. Methyl mercury was added to aliquots of sperm suspensions in BWW medium in doses of 10, 5, 2, and 1 ppm. After 3 hours, the speed relative to the corresponding control value was 35 percent, 59 percent, 59 percent, and 92 percent at doses of 10, 5, 2, and 1 ppm respectively. The percentage of motile spermatozoa decreased significantly at 10 ppm. Microscopic observation detected abnormal motility at 5 and 10 ppm, especially after 20–40 minutes. Head movement increased from side to side, and many spermatozoa developed coiled tails. In an in vivo study, morphological abnormalities of sperm tail in semen increased with methyl mercury treatment (Figure 6.9).

Embryopathic Effects

Of the several toxic trace metals, methyl mercury is the one that is most clearly established as being a teratogen for humans and experimental animals. The poisonings in Japan and Iraq established that mercury is a human teratogen in relatively high doses, with major effects on the developing nervous system. A cerebral-palsy-like clinical syndrome resulted. Autopsies by Takeuchi on three fetal deaths (Kutsuma 1968) revealed a decreased number of nerve cells in the cerebral cortex and a generalized hypoplasia of the cerebellum. Total brain weight was markedly decreased. Choi et al. (1978) autopsied two fetal brains from fetal deaths in Iraq. High levels of maternal mercury exposure (Marsh et al. 1981) were associated with abnormal neuronal migration, and deranged organization of brain centers and

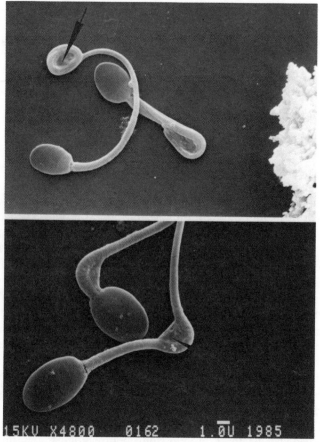

Figure 6.9. Macaque spermatozoa. The two at the bottom are kinked (*see arrow*) at site of persistent cytoplasm near head. The two at the top have coiled tails. At 5–10 ppm MeHg exposure in vitro, approximately one-third of the sperm will have this abnormal morphology. (Scanning electron microscopy photographs.)

layers were described. After the period of congenital exposure, the women in Japan and Iraq produced offspring that tended to be smaller than normal, but many uncontrolled variables make the human data difficult to interpret. In laboratory rodents, there is a dose-related decrease in size and weight of offspring congenitally exposed to methyl mercury.

Because the studies in human cases were retrospective, the specific details concerning the doses and duration of methyl mercury intake, blood mercury levels, and clinico-toxico-neuropathological relationships could not be documented precisely. Most studies in animal experiments have been prospective, so that toxicological data have been easily obtained, but marked differences between species have made it difficult to see the effect of chronic exposure of organic mercury on the developing nervous system. For example, small rodents and cats, which have been commonly used for acute experiments, have a short gestational period that makes chronic mercury exposure to fetuses difficult to control in these species. Because of a longer gestational period of 158–164 days, similarity of placentas, and their close phylogenetic relationship to humans, macaques are virtually indispensable for experiments involving chronic exposure to mercury in utero.

We have examined the physical and behavioral development of offspring born to macaque females with blood levels of mercury between 0.5 and 2.0 ppm and have found some interesting structural and functional changes not reported at the lower dose levels in the human cases. At any of the given maternal mercury blood levels within the range study, maternal level was lower than the fetal umbilical cord blood by a ratio of 1 : 1.5–2.0. Our observations on the physical characteristics of the offspring for male and female newborns reveal that continuous low-level exposure of the mother producing blood levels below the toxic level was not associated with specific gross malformations other than those of the central nervous system. The length of gestation was comparable in experimental and control groups.

At blood levels of 2.5 ppm, there were characteristic anatomic malformations in the brain consistent with those described in the human cases. The results of our experiments confirm and amplify previous observations on human organic mercury intoxication in Japan, Iraq, and the United States and in extensive animal experiments.

Three of our female monkeys exposed to methyl mercury produced offspring with severe brain anomalies (Figure 6.10). They received 100–110 μg/kg per day. At this dose, mild clinical neurotoxicity generally occurred in adult rhesus monkeys after 8–10 months of exposure (long after the birth of the infant). This is very near the clinical threshold of exposure. From our past observations, we expected that the mothers would not become symptomatic during their pregnancies with this dose.

The blood mercury levels were very similar in the three pregnancies: they remained between 1.5 and 2.5 ppm during the second and third trimesters, with peak levels in the late second or early third trimester. The blood mercury levels in all three newborns were higher than those of their respective mothers at birth. The differences among the three animals reflect the difference in ages at sacrifice. Case 1, surviving for 18 months without further exposure to mercury, showed practically no mercury in all sample sites of the nervous system, whereas case 2, who was only 2 weeks old, showed almost uniformly high levels except in the occipital lobe. The tissue mercury levels in case 3 were intermediate, this animal surviving 7 months. This animal also showed significant variations in the mercury levels in different sites of the central nervous system, still high in the cerebrum but practically none in the

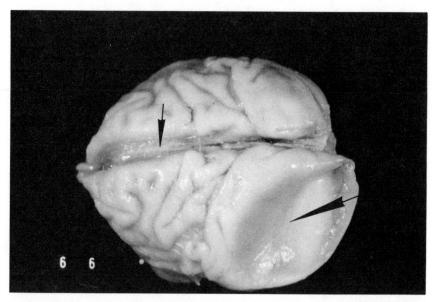

Figure 6.10. Macroscopic view of brain of an infant congenitally exposed to methyl mercury, showing generalized brain hypotrophy with small gyri and wide sulci between cerebral hemispheres (*small arrow*), and large cyst at left occipital pole (*large arrow*).

cerebellum. In view of previous observations that macaque monkeys (Shaw et al. 1980) and squirrel monkeys (Berlin et al. 1975*a*) show no changes in the cerebellum in chronic organic mercury encephalopathy, this is intriguing. The tissue mercury levels in cases 2 and 3 suggest that the clearance is more rapid from the cerebellum than from the cerebrum, but further studies must determine whether this explains the sparing of the cerebellum in nonhuman primates.

The mothers of the three macaque infants did not show signs of neurotoxicity during pregnancy, but the mother of case 1 developed difficulty with grasping and weakness of her legs after delivery of the infant. Similarly, humans have shown little or no evidence of neurotoxicity during pregnancy, but the appearance of neurotoxic symptoms after delivery has been observed both in humans and in animals and suggests that the pregnancy protects from neurotoxicity. By contrast, 31 pregnant women in an Iraq epidemic showed severe symptoms of neurotoxicity with a high mortality rate, suggesting that they had been exposed to higher doses or a different form of mercury (Amin-Zaki et al. 1974).

No clinical abnormalities were detected at birth in any of our three macaque infants; only after a week did signs appear. Human infants with congenital Minamata disease have also been considered to be normal at birth and generally require 3–6 months, or even longer, before they show progressive symptoms and signs of cerebral palsy, seizures and mental retardation. The difference in the length of this latent period between the two species can probably be explained by the different pace of postnatal psychomotor development.

Skull deformity, such as microcephaly and flattened skull vault, as seen in two of our cases (1 and 3), has also been observed in human patients in Minamata and is a secondary effect resulting from the markedly degenerated and hypoplastic brain. Our other case was sacrificed at age 2 weeks, when he suddenly and unexpectedly developed respiratory difficulty. Amin-Zaki et al. (1974) reported a similar case who died unexpectedly on the 33rd day of life, having been born from a mother showing neurotoxic symptoms after consuming methyl mercury contaminated bread during the first trimester. The pathological findings on this baby were subsequently reported by Choi et al. (1978) as showing developmental abnormalities characterized by heterotopic neurons in the cerebral and cerebellar white matter and disorganized cerebral cortex. These findings are quite different from ours.

Our case 1 was blind, quadriplegic, and had frequent seizures characterized by twitching and kicking movements of the spastic limbs for most of her 18 months of life. Our case 3 showed less severe but still very obvious motor abnormalities characterized by paroxysmal rhythmic jerking of the whole body, inability to stand or walk, and difficulty grasping or releasing grasp from the walls of the cage. However, this animal was able to move around by crawling and hopping. Based on long-term observations on 40 cases of congenital Minamata disease, Harada (1977) concluded that these patients could be categorized as having cerebral palsy of very variable types, indistinguishable from those caused by factors other than organic mercury poisoning. In general, mental symptoms, cerebellar symptoms, and strabismus were more common in patients with congenital Minamata disease, but none of these signs can be used as a specific diagnostic criterion.

We have observed two types of morphological changes in the brains of these three monkey infants. The brains of cases 1 and 3, who were sacrificed at age 18 months and 7 months respectively, were essentially identical, even though the clinical manifestations were quite different in both animals. Both showed diffuse sclerotic atrophy of the cerebral cortex, subcortical white matter, and basal ganglia with preservation of the medial thalamus, brain stem, and cerebellum. The cerebral cortical degeneration was most marked in the occipital lobes, with concomitantly marked dilatation of the occipital horn and trigone of the ventricles. Case 2, who was sacrificed at age 2 weeks, was quite different. No gross microcephaly was present. In fact, the weight of the cerebrum of this 2-week-old animal was more than three times greater than that of the other two older animals. Microscopic lesions were striking but somewhat different, characterized by multiple foci of neuronal degeneration, gliosis and calcification of the deeper layers of the cerebral cortex (especially at the depths of sulci) and basal ganglia, and gliosis and calcification of the cerebral white matter. The brain stem and cerebellum were uninvolved, as in the other two cases and as in adult rhesus monkeys.

For the following reasons, the differences in morphological characteristics between case 2 and cases 1 and 3 most likely represent different temporal stages of the same pathological process. (1) Case 2 was only 2 weeks old, whereas cases 1 and 3 were 18 months and 7 months old respectively. (2) Many of the histological lesions in case 2 were still active in showing karyorrhexis, eosinophilia of neurons, and hypertrophic astrocytes, as well as older lesions represented by microcystic degeneration and calcification. Atrophy, gliosis, and calcification are indicative of the end-stage of cell and tissue loss and characterized the findings in cases 1 and 3. (3) Arterial changes represented by intimal fibrosis, medial degeneration, calcification of the internal elastica lamina, and stenosis of the lumen are indicative of old lesions and were seen only in cases 1 and 3 but not in case 2.

It is generally accepted that the fetal nervous system has a greater affinity for organic mercury than the adult nervous system. Is this a function of affinity per se, or is it a reflection of the stronger blood-brain barrier in the adult? With a stronger affinity, the immature nervous system would release mercury more slowly, causing the destructive process to be more prolonged. Although we do not have data showing the duration of carryover brain damage after the cessation of methyl mercury exposure in the adult nervous system, the progressiveness of the neurological symptoms for months or years after termination of exposure to organic mercury in human congenital Minamata disease seems to support this idea. Abnormal neuronal migration suggestive of developmental anomaly as described by Choi et al. (1978) was not observed in our animals.

There is a trend toward lower birth weights, shorter crown/rump length, microcephaly, and other physical parameters of decreased size. However, one must be cautious in interpreting these data, because, as indicated, we separate the offspring and the male and female, which have an inherent difference in size in macaque monkeys. We have also found behavioral changes in the offspring, which are being reported separately (Burbacher et al. 1986; Gunderson et al. 1986) and are not an appropriate subject for this chapter.

Pursuing the cause for the reduced birth weights in methyl mercury exposed rodent embryos and fetuses, we have studied the mitotic rate and cell cycle in vitro and in vivo. Flow cytometry has revealed that the cell cycle is impeded in the G2 phase, which includes the first half of mitosis (to metaphase). The effects of methyl mercury on cell cycle kinetics were investigated by Vogel in my laboratory (Vogel et al. 1986) to help identify its mechanisms of action. Flow cytometric analysis of normal human fibroblasts grown in vitro in the presence of BrdUrd allowed quantitation of the proportion of cells in G1, S, G2, and the next G1 phase. This technique provides a rapid and easily performed method of characterizing phase lengths and transition rates for the complete cell cycle. After first exposure to methyl mercury, the cell cycle time was lengthened due to a prolonged G1. At 3 μM methyl mercury, the G1 phase length was 25 percent longer than the control. The G1/S transition rate was also decreased in a dose-related manner. Confluent cells exposed to methyl mercury and replated with methyl mercury respond the same as cells that have not been exposed to methyl mercury before replating. Cells exposed for long times to methyl mercury lost a detectable G1 effect and instead showed an increase in the G2 percentage, which was directly related to methyl mercury concentration and length of exposure. After 8 days at 5 μM methyl mercury, 45 percent of the population was in G2. The G2 accumulation was reversible up to 3 days, but at 6 days the cells remained in G2 when the methyl mercury was removed. Cell counts and viability indicated that there was not a selective loss of cells from the methyl mercury. Methyl mercury has multiple effects on the cell cycle, which include a lengthened G1 and decreased transition probability after short-term exposure of cycling cells and a G2 accumulation after a longer-term exposure. There were no detectable S phase effects. It appears that mitosis (the G2 accumulation) and probably synthesis of some macromolecules in G1 (the lengthened G1 and lowered transition probability) are particularly susceptible to methyl mercury.

Similarly, our mitotic counts indicate an increase in the number of cells in this early phase. Further pursuit of the phenomenon on the biochemical level indicates that methyl mercury binds to the sulfhydryl groups of tubulin that form the microtubules of the mitotic spindle and thus impedes their assembly and accelerates their disassembly (Vogel et al. 1985). This represents one of several possible mechanisms of action of methyl mercury on the development of the nervous system.

Summary

The lesions of methyl mercury intoxication vary with the blood level and chemical form of mercury. At high exposure levels, gross and microscopic changes are seen principally in the liver, kidneys, and brain in the adult. At lower levels of exposure, microscopic and ultrastructural lesions can be seen in these organs and also in the intestine, heart, and spermatozoa. At even lower levels, the reproductive outcome is adversely affected, and the characteristics of the offspring are altered with respect to birth weight (possibly), brain structure, and function.

Acknowledgments

The authors express their appreciation to the numerous participants who contributed to the primate studies referred to here: Drs. Chen, Finocchio, Luschei, Vogel, and Mohamed. The primate research was supported by the National Institute of Environmental Health Sciences, grants ES00677 and ES07032.

References

Aaronson, R. M., and Spiro, H. (1973). Mercury and the gut. *Dig Dis* 18:583–594.

Al-Damluji, S. F. (1976). Organic mercury poisoning in Iraq: History prior to the 1971–1972 outbreak. *Bull WHO* 53(Suppl.):11–13.

Al-Saleem, T. (1976). Levels of mercury and pathological changes in patients with organomercury poisoning. *Bull WHO* 53(Suppl.):99–104.

Amin-Zaki, L.; Elhassani, S.; Majeed, M.; Clarkson, T. W.; Doherty, R. A.; and Greenwood, M. (1974). Intrauterine methylmercury poisoning in Iraq. *Pediatrics* 54:587–595.

Bakir, F.; Damluji, S. F.; Amin-Zaki, L.; Murtadha, M.; Khalidi, A.; Al-Rawi, N. Y.; Tikriti, S.; Dhahir, H. I.; Clarkson, T. W.; Smith, J. C.; and Doherty, R. A. (1973) Methylmercury poisoning in Iraq. *Science* 181:230–242.

Berlin, M.; Carlson, J.; and Norseth, T. (1975a). Dose dependence of methylmercury metabolism: A study of distribution, biotransformation, and excretion in the squirrel monkey. *Arch Environ Health* 30:307–313.

Berlin, M.; Grant, C. M.; Hellberg, J.; Hellstrom, J.; and Schutz, A. (1975b). Neurotoxicity of methylmercury in squirrel monkeys. *Arch Environ Health* 30:340–348.

Burbacher, T. M.; Grant, K. S.; and Mottet, N. K. (1986). Environmentally induced deficits in primate cognition: Methylmercury retards object permanence development. *Dev Psych* 22:1–7.

Burbacher, T. M.; Monnett, C.; Grant, K. S.; and Mottet, N. K. (1984). Methylmercury exposure and reproductive dysfunction in the nonhuman primate. *Toxicol Appl Pharmacol* 75:18–24.

Chang, L. W.; Reuhl, K. R.; and Lee, G. N. (1977). Degenerative changes in the developing nervous system as a result of in utero exposure to methylmercury. *Environ Res* 14(3):414–423.

Chen, W.-J.; Body, R. L.; and Mottet, N. K. (1983). Biochemical and morphological studies of monkeys chronically exposed to methylmercury. *J Toxicol Environ Health* 12:407–416.

Choi, B. H.; Laphan, L. W.; Amin-Zaki, L.; and Al-Saleem, T. (1978). Abnormal neuronal migration, deranged cerebral cortical organization, and diffuse white matter astrocytosis of human fetal brain. *J Neuropathol Exp Neurol* 37:719–733.

Clarkson, T. W. (1971). Epidemiological and experimental aspects of lead and mercury contamination of food. *Food Cosmet Toxicol* 9:229–243.

Clarkson, T. W.; Kershaw, T. G.; and Dhahir, P. H. (1980). The relationship between blood levels and dose of methylmercury in man. *Arch Environ Health* 35:28–35.

Cowan, M. J.; Giddens, W. E.; and Reichenbach, D. D. (1983). Selective myocardial cell necrosis in non-human primates. *Arch Pathol Lab Med* 107:34–39.

Crooker, A. R.; Johnson, D. E.; and Mottet, N. K. (1984). Mercury in primate Paneth cells following methylmercury hydroxide ingestion. *Proc Electron Microscop Soc Am* 42:290–291.

Desnoyers, P. A., and Chang, L. W. (1975). Ultrastructural changes in the liver after chronic exposure to methylmercury. *Environ Res* 10:59–75.

Finocchio, D. V.; Luschei, E. S.; Mottet, N. K.; and Body, R. L. (1980). Effects of methylmercury on the visual system of rhesus monkeys (*Macaca mulatta*), I: Pharmacokinetics of chronic methylmercury related to changes in vision and behavior. In *Neurotoxicity of the Visual System,* edited by W. H. Merigan and B. Weiss, pp. 113–121. New York: Raven Press.

Fowler, B. A. (1972). Ultrastructural evidence for nephropathy induced by long-term exposure to small amounts of methylmercury. *Science* 175:780–781.

Fowler, B. A.; Brown, H. W.; Lucier, G. W.; and Beard, M. E. (1974). Mercury uptake by renal lysosomes of rats ingesting methylmercury hydroxide. *Arch Pathol* 98:297–301.

Fowler, B. A., and Woods, J. S. (1977). Transplacental toxicity of methylmercury to fetal rat liver mitochondria. *Lab Invest* 36:122–130.

Garman, R. H.; Weiss, B.; and Evans, H. L. (1975). Alkylmercury encephalopathy in the monkey. *Acta Neuropathol* (Berl) 32:61–74.

Goldblatt, S. (1928). Acute mercurial intoxication: A report of thirty-eight cases. *Am J Med Sci* 176:645–654.

Goyer, R. A. (1985). Urinary system. In *Environmental Pathology,* edited by N. K. Mottet, pp. 301–303. New York: Oxford University Press.

Gritzka, T. L., and Trump, B. F. (1968). Renal tubular lesions caused by mercuric chloride. *Am J Pathol* 52:1225–1277.

Gunderson, V.; Grant, K. S.; Burbacher, T. M.; Fagan, J.; and Mottet, N. K. (1986). Low level prenatal methylmercury exposure retards visual recognition memory in infant Macaques. *Child Dev* 57:1076–1083.

Harada, Y. (1977). Congenital Minamata disease. In *Minamata Disease: Methyl Mercury Poisoning in Minamata and Niigata, Japan,* edited by T. Tsubaki and K. Irukayama. New York: Elsevier.

Hunter, D.; Bomford, R. R.; and Russell, D. S. (1940). Poisoning by methylmercury compounds. *Q J Micro Sci* 9:193–213.

Hunter, D., and Russell, D. S. (1954). Focal cerebral and cerebellar atrophy in a human subject due to organic mercury compounds. *J Neurol Psychiatry* 17:235–241.

Ikeda, Y.; Tobe, M.; Kobayashi, K.; Suzuki, S.; Kawasaki, Y.; and Yonemaru, H. (1973). Long-term toxicity study of methylmercuric chloride in monkeys. *Toxicol* 1:361–375.

Joiner, F. E., and Hupp, E. W. (1978). Behavioral observations in squirrel monkeys (*Saimiri sciureus*) following methylmercury exposure. *Environ Res* 16:18–28.

Jolili, M. A., and Abbasi, A. H. (1961). Poisoning by methylmercury toluene sulphonanilide. *Br J Ind Med* 18:303–308.

Kershaw, T. G.; Dhahir, P. H.; and Clarkson, T. W. (1980). The relationship between blood levels and dose of methylmercury in man. *Arch Environ Health* 35:28–35.

Kutsuma, M., ed. (1968). *Minamata Disease.* Kumamoto, Japan: Kumamoto University Press.

Luschei, E.; Mottet, N. K.; and Shaw, C.-M. (1977). Chronic methylmercury exposure in the monkey (*Macaca mulatta*): Behavioral tests of peripheral vision, signs of neurotoxicity, and blood concentration in relation to dose and time. *Arch Environ Health* 32:126–131.

Madsen, K. M., and Christensen, E. I. (1978). Effects of mercury on lysosomal protein digestion in the kidney proximal tubule. *Lab Invest* 38:165–174.

Magos, L.; Bakir, K. F.; Clarkson, T. S.; Al-Jawad, A. M.; and Al-Soffi, M. H. (1976). Tissue levels of mercury in autopsy specimens of liver and kidney. *Bull WHO* 53(Suppl.):93–97.

Marsh, D. O.; Myers, G. J.; Clarkson, T. W.; Amin-Zaki, L.; Tikriti, S.; Majeed, M. A.; and Dabbagh, A. R. (1981). Dose-response relationship for human fetal exposure to methylmercury. *Clin Tox* 18:1311–1318.

Mohamed M.; Burbacher, T. M.; and Mottet, N. K. (in press). The effects of methylmercury on primate sperm structure and function. *Acta Pharmacol Toxicol.*

Mohamed, M.; Lee, W. I.; Burbacher, T. M.; and Mottet, N. K. (1986). Laser light-scattering study of the toxic effects of methylmercury on sperm motility. *J Androl* 7:11–15.

Mottet, N. K. (1974). Some subtle lesions of methylmercury intoxication. *Lab Invest* 30:384–385. (Abstract)

Mottet, N. K., and Body, R. L. (1974). Mercury burden of human autopsy organs and tissues. *Arch Environ Health* 29:18–24.

——— (1976). Primate Paneth cell degeneration following methylmercury hydroxide ingestion. *Am J Pathol* 84:93–102.

Mottet, N. K.; Shaw, C. M.; and Burbacher, T. M. (1985). Health risks from increases in methylmercury exposure. *Environ Health Perspect* 63:133–140.

Moutinho, M. E.; Tompkins, A. L.; Rowland, T. W.; Banson, B. B.; and Jackson, A. H. (1981). Acute mercury vapor poisoning. *Am J Dis Child* 135:42–44.

Natelson, E. A.; Blumenthal, B. J.; and Fred, H. L. (1971). Acute mercury vapor poisoning in the home. *Chest* 59:677–678.

National Academy of Sciences (1978). *Mercury in the Environment.* Washington, D.C.: Environmental Studies Board, National Research Council.

Pazderova, J.; Jirasek, A.; Mraz, M.; and Pechan, J. (1974). Post-mortem findings and clinical signs of dimethylmercury poisoning in man. *Arch Arbeitsmed* 33:323–328.

Piotrowski, J. K., and Inskip, M. J. (1981). *Health Effects of Methylmercury.* MARC Report 24. London: U.N. Environmental Programme, Monitoring and Assessment Research Centre, Chelsea College, University of London.

Popescu, H. I. (1978). Poisoning with alkylmercury compounds (letter to the editor). *Br Med J* 1:1347.

Reichenbach, D. D. (1985). Cardiovascular system. In *Environmental Pathology,* edited by N. K. Mottet, pp. 356–368. New York: Oxford University Press.

Reynolds, W. A., and Pitkin, R. M. (1975). Transplacental passage of methylmercury and its uptake by primate fetal tissues. *Proc Soc Exp Biol Med* 148:523–526.

Rice, D. C., and Gilbert, S. G. (1982). Early chronic low-level methylmercury poisoning in monkeys impairs spatial vision. *Science* 216:759–761.

Shaw, C.-M.; Mottet, N. K.; Body, R. L.; and Luschei, E. S. (1975). Variability of neuropathologic lesions in experimental methylmercury encephalopathy in primates. *Am J Pathol* 80:451–470.

Shaw, C.-M.; Mottet, N. K.; and Chen, W.-J. (1980). Effects of methylmercury on the visual system of rhesus macaque (*Macaca mulatta*), II: Neuropathological findings (with emphasis on vascular lesions in the brain). In *Neurotoxicity of the Visual System,* edited by W. H. Merigan and B. Weiss, pp. 123–134. New York: Raven Press.

Shaw, C.-M.; Mottet, N. K.; Luschei, E. S.; and Finocchio, D. F. (1979). Cerebrovascular lesions in experimental methylmercurial encephalopathy. *Neurotoxicology* 1:57–74.

Su, J. Y., and Chen, W.-J. (1979). The effects of methylmercury on isolated cardiac tissues. *Am J Pathol* 95:753–763.

Takeuchi, T., and Eto, K. (1977). Pathology and pathogenesis of Minamata disease. In *Minamata Disease,* edited by T. Tsubaki and K. Irukayama, chap. 2, pp. 103–141. New York: Elsevier.

Tamashiro, H.; Akagi, H.; Arakaki, M.; Futatsuka, M.; and Roht, L. (1984). Causes of death in Minamata disease: Analysis of death certificates. *Int Arch Occup Environ Health* 54:135–146.

Tsubaki, T., and Irukayama, K., eds. (1977). *Minamata Disease.* New York: Elsevier.

Turner, M. D.; Marsh, D. O.; Smith, J. C.; Inglis, J. B.; Clarkson, T. W.; Rubio, C. E.; Chiriboga, J.; and Chiriboga, C. C. (1980). Methylmercury in populations eating large quantities of marine fish. *Arch Environ Health* 35:367–378.

Verity, M. A., and Brown, W. J. (1970). Hg^{2+}-induced kidney necrosis. *Am J Pathol* 61:57–74.

Vitulli, W. F. (1974). Mercury effects from chronic and acute doses on fixed interval operant behavior of female squirrel monkeys. *Psychol Rep* 35:3–9.

Vogel, D. G.; Margolis, R. L.; and Mottet, N. K. (1985). The effects of methylmercury binding to microtubules. *Toxicol Appl Pharmacol* 80:473–486.

Vogel, D. G.; Rabinovitch, P. S.; and Mottet, N. K. (1986). Methylmercury effects on cell cycle kinetics. *Cell Tissue Kinet* 19:227–242.

Ware, R. A.; Burkholder, P. M.; and Chang, L. W. (1975). Ultrastructural changes in renal proximal tubules after chronic organic and inorganic mercury intoxication. *Environ Res* 10:121–140.

Willes, R. F.; Truelove, J. G.; and Nera, E. A. (1978). Neurotoxic response of infant monkeys to methylmercury. *Toxicol* 9:125–135.

SEVEN

Sensory Deficits Caused by Exposure to Methyl Mercury

Zoltan Annau and Christine U. Eccles

The first detailed description of methyl mercury intoxication, as well as the first animal experimentation using this chemical, was provided by Hunter, Bomford, and Russell in 1940. A variety of organic mercury compounds had been used since 1914 as seed dressings, and the four cases described by these authors were workers in a factory who had handled mercury, methyl iodide, and methyl mercury iodide in the manufacturing of seed fungicides. The men wore protective dust masks and gloves as well as goggles, but despite these precautions they came down with severe methyl mercury poisoning. The cases had a similarity in symptomatology that has by now become the landmark of intoxication with methyl mercury compounds. The symptoms started with numbness in the fingers and toes that spread to the hands and feet. This was followed by muscle weakness and clumsiness in walking and handling objects with the fingers. As the intoxication developed, the victims had difficulty understanding speech, although their auditory acuity was not impaired. Peripheral vision became impaired as well, and they did not see moving objects in their field of vision; one worker was almost run over by a car while crossing a street. A change in personality was noted, and the victims became irritable. At the height of the intoxication they became totally ataxic and could not feed themselves, and their speech became incoherent and spasmodic.

The neurological examination showed that, while some of the reflexes were normal, there was great loss of sensory capacity. In one case there was gross impairment of two-point discrimination in the fingertips, and the subject could not tactually discriminate objects placed in his hands.

Hunter, Bomford, and Russell proceeded to administer methyl mercury iodide or nitrate to rats (1 mg and then 2 mg per day) and exposed one monkey to the iodide vapor (concentration not given). The rats showed the development of ataxia, and the monkey showed behavioral abnormalities that more closely resembled what the authors had observed in the human victims. Pathological examination of the rats revealed severe degeneration of the peripheral nerves, the posterior spinal roots, and the trigeminal nerves. The monkey showed similar degeneration of the myelin sheath in the peripheral nerves examined. In addition, there was evidence of frontal and occipital cortical damage, although the cerebellar cortex seemed unaffected.

In a subsequent paper, Hunter and Russell (1954) described the cortical and cerebellar damage following the autopsy of one of the four victims described in their earlier paper. This person had shown some recovery from the methyl mercury intoxication, although he had lost vision in one eye and had remained somewhat ataxic. Examination of the brain revealed gross loss of neurons in the visual cortex as well as in the granule cell layer of the cerebellum.

These two papers provided a guideline for subsequent researchers and for clinicians interested in organic mercury poisoning, and in fact the "Hunter-Russell syndrome" became the term for describing this type of mercury intoxication. Despite the relatively well established literature on organic mercury toxicity, the first major episode of methyl mercury intoxication in Minamata, Japan, went undiagnosed for several years. Although it is not the purpose of this chapter to provide yet another account of this episode, it should be noted that in the tabulation of symptoms experienced by the inhabitants of this small fishing village, signs of sensory disturbances were prominent and persistent. Thus, Takeuchi (1972, 1985) and Harada (1978) listed disturbances of sensation and visual constriction at the top of a list of symptoms, with 85 percent of the patients identified by Harada also having hearing impairment. What is equally important is that in a follow-up of some of these patients in 1972, there seemed to be no improvement in the sensory symptoms, and some worsening of the neuromuscular problems. Gerstner and Huff (1977) indicated that the patients also experienced gustatory impairment that may have played a major role in their decreased food intake. While there were some interesting differences in the symptoms of mercury-intoxicated Iraqis following the outbreak of poisoning in 1972, on the whole the sensory disturbances dominated the neurological impairments of this population as well (Bakir et al. 1973; Rustam and Hamdi 1974).

The sensory system that has been investigated most intensively in animal research is the visual system. The constriction of the visual field experienced by humans without apparent damage to the retina led to many studies designed to investigate dose-effect relationships both in terms of behavioral changes and in terms of neuropathological alterations in the visual system.

In order to obtain data as similar as possible to human mercury exposures, researchers at the University of Rochester chose monkeys as the experimental subjects. The stumptail macaque (*Macaca arctoides*) was trained on two visual discrimination tasks. On the form-discrimination task, a circle, triangle, or square was projected onto a rear-illuminated key. Pressing the key with the square resulted in a sip of fruit juice; pressing either of the other keys (whose position was randomized) terminated the trial and postponed the next trial for 10 seconds. The second task was a brightness-discrimination task in which only one of the three keys was illuminated and the monkey had to press that key. The luminance of the key was adjusted to four different levels.

In order to raise blood mercury levels rapidly, the animal was treated with

1 mg/kg priming doses of methyl mercury mixed into the food at 5-day intervals. When blood levels had reached 2.5 μg/ml, the animal was switched to 0.5 mg/kg once a week. Blood levels peaked at 3.0 μg/ml after 13 weeks, and then stabilized at approximately 2.5 μg/ml thereafter.

The control monkey's performance remained stable for 34 weeks. The animal treated with methyl mercury was stable for 12 weeks, and then it began to show a decline in accuracy on the form-discrimination task at the lowest level of luminance. Following a period of improvement (weeks 18–22) the performance deteriorated even at the higher luminance levels. After 28 weeks, performance deteriorated markedly on the form discrimination (33 percent of control), although the brightness discrimination remained above chance at the highest luminance levels, indicating that the monkey was not blind (Evans et al. 1975). Additional measures taken during the experiments revealed that the response latency of the intoxicated monkey remained stable until it had difficulty seeing the dim stimuli and was making more errors on the form-discrimination task.

The loss of touch sensation (hypesthesia) was tested in the animal by making it reach for a marshmallow through a hole in the cage wall without being able to guide its hand visually. At 21 weeks of exposure, the monkey started to miss the marshmallow and was also sometimes unable to distinguish marshmallows from other objects. Although these measures of impairment were not as objective as the form-discrimination task, they reflected the similarity of primate and human intoxications.

In a subsequent paper, Garman, Weiss, and Evans (1975) described the neuropathology of both squirrel monkeys and the macaque described above, following a variety of mercury-dosing regimens that were maintained from 30 to 365 days before sacrifice. Initially, neuronal loss was most severe in laminae 2 and 3 of the cortex, but could be found in all laminae. Some areas were devoid of neurons. The most damaged area was in the striate cortex within the calcarine fissure. Parts of the temporal and parietal cortex around the Sylvian fissure were also severely damaged. There was also some evidence through the appearance of glial cells that cerebellar damage would have resulted from more prolonged treatment. There was no evidence of damage in the spinal cord or peripheral nerves.

These two studies taken together show that at blood levels of 2–3 μg/ml and relatively short exposure periods, severe neurological impairment can be observed that correlates well with the development of quantifiable pathology. One note of caution made by these authors was that not all monkeys developed neurological signs within a treatment schedule, indicating individual susceptibility to methyl mercury intoxication in animals.

Using a somewhat different approach, Berlin et al. (1975) used squirrel monkeys trained on the Wisconsin General Test apparatus to determine the impairment caused by methyl mercury. In this test, the animal had to pull one of two chains to reach a stimulus object. The correct choice was rewarded with a raisin. In addition, in order to measure their critical fusion intensity (CFI), the monkeys were trained to respond to a flickering light by touching a panel. Methyl mercury hydroxide was administered through a stomach tube weekly in doses varying from 0.2 to 0.8 mg.

After a total dose of 5 mg/kg, the monkeys developed sudden neurological disturbances at around 30 days of treatment, which eventually resulted in total blindness. The dosing of other animals was adjusted to reach blood levels of 1.5 μg/g at 20, 50, 80, and 120 days. The first two groups showed neurological signs within 10 days of reaching peak blood levels. The latter two groups showed these signs when they reached the desired blood levels. There was a marked deterioration on the task, which appeared to result from the inability of the monkeys to locate the stimuli in their visual field as well as a clumsiness in manipulating the chain and picking up the reward. The critical fusion intensity test proved to be extremely sensitive in that all monkeys showed increased CFI before neurological impairment and at blood levels of 1.2 μg/g. The pathological observations in this study confirmed the observations of the Rochester group in that there was severe damage to the visual areas of the cortex and no damage to peripheral nerves (Garman et al. 1975). The brain-blood mercury ratio in the monkeys was found to be 5.6 to 1. Attempts to correlate the extent of cortical damage with the length of exposure were possible up to 90 days of exposure, but not beyond. Longer exposure did not seem to extend the damage.

In a more sophisticated approach to measuring changes in flicker sensitivity, Merigan (1979) described a procedure where the monkey was placed in a chair and faced two oscilloscope displays controlled by computer. The illuminated screen of one of the screens was flickered, and the animal had to indicate its observance of this by touching a panel on the same side as the flickering stimulus. Both frequency and the modulation depth of the stimulus were controlled by the computer. In addition, the luminance level was controlled by filters placed over the screen.

The results showed that methyl mercury intoxication greatly reduced the ability of the monkey to perceive high-frequency flicker (above 10–15 Hz) at low levels of luminance. At high luminance levels the monkey could respond up to 45 Hz, compared with 70 Hz for the control animal.

An interesting finding reported by Merigan et al. (1984) was that monkeys exposed to methyl mercury until they had a definite constriction of their visual fields (blood levels of 1.56 and 2.08 ppm) showed recovery over a period of 20–30 weeks following cessation of dosing. Examination of the visual cortex of these two animals failed to reveal any sign of damage. The authors were unable to offer an explanation for the lack of measurable neuropathology (at least at the light microscope level), nor could they explain the apparent total recovery of visual function upon termination of treatment.

Since blood levels of mercury in at least one of the animals was in the range where clear neuropathology can be expected, and indeed was seen in other animals in this study, the reason for the recovery and lack of neuropathology remains to be elucidated. In terms of human exposures, there are similar reports of transitory changes in visual function (Iwata 1973), although there is more compelling evidence that the changes are irreversible. Mukuno, Ishikawa, and Okamura (1981) reported on the results obtained by testing patients from Minamata who had been exposed to methyl mercury 15–25 years earlier. Their spatial contrast sensitivity was measured by the Arden grating chart, and their visual acuity, visual field, and visual evoked potentials were also measured. All mercury-exposed persons were different from controls in terms of their Arden test scores. The difference between the groups increased as the spatial frequency increased in the test. Twelve people had their visual evoked potentials recorded. In seven, the potentials were unrecordable. The other five all showed abnormal evoked potentials, especially at high-stimulus frequencies. There was no correlation between the Arden score and visual acuity or visual field measures. The authors concluded that in future measurements of intoxication the Arden test score and the visual evoked potentials could be used as sensitive indicators of toxicity.

The visual evoked potential has in fact been used in some studies to detect subclinical intoxication. Dyer, Eccles, and Annau (1978) exposed rats in utero on day 7 of gestation to 5 mg/kg of methyl mercury chloride administered to the mother. This dose of mercury did not cause any teratological effect in the offspring. On day 65 of age, the female offspring were implanted with skull electrodes, and flash evoked potentials were recorded in unanesthetized animals. The effect of mercury treatment in utero was to increase the P1–N1 amplitudes significantly, and these differences became greater as the intensity of the light stimulus was increased. The amplitudes of the other peaks did not change significantly. Both P2 and N2 latencies were significantly shorter in the animals exposed to the mercury.

These results indicated that a single in utero exposure to methyl mercury had long-lasting effects on visual function. The authors speculated that the changes in conduction velocity (latency) may have been due to specific damage to slow conducting fibers and the alterations in amplitudes attributable to functional changes in the reticulostriate system. No neuropathological measures or other functional (behavioral) measures were taken in order to confirm these hypotheses.

Mattsson et al. (1981) administered 500 μg/kg per day of methyl mercury chloride to adult beagle dogs. Visual evoked potentials were recorded daily. After 1 week of dosing, subtle alterations in the evoked potential appeared. A parallel group of animals had blood concentrations of 0.74 μg/ml and brain concentrations of 1.28 μg/g in the visual cortex. Following this early change, no further alterations in the evoked potentials were noted, despite continued dosing, until a rapid decline set in at 5–8 weeks of dosing. At this time, severe neurological signs were also present. The authors suggest that during the "silent" phase of intoxication, that is, before overt neurological signs, neurons in the visual cortex may undergo physiological dysfunction rather than irreversible damage. This suggestion would be in agreement with the data of Merigan et al. (1984), who showed total recovery of function following mild intoxication.

Although hearing deficits are among the salient features of methyl mercury intoxication in humans, few animal studies have been addressed to this issue. Falk, Klein, and Haseman (1974) treated guinea pigs with 2 mg/kg of methyl mercury hydroxide five times a week. Four groups of animals were treated either for 1 week, 2 weeks, 4 weeks, or 6 weeks before termination and histological examination. Weight loss and reduced activity after 4 weeks of treatment were the only signs of intoxication. Examination of the auditory system revealed that the treatment had damaged the outer hair cells, with most of the damage occurring at 2.5 turns from the base of the cochlea and at the inner row at 3.5 turns. There seemed to be no damage in the auditory nerve or in the stria vascularis. There also seemed to be no correlation between duration of treatment and extent of damage. The authors concluded that the reported incidence of high frequency hearing loss in human victims of mercury poisoning agreed with the neuropathological findings in their animal model. Central lesions of auditory structures may account for the additional deficits seen in humans, such as inability to comprehend speech.

Anniko and Sarkady (1978) carried out a somewhat similar study, in which guinea pigs were exposed to both acute and chronic treatment with mercury chloride. Although this was not an organic form of the mercury, and therefore the results may not necessarily be comparable to the studies reviewed in this chapter, some of the findings confirm the results of Falk, Klein, and Haseman (1974). Total doses ranged from 10 to 90 mg/kg administered over 1–49 days. Most of the damage seen resulted from the acute treatment and consisted of hair-cell loss in the second and third turns of the cochlea. In addition to these findings, the authors also reported that the chronic treatment resulted in significant damage to the cochlear nerves (demyelination). Whether this latter result can be attributed to the chronic treatment or to the inorganic form of the mercury remains to be resolved.

A novel method for detecting sensory deficits was employed by Wu et al. (1985). Using auditory and electric shock startle stimuli, and using a noise, a silent period, or a cutaneous stimulus as the prestimulus to modulate the startle response, the authors exposed rats to high doses of mercury. The animals were given either 13.3, 40.0, or 50.0 mg/kg of methyl mercury chloride injected over a period of 5 days. These rather toxic doses resulted in weight loss and death in the high-dose animals over a period of weeks.

Animals that had received 50 mg/kg showed a significant reduction in the inhibition of the startle response elicited by the prestimulus. Histological examination of these animals showed the expected damage in peripheral nerves. Animals that had received the two lower doses showed either no effect at the lowest dose, or a significant reduction in startle inhibition by the prestimulus over a period of 7 weeks of testing. Testing of the high-dose animals was terminated at this time because of loss of animals.

While this approach to neurotoxicity testing may offer a rapid method for detecting sensory loss, the extremely high doses of mercury used in this study make it difficult to determine whether more subtle and earlier alterations in function can be detected.

Attempts to relate pathological changes in the peripheral nervous system with electrophysiological alterations have also been made. Somjen, Herman, and Klein (1973) administered either 10 mg/kg of methyl mercury hydroxide daily for 7 days, or 2 mg/kg for 3–4 weeks. The animals were treated until they developed overt neurological signs of intoxication. The conduction velocity of the compound action potential resulting from stimulation of the sciatic nerve was significantly reduced in animals exposed to mercury. There was also a reduction of amplitude. Intracellular recording of sensory ganglion cells showed prolonged and abnormal spikes, indicating a delayed repolarization. The authors concluded that mercury poisoning affects sensory cells first, and this is followed by degeneration of the axons. Using a biochemical approach to the study of mercury intoxication, Cavanagh and Chen (1971) also arrived at this conclusion.

Le Quesne et al. (1974) conducted an electrophysiological study of peripheral nerve status on 19 patients exposed to methyl mercury in Iraq. These subjects had been exposed to the mercury approximately 4 months before the measurements and had a wide range of neurological symptoms. Sensory nerve conduction velocities recorded from the median nerve fell into the normal range. Additional conduction velocity measures were taken from the lateral popliteal nerve, and these were also normal. The authors concluded from the study that despite the severe neurological symptoms, such as abnormal two-point discrimination, defective position sensation, and reduced pain thresholds, the peripheral nerves were functioning normally and the indication was that these alterations were due to central damage. It is interesting to note that while these experimenters found no alteration in vibratory sensitivity, Tsubaki et al. (1977) reported a significant loss in this sensory modality in Minamata victims.

Despite the findings of intact peripheral nerves in humans, most animal models of mercury intoxication using the rat have shown extensive degeneration of peripheral nerves. Thus, Klein et al. (1972), Herman et al. (1973), and Miyakawa et al. (1970) all demonstrated severe peripheral nerve damage following methyl mercury exposure. Because of the discrepancy between rat

Tsubaki, T.; Shirakawa, K.; Hirota, K.; and Kanbayashi, K. (1977). Neurological aspects of methylmercury poisoning in Niigata. In *Minamata Disease,* edited by T. Tsubaki and K. Irukayama, pp. 145–165. New York: Elsevier.

Wu, M. F.; Ison, J. R.; Wecker, J. R.; and Lapham, L. W. (1985). Cutaneous and auditory function in rats following methyl mercury poisoning. *Toxicol Appl Pharmacol* 79:377–388.

EIGHT

Prenatal Exposure to Methyl Mercury

Christine U. Eccles and Zoltan Annau

The research that followed the major outbreaks of methyl mercury poisoning in Japan and Iraq constitutes classic studies in environmental toxicology. Clinical and experimental studies have provided what may be the best documentation of the particular sensitivity of the developing organism to the effects of organic mercury (see review by Chang and Annau 1984). Information on dose-response relationships, body burdens, and excretion rates has come from studies on the Iraqi population exposed to methyl mercury (Bakir et al. 1973; Marsh et al. 1980). Studies in Japan, on the other hand, have yielded important documentation of the neuropathology associated with exposure to methyl mercury (Takeuchi and Eto 1977).

The important neurological features of "congenital" or "fetal" Minamata disease can be distinguished from the adult form of the disease in several ways. First, the neuropathology seen in the congenital cases is more widely distributed and diffuse than the localized lesions of the calcarine and precentral cortical areas described for the adult form. In the cerebellum, the Purkinje cells and the molecular layer, as well as the granule cell layer, reveal severe degeneration equally distributed throughout the cerebellar hemispheres and the vermis (Matsumoto et al. 1964). Generally, the degree of atrophy present is more severe than in the adult form. Evidence of malformation and lack of development has also been reported. Examples of these types of changes are abnormal architecture of cells in the cerebrum and cerebellum, poorly myelinated areas, hypoplasia of the corpus callosum, and the presence of matrix cells lining the ventricular walls. These neuropathological findings are reflected by the grossly abnormal neurological and behavioral development of these victims. Initial signs of toxicity became apparent in infants several weeks to months after birth (Harada 1977). The earliest signs were delayed movement, failure to follow visual stimuli, uncoordinated suckling and swallowing, and convulsions. As victims grew older, primitive reflexes remained and flaccid or spastic paralysis developed. Indicators of normal motor development, such as grasping, crawling, standing, and walking, were either delayed or never achieved. Prenatal exposure to methyl mercury also resulted in severe mental deficiency and retardation in 100 percent of the patients diagnosed. This was not characteristic of the adult syndrome found in Minamata Bay, or that described earlier by Hunter and Russell (1954).

Japanese investigators have also described a third subgroup of patients that had been exposed to methyl mercury during early childhood (Takeuchi et al.

1979). Like those seen after in utero exposure, the clinical symptoms observed in this group are more severe than those observed in adults and include muscular rigidity, ankle clonus, pathological reflexes, blindness, deafness, and convulsions. The complete loss of motor and mental functions, or decortication syndrome, is correlated with severe and widespread lesions of the cerebral cortex similar to those described for fetal Minamata disease. Neuronal loss in excess of 50 percent has been found over widespread areas of the cerebral cortex.

Placental Transfer

The human neuropathology and behavioral alterations seen in both Japan and Iraq raised considerable interest in defining the kinetics of absorption, distribution, and excretion and in dose-response relationships of methyl mercury intoxication. One of the most interesting findings at Minamata was that asymptomatic mothers gave birth to children with severe irreversible mental retardation. Some of the first experimental inquiries addressed the issue of placental transfer and maternal/fetal concentration ratios.

Experimental studies on placental transfer of methyl mercury and its distribution in the fetus have contributed to our understanding of in utero methyl mercury poisoning. Relative relationships between maternal and fetal tissue levels of mercury measured in experimental animals are similar to those observed in humans. The extent to which accumulation will occur depends on the amount given to the mother, quantitative rates of transfer to and from the fetus, the period of gestation in which it is administered, and the length of time between administration and analysis of the tissue sample (Mirkin 1976).

Placental transfer and fetal accumulation of methyl mercury has been documented in the rat (Yang et al. 1972; Null et al. 1973; Wannag 1976), mouse (Olson and Massaro 1977; Berlin and Ulberg 1963), guinea pig (Kelman and Sasser 1977), and macaque monkey (Reynolds and Pitkin 1975). Reynolds and Pitkin showed that in the monkey the placenta partially impedes the passage of methyl mercury from mother to fetus. When methyl mercury was injected into the maternal circulation, the maternal-fetal blood mercury ratio was about 10 : 1 for the first 5 hours after administration. Conversely, fetal administration of methyl mercury yielded a fetal-maternal blood mercury ratio of 25 : 1, indicating that movement of methyl mercury from fetus to mother occurred less readily than movement in the opposite direction. The authors suggest that this may account for the increased danger to the fetus during chronic exposure.

The quantity of methyl mercury transferred between mother and fetus depends on the developmental stage of the placenta. As the placenta matures, the depth of tissue layers interposed between the fetal capillaries and the maternal blood supply varies. In the rodent placenta, the relative permeability of the placenta to the drug phenytoin, for example, is biphasic. Transfer of the drug is maximum in early and late stages and is reduced during mid-gestation (Stevens and Harbison 1974). A similar phenomenon has been observed after administration of methyl mercury. Olson and Massaro (1977) administered a single dose of methyl mercury (5 mg/kg) to pregnant mice on day 7, 10, 11, 12, or 13 of gestation. They measured fetal mercury concentration increasing in proportion to maternal blood levels as methyl mercury was given at later gestational stages. Peak fetal mercury concentrations were reached 3 days after administration. Increased fetal sequestration of methyl mercury during the later stages of gestation was associated with but not known to be dependent on an increase in maternal liver net elimination rate.

Olson and Massaro also contrasted in utero exposure and suckling exposure by cross-fostering. Several litters of pups that received methyl mercury in utero were reared by saline-treated mothers. Much more of the methyl mercury was derived from prenatal exposure than from postnatal exposure. The tissue levels of mercury on postpartum day 10 in the offspring of methyl mercury treated mothers cross-fostered to saline-treated mothers were between 15 and 30 times higher than those in the conversely cross-fostered offspring.

Fetal brain levels were measured after administration of methyl mercury to pregnant rats and were found to be approximately twice as high as maternal brain levels (Yang et al. 1972; Null et al. 1973). Brain levels of mercury in nonpregnant female rats were measured and were found to be 1.1–1.4 times higher than those measured in pregnant females (Null et al. 1973). The reason for this difference is unknown, but the authors suggest that it may be induced by hormonal changes of pregnancy. An alternative hypothesis is that the fetus may act as a "sink" sequestering the mercury away from the mother. Recent reviews have referred to the possibility that the pregnant female may be relatively resistant to methyl mercury toxicity (Shimai and Satoh 1985; Junghans 1983).

The prenatally or postnatally exposed neonate may be at additional risk due to prolonged retention of mercury. This effect has been noted experimentally in mice and rats and probably occurs in humans (Amin-Zaki et al. 1979; Choi et al. 1978; Thomas et al. 1982). The immaturity of the glutathione-dependent biliary excretion system seems to be responsible for the neonate's inability to excrete methyl mercury (Thomas et al. 1982).

Nonneural Effects

The accumulation of methyl mercury in fetal organs can lead to various teratogenic or embryocidal effects. The degree to which these effects are manifested depends on the species and strain of the animal tested, the size and number of doses administered, and the time of gestation in which exposure occurs.

One of the most commonly observed effects of prenatal exposure to methyl mercury is intrauterine death, usually revealed by fetal resorption or stillbirth. High rates of fetal mortality are produced when methyl mercury is administered during the period of organogenesis. In rodents, this sensitive period is generally the second week of gestation. In the golden hamster, about half the fetuses were resorbed after a single 8 mg/kg dose of methyl mercury was given on gestational day 5, 8, or 9 (Harris et al. 1972). Administration of an 8 mg/kg dose of methyl mercury on day 8 of gestation produced a markedly reduced rate of weight gain, which was associated with a 50 percent resorption rate (Eccles and Annau 1982*a*). A lower dose of methyl mercury (5 mg/kg) did not alter normal maternal weight gain and did not result in an increased rate of resorption.

Differences among strains of a species were reported by Spyker and Smithberg (1972) and Su and Okita (1976). Spyker and Smithberg treated mouse strains 129/SvSl and A/J with 0, 2, 4, or 8 mg/kg of methyl mercury on one of days 6–12 of gestation. They found that the resorption rate was dependent on strain, dose, and day of treatment. Mice of the 129/SvSl strain were more susceptible to the embryocidal effects of methyl mercury than A/J mice. The resorption rate in strain 129/SvSl was between 80 and 100 percent when the highest dose, 8 mg/kg, was given to the mother on one of days 9–13. When methyl mercury was given on day 6, 7, or 8, the rate of resorption was only 12 percent. Inversely, strain A/J showed a marked increase in congenital defects without a significant increase in resorptions on any of the treatment days.

Su and Okita (1976) also observed strain specificity with respect to the embryolethal effects of methyl mercury. In their study, the CD strain of mouse was apparently less sensitive to fetotoxic effects than the C57BL/6J or 129/SvSl strain. In the C57BL/6J mice, 57 percent of the fetuses were resorbed when pregnant mice were given 8 mg/kg on day 10 of gestation. The incidence of resorption in 129/SvSl mice increased when 12 mg/kg was administered on day 10. In this case, 33 percent of the total number of fetuses were resorbed and all the litters in this group contained resorbed fetuses. Teratogenic effects were found in all strains tested, but procedural inconsistencies (e.g., variations in route of exposure and dose) preclude drawing further conclusions regarding strain specificity from these data.

Congenital defects that have been reported following methyl mercury exposure include cleft palate, clubfoot, hydrocephaly, and eye and brain defects (Spyker and Smithberg 1971; Harris et al. 1972; Su and Okita 1976). These malformations are most likely to occur when treatment takes place during the period of organogenesis. In mice, various forms of cleft palate predominate (Spyker and Smithberg 1971; Su and Okita 1976), while clubfoot is the most frequently occurring malformation reported in hamsters (Harris et al. 1972). Su and Okita (1976) observed a remarkable 97 percent incidence of cleft palate in fetuses whose mothers received daily 5 mg/kg doses on days 7–12 of gestation, demonstrating that multiple doses may produce a more dramatic effect than a single large dose.

Although the fetal liver and kidney accumulate methyl mercury to a great extent, damage to these organs is not necessarily expected, in view of the relative insensitivity of the adult liver and kidney to the effects of alkyl mercury. Ware et al. (1974) found a consistent pattern of liver injury in neonatal rat pups treated with 2, 3, or 4 mg/kg on day 9 of gestation. The extent and severity of damage depended on the dose. Under light microscopy, vacuolation, an increase in lysosomal profiles, and some cellular necrosis appeared in the hepatocytes. Mitochondrial degeneration, dilatation of the endoplasmic reticulum, and extrusion of hepatocyte cytoplasm were seen in electron micrographs. Fowler and Woods (1977) observed morphological and functional aberrations in the neonatal rat liver after prenatal exposure to methyl mercury throughout gestation. A single 4 mg/kg dose on day 8 of pregnancy resulted in degenerative changes in the proximal convoluted tubule, and hyperplasia in the distal convoluted tubule, of the neonatal rat kidney (Chang and Sprecher 1976). A thickening of the epithelial lining and a higher mitotic index were found in the distal tubules of pups treated with methyl mercury. Although generally considered a mitotic inhibitor, mercury has been reported to stimulate cell growth and proliferation under certain conditions (Chang et al. 1976). Hyperplastic changes have not been observed in the renal tubules of adult animals after mercury exposure, suggesting that immature cells may be more sensitive to stimulation than adult cells.

An unusual type of functional teratogenesis induced by methyl mercury was reported by Robbins et al. (1978). This group measured a delayed depression in cytochrome-P450-dependent enzyme systems in the livers of adult male rats that had been exposed prenatally to methyl mercury on day 0 or day 7 of gestation. The effect was not apparent until the animals were 6 months old. Decreased cytochrome P450 levels were not observed in microsomes obtained from immature males or females or from rats treated on day 14 of gestation. This study suggests that appearance of functional teratogenesis may be delayed and that the stage of development in which exposure occurs may be critical.

The Effects of Methyl Mercury on the Developing Nervous System

Because of the predominantly neurological defects observed in humans after prenatal and neonatal exposure to methyl mercury, much of experimental animal research in this area has been directed toward the developing nervous system. In contrast to other organ systems, the mammalian central nervous system continues to undergo rapid development throughout late gestation and the neonatal period. The series of events that occur parallel to development of the central nervous system are very similar from species to species. The major difference is the extent of maturation of the brain at the time of birth. The brains of most species are morphologically and functionally immature at birth and increase in size and complexity during the postnatal period (Mirkin 1976).

Four major periods of development proceed more or less sequentially in all areas of the brain (Jacobson 1978). The first period is one of intense cell proliferation and migration. Rapidly dividing cells and migrating cells are particularly susceptible to the destructive effects of radiation, viruses, and cytotoxic chemicals. Growth of the nucleus, cell body, axons, and dendrites occurs during the second period, in a process that is directional and specific and indicative of differentiation. This is followed by synaptogenesis, during which period neural connections are established. Manipulation of the environment of developing dendrites may be another mechanism by which chemicals can alter neural function. Finally, there is the period of glial cell growth, an event associated with the development of the blood-brain barrier. Exposure to methyl mercury may interfere with any of these stages of brain development and result in early behavioral abnormalities as well as long-term deficits. Whether any of these processes are specifically affected by methyl mercury has been addressed in only a few experimental studies (Sager et al. 1982; Rodier et al. 1984). Early postnatal exposure to methyl mercury in the mouse, for example, produced mitotic arrest at 24 hours after dosing, as reflected by a decrease in the percentage of late mitotic figures in the cerebellum and no change in total mitotic figures (Sager et al. 1982). More recently, the same group has demonstrated a similar but less marked effect after treatment on day 12 of gestation in the developing hippocampus and cortex. An interesting difference in the results of these two studies is that later treatment (postnatal day 2) was associated with cell loss over the 48-hour exposure period, and the earlier treatment was not.

Prenatal exposure to methyl mercury in the cat characteristically results in incomplete granular cell layer formation in the cerebellum as well as abnormal cytoarchitecture in cerebral neurons (Khera 1973). Methyl mercury given to kittens during the postnatal period of brain development produced degenerative changes in the internal granule cell layer, some loss of Purkinje cells, and abnormal myelination (Khera et al. 1974). In mice, Khera and Tabacova (1973) observed a delayed migration of the external granule cell layer after a dose of 1 mg/kg per day on gestational days 6–17. There were fewer cells in the external granule layer, and the molecular layer was poorly defined.

Ultrastructural changes in the brains of rats and mice fed low doses of methyl mercury prenatally were reported by Chang et al. (1977; see Chapter 5, by Chang, in this volume). Accumulations of lysosome-like dense bodies were observed in the Purkinje cells and granule cells. The rough endoplasmic

Table 8.1   Neuropathology produced by developmental exposure to methyl mercury

Exposure	Species	Effect Reported	Reference
Prenatal	Rat, mouse	Ultrastructural changes in Purkinje and granule cells of cerebellum; disturbed myelin formation.	Chang et al. 1977 Reuhl and Chang 1979
Prenatal	Mouse	Delayed migration of external granule cell layer.	Khera and Tabacova 1973
Postnatal	Cat	Degenerative changes in internal granule cell layer; loss of Purkinje cells; abnormal myelination.	Khera et al. 1974
Prenatal	Cat	Incomplete granular layer in cerebellum; abnormal cytoarchitecture in cerebrum.	Khera 1973
Prenatal	Mouse	Mitotic arrest in hippocampus and cortex.	Rodier et al. 1984
Postnatal	Mouse	Mitotic arrest in cerebellum.	Sager et al. 1982

reticulum in Purkinje cells was abnormal, and axons frequently displayed incomplete myelination. Disturbed myelin formation and degenerating axons are among the toxic changes that persisted in adult animals (Reuhl and Chang 1979).

The neuropathological studies, when considered together, suggest that methyl mercury produces two types of effects in the developing nervous system (see Table 8.1). One is on specific developmental processes (i.e., cell mitosis and migration); the other is a toxic degenerative effect resulting in cell death or structural damage. The time-dependency and dose-dependency of these effects and their relative importance to long-term consequences of developmental exposure need further investigation.

Although several neuropathological changes occur with overt methyl mercury intoxication, biochemical, neurophysiological, and behavioral changes may occur at low dose levels in the absence of histopathology or marked physical debilitation. Many of the biochemical consequences of exposure to methyl mercury during gestation or the neonatal period are reviewed in other chapters in this book (Chapter 9, by Thomas and Syversen, and Chapter 10, by Komulainen and Tuomisto).

The electrophysiological consequences of prenatal exposure to methyl mercury have been examined in a study employing the visual evoked potential as a measure of the central nervous system's functional status. Peak-to-peak latencies of the early components were decreased in rats exposed to methyl mercury throughout gestation (Zenick 1976). Dyer et al. (1978) administered a single dose of 0 or 5 mg/kg of methyl mercury to pregnant rats on day 7 of gestation and recorded the flash-evoked potential in unanesthetized adult female offspring. In partial agreement with work by Zenick, latencies of several of the components of the evoked potential were shorter in

Table 8.2   Behavioral effects of developmental exposure to methyl mercury

Exposure	Species	Effect Reported	Reference
Prenatal	Mouse	Abnormal swimming behavior.	Spyker et al. 1972
Prenatal	Mouse	Decreased locomotor activity.	Su and Okita 1976
Prenatal	Mouse	Decreased latency to onset of flurothyl-induced seizures.	Su and Okita 1976
Prenatal	Rat	Increased susceptibility to audiogenic seizures.	Menashi et al. 1982
Prenatal	Mouse	Impaired acquisition of two-way active avoidance; impaired retention of passive avoidance task; no motor impairment.	Hughes and Annau 1976
Prenatal	Rat	More errors in a water escape T-maze; no motor impairment.	Zenick 1974
Prenatal	Rat	Impaired acquisition and reacquisition of two-way active avoidance; no motor impairment.	Eccles and Annau 1982*b*
Prenatal	Rat	Impaired learning in two-way active avoidance.	Tanimura et al. 1981
Prenatal	Rat	Fewer avoidances and escapes in a lever press active avoidance task; fewer responses during acquisition period of continuous reinforcement task.	Schalock et al. 1981
Prenatal	Rat	Altered response to *d*-amphetamine.	Hughes and Sparber 1978
Prenatal	Rat	Altered response to *d*-amphetamine.	Eccles and Annau 1982*b*
Prenatal	Rat	Earlier eye-opening; enhanced clinging ability.	Sobotka et al. 1974
Prenatal	Rat	Increased activity levels in neonates.	Eccles and Annau 1982*a*
Prenatal	Rat	Apomorphine-induced stereotypy in 15-day-old pups.	Cuomo et al. 1984

the rats exposed to mercury. One possible explanation for this is that shorter latencies may be the result of selective destruction of small neurons with slow conduction velocities. This hypothesis is supported by neuropathological studies demonstrating selective loss of small neurons after exposure to methyl mercury (Chang et al. 1977; Carmichael et al. 1975). Peak-to-peak amplitudes were increased in early components of the evoked potential in animals exposed to methyl mercury. The visual system is clearly sensitive to perturbation by methyl mercury administered during development. Unfortunately, studies of critical periods and dose-dependency of these effects have not been reported.

Behavioral abnormalities occur after developmental exposure to methyl mercury. Although this area of research is relatively unexplored in clinical situations, its potential has been demonstrated in animal models (see Table 8.2). Spyker, Sparber, and Goldberg (1972) demonstrated that obvious neurological impairment is not necessary in order to detect effects induced by methyl mercury. In their study, 129/SvSl mice treated with 3.2 mg/kg of methyl mercury dicyandiamide on day 7 or 9 of gestation were not different from controls with respect to brain weight, protein content, choline acetyltransferase, or cholinesterase. But differences were detected in some parameters of open field activity and swimming behavior. Methyl mercury treated mice remained in the center square of an open field longer than controls and took more steps in a backward direction during the test session. In the swimming test, more than half the treated mice showed intermittent periods of apparent neuromuscular incoordination, floating in a vertical position and swimming with excessive movement. The deviant swimming behaviors were interpreted as "signs of neuromuscular impairment." The possibility that the abnormal responses may have been a reflection of a failure to habituate to a novel situation or maladaptive responses to stress was not considered. Mottet (1974), using rats, did not report differences in swimming behavior between methyl mercury treated groups and controls.

Su and Okita (1976) administered 0, 6, 8, or 12 mg/kg of methyl mercury to 129/SvSl mice and observed behavioral changes in the offspring of treated mothers. In the open field test, 23-day-old and 33-day-old treated offspring took longer to leave the center square, and at the highest dose they traversed a fewer number of peripheral squares. Measurements of spontaneous locomotor activity at 24, 44, and 64 days of age revealed significantly lower locomotor activity in the 8 mg/kg and 12 mg/kg groups at 24 days. Only in the 12 mg/kg group was this effect still present at 64 days.

Su and Okita's study also investigated convulsive behavior induced by flurothyl inhalation. A decreased latency to onset of maximal clonic-tonic convulsion and decreased latency to death as a result of the convulsion were measured in the treated mice when compared with controls. However, fewer mercury-treated mice displayed an earlier stage of convulsion—the preliminary clonic convulsion. A study by Menashi et al. (1982) also reported increased susceptibility to audiogenic seizures induced by a bell in rats exposed to methyl mercury on day 8 of gestation. Since flurothyl inhalation and audiogenic seizure induction do not allow adequate stimulus control, definite statements regarding seizure susceptibility of rats treated with methyl mercury cannot be made.

Hughes and Annau (1976) administered doses of methyl mercury ranging from 0 to 10 mg/kg to CFW mice on day 8 of gestation and tested the offspring in five different behavioral paradigms (open field, two-way active avoidance, passive avoidance, conditioned suppression, and water escape). A cross-fostering procedure was employed in some treatment groups to test whether the deficits present were due mainly to prenatal exposure or to postnatal exposure via suckling. Results indicated that the major effects observed were due to in utero exposure of the mice. This finding is expected based on studies of methyl mercury distribution in cross-fostered mice (Olson and Massaro 1977). In contrast to other studies (Su and Okita 1976), how-ever, the study of Hughes and Annau failed to demonstrate a motor impair-ment in treated mice, as indicated by movement in an open field, by time to enter a compartment with a water spigot, or by measurements of escape latencies in a water escape test and the two-way avoidance task.

The behavioral effects of prenatal exposure to methyl mercury are seen most consistently in tests of learning—specifically, active avoidance and passive avoidance tasks. Offspring of mice receiving 3 and 5 mg/kg required more trials to reach a criterion of 10 consecutive avoidances from shock in a two-way avoidance task (Hughes and Annau 1976). In the passive avoidance task, control and treated groups learned to avoid shock at a similar rate, but treated groups demonstrated impaired retention when retested after the shock circuit was deactivated. The results indicated that the animals treated with methyl mercury displayed a cognitive deficit rather than a motor impairment.

Similar results have been reported by others. Zenick (1974), for example, found that rats exposed prenatally made more errors in a water escape T-maze, but that there were no differences in swimming ability, as shown by similar values obtained for escape latencies in the control and treated groups. In a more recent study by Eccles and Annau (1982*b*), Long-Evans hooded rats displayed a marked deficit in two-way shuttle box avoidance acquisition and reacquisition after treatment with methyl mercury on day 15 of gestation. In the rats treated on day 8 of gestation, a small but significant deficit was observed only in the reacquisition phase of testing. Parameters that might reveal a motor deficit in these animals, such as escape latencies and intertrial crossings, were not different from controls for either treatment day.

In an avoidance task in which rats were required to press a lever to avoid or escape shock, the group exposed to 10 mg/kg of methyl mercury on day 4 of gestation took longer to reach the avoidance criterion, emitted fewer avoidance responses, and made fewer escape responses (Schalock et al. 1981). Similarly, in a test of appetitive learning (continuous reinforcement) this group made fewer responses during acquisition, more responses during extinction, and fewer responses during reacquisition. Although impaired per-formance was exhibited by animals exposed to methyl mercury in both tests, this group, in contrast to the studies described above, displayed decreased activity levels, compared with controls.

In cases of low-level mercury exposure where the behavioral effects of methyl mercury may not be overtly discernible, the administration of psycho-tropic drugs with known behavioral effects has proven useful as a testing tool. Several studies have shown that animals treated with methyl mercury do not display the same responses as control animals to drugs that disrupt cate-cholamine function (Hughes and Sparber 1978; Eccles and Annau, 1982*b;* Cuomo et al. 1984). This differential sensitivity to catecholaminergic drugs might be expected, considering the long-lasting effects on catecholamine neurotransmitter systems that have been reported after perinatal exposure to methyl mercury (Taylor and DiStefano 1976; Bartolome et al. 1984). Motor activity measures revealed shifts in the dose-response curve for d-amphetamine after treatment with methyl mercury (8 mg/kg) on day 8 of gestation. In a study that employed the same dose and day of methyl mercury treatment (Cuomo et al. 1984), apomorphine-induced stereotypy was elicited in 15-day-old methyl mercury exposed pups. Control pups did not exhibit stereotypical responses to the drug until 22 days of age. At 22 days of age, however, pups exposed to methyl mercury demonstrated an enhanced response to apomorphine, as compared with control animals. These behavioral effects were paralleled by neurochemical data indicating that the number of ^{3}H-spiroperidol binding sites was significantly increased in rats pretreated with methyl mercury at 22 days of age. However, an increase in binding sites was not detected in 15-day-old treated pups.

A small number of investigators have examined neonatal behaviors after prenatal exposure. In addition to finding neurochemical changes, Sobotka et al. (1974) reported altered patterns of behavioral development. Treated pups were free from overt signs of toxicity, although body weights were slightly reduced at the highest dose. Rather than delayed development, these investigators observed earlier eye-opening and a transient period of enhanced clinging ability. Results were interpreted as reflections of compressed development of the central nervous system. A shortened time period for brain development may permanently affect behavioral flexibility and the behavioral repertoire of the adult organism (Schapiro 1968). These findings leave open the possibility that methyl mercury could interact with the neonatal endocrine system, thereby critically influencing brain maturation.

Neonatal activity measurements taken over the course of the preweaning period reflect the functional development of the brain. To some degree, ontogenetic changes in locomotor activity reflect different rates of maturation of several neurotransmitter systems (Campbell and Mabry 1973; Campbell et al. 1969; Murphy et al. 1979). Neonatal locomotor behavior has been used as a sensitive indicator of developmental exposure to methyl mercury (Eccles and Annau 1982a). A dose of 5 mg/kg on day 8 of gestation produced an elevation in activity on postnatal day 4, whereas 8 mg/kg on the same treatment day elevated activity on postnatal day 8. Treatment with methyl mercury later in gestation (i.e., day 15) resulted in increased activity levels on postnatal days 8 and 15. These results could be explained by increased levels of catecholaminergic function or decreased function of transmitters that mediate behavioral inhibition.

An unusual test of neonatal behavior has been explored by Adams et al. (1983). Ultrasonic vocalization patterns of rat pups treated prenatally with methyl mercury on gestation day 7 were recorded on postnatal days 7, 9, and 11. Effects of methyl mercury were not detected, but data analysis revealed significant effects of age and test condition (clean bedding vs. home cage bedding). Although no treatment effects were obtained, this study provides useful information regarding variables that must be considered when applying this method.

Time and duration of treatment play an important role in determining the nature of the effects observed. Treatment early in gestation is associated with a high rate of fetal mortality and gross teratology. Exposure later in gestation is manifested by neurological and/or behavioral effects. Eccles and Annau have shown that the nature and degree of behavioral effects observed also vary with the day of gestation in which methyl mercury is administered (Eccles and Annau 1982*a*, 1982*b*). Chemicals that can specifically interfere with proliferating cell systems (e.g., azacytidine, methazoxymethanol) have also been used to demonstrate that disruption of brain development at critical time periods can produce distinct behavioral profiles that may be correlated with time of treatment (Kabat et al. 1985; Rodier et al. 1979). Administration of methazoxymethanol on day 15 of gestation produces a relatively specific loss of cerebral interneurons in layers II–IV (Johnston and Coyle 1980). This loss is reflected by a deficiency in GABAergic markers such as glutamic acid decarboxylase (GAD) (Johnston and Coyle 1980). A study by O'Kusky and McGeer (1985) has recently shown that postnatal administration of methyl mercury to rats also produces a selective decrease in GAD activity in the cerebral cortex and neostriatum. These neurochemical changes were accompanied by relatively severe neurological impairment consisting of visual disturbances, hypertonia, anteroflexion of the head and neck, and hyperreflexia. Morphological changes include degeneration of GABAergic stellate neurons in layer IV of the visual cortex. High doses of methyl mercury (5 mg/kg per day) were used to produce these effects, but the data suggest that some aspects of methyl mercury toxicity may be mimicked by a lesion produced by an antimitotic and that a cerebral-palsy-like syndrome similar to that observed in humans may be produced by methyl mercury in a rat model.

Results from the collection of studies reviewed above are difficult to pull together in a general discussion of common findings and conclusions. The experiments have been performed over a relatively long period of time and represent a wide variety of animal models and test methods. Selection of appropriate animal models for examining methyl mercury's effects on the developing nervous system is an important issue that has not been adequately addressed. The developmental period in which treatment occurs is an important variable when considering an agent like methyl mercury. Differences in age of exposure in humans clearly lead to differences in the neuropathology produced. The rat brain undergoes rapid development in the second and third weeks of gestation and in the first two postnatal weeks. In these periods, methyl mercury can exert damaging effects on developing structures, or degenerative effects on cell groups already formed. A hypothesis often stated but not tested is that developing neurons may be differentially sensitive to exposure to methyl mercury. The question of whether regional vulnerabilities exist in the developing nervous system goes a step further and remains to be answered.

Despite the unresolved questions, the human episodes of methyl mercury intoxication, as well as the experimental animal literature, clearly indicate that doses of methyl mercury that are not toxic to the mother can produce significant damage to the central nervous system of offspring. This damage in animal models is most readily seen in the developing motor systems in the early postnatal period and in cognitive functions in the adult organism. The use of pharmacological challenges has also revealed subtle alterations in nervous system function that cannot be readily detected. In experimental studies, these methods continue to be useful as means of addressing mechanistic questions in the intact animal. Furthermore, such tests have not yet been applied in human situations, where they may be useful as probes in uncovering cases of subclinical neurotoxicity.

References

Adams, J.; Miller, D. R.; and Nelson, C. J. (1983). Ultrasonic vocalizations as diagnostic tools in studies of developmental toxicity: An investigation of the effects of prenatal treatment with methylmercuric chloride. *Neurobehav Toxicol Teratol* 5:29–34.

Amin-Zaki, L.; Elhassani, S.; Majeed, M. A.; Clarkson, T. W.; Doherty, R. A.; and Greenwood, M. (1974). Intra-uterine methylmercury poisoning in Iraq. *Pediatrics* 54:587–595.

Amin-Zaki, L.; Elhassani, S.; Majeed, M. A.; Clarkson, T. W.; Doherty, R. A.; Greenwood, M. R.; and Giovanoli-Jakubezak, T. (1976). Perinatal methylmercury poisoning in Iraq. *Am J Dis Child* 130:1070–1076.

Amin-Zaki, L.; Majeed, M. A.; Elhassani, S. B.; Clarkson, T. W.; Greenwood, M. R.; and Doherty, R. A. (1979). Prenatal methyl-mercury poisoning. *Am J Dis Child* 133:172–177.

Bakir, F.; Damluji, S. F.; Amin-Zaki, L.; Murtadha, M.; Khalidi, A.; Al-Rawi, N. Y.; Tikriti, S.; Dhahir, H. I.; Clarkson, T. W.; Smith, J. C.; and Doherty, R. A. (1973). Methyl mercury poisoning in Iraq. *Science* 181:230–241.

Bartolome, J.; Whitmore, W. L.; Seidler, F. J.; and Slotkin, T. (1984). Exposure to methyl mercury in utero: Effects on biochemical development of catecholamine neurotransmitter systems. *Life Sci* 35:657–670.

Berlin, M., and Ulberg, S. (1963). Accumulation and retention of mercury in the mouse. *Arch Env Health* 6:610–616.

Campbell, B. A.; Lytle, L. D.; and Fibiger, H. C. (1969). Ontogeny of adrenergic arousal and cholinergic inhibitory mechanisms in the rat. *Science* 166:635–637.

Campbell, B. A., and Mabry, P. D. (1973). The role of catecholamines in behavioral arousal during ontogenesis. *Psychopharmacologia* 31:253–264.

Carmichael, N.; Cavanagh, J. B.; and Rodda, R. A. (1975). Some effects of methyl mercury salts on the rabbit nervous system. *Acta Neuropath* 32:115–125.

Chang, L. W., and Annau, Z. (1984). Developmental neuropathology and behavioral teratology of methyl mercury. In *Neurobehavioral Teratology,* edited by J. Yanai, pp. 405–432. Amsterdam: Elsevier.

Chang, L. W.; Mak, L. L. M.; and Martin, A. H. (1976). Effects of methyl mercury on limb-regeneration of newts. *Environ Res* 11:305–309.

Chang, L. W.; Reuhl, K. R.; and Spyker, J. M. (1977). Ultrastructural study of the latent effects of methyl mercury on the nervous system after prenatal exposure. *Environ Res* 13:171–185.

Chang, L. W., and Sprecher, J. A. (1976). Degenerative changes in the neonatal kidney following in utero exposure of methyl mercury. *Environ Res* 11:392–406.

Choi, B. H.; Lapham, L. W.; Amin-Zaki, L.; and Saleem, T. (1978). Abnormal neuronal migration, deranged cerebral cortical organization, and diffuse white matter astrocytosis of human fetal brain: A major effect of methylmercury poisoning in utero. *J Neuropathol Exp Neurol* 37:719–733.

Cuomo, V.; Ambrosi, L.; Annau, Z.; Cagiano, R.; Brunello, N.; and Racagni, G. (1984). Behavioral and neurochemical changes in offspring of rats exposed to methyl mercury during gestation. *Neurobehav Toxicol Teratol* 6:249–254.

Dyer, R. S.; Eccles, C. U.; and Annau, Z. (1978). Evoked potential alterations following prenatal methyl mercury exposure. *Pharmacol Biochem Behav* 8:137–141.

Eccles, C. U., and Annau, Z. (1982a). Prenatal methyl mercury exposure, I: Alterations in neonatal activity. *Neurobehav Toxicol Teratol* 4:371–376.

—— (1982b). Prenatal methyl mercury exposure, II: Alterations in learning and psychotropic drug sensitivity in adult offspring. *Neurobehav Toxicol Teratol* 4:377–382.

Fowler, B. A., and Woods, J. S. (1977). The transplacental toxicity of methyl mercury to fetal rat liver mitochondria: Morphometric and biochemical studies. *Lab Invest* 36:122–130.

Harada, Y. (1977). Congenital Minamata disease. In *Minamata Disease: Methyl Mercury Poisoning in Minamata and Niigata, Japan,* edited by T. Tsubaki and K. Irukayama. New York: Elsevier.

Harris, S. B.; Wilson, J. G.; and Printz, R. H. (1972). Embryotoxicity of methyl mercury chloride in golden hamsters. *Teratology* 6:139–142.

Hughes, J. A., and Annau, Z. (1976). Postnatal behavioral effects in mice after prenatal exposure to methyl mercury. *Pharmacol Biochem Behav* 4:385–391.

Hughes, J. A., and Sparber, S. B. (1978). *d*-Amphetamine unmasks postnatal consequences of exposure to methyl mercury in utero: Methods for studying behavioral teratogenesis. *Pharmacol Biochem Behav* 8:365–375.

Hunter, D., and Russell, D. S. (1954). Focal cerebral and cerebellar atrophy in a human subject due to organic mercury compounds. *J Neurol Neurosurg Psychiat* 17:235–241.

Jacobs, J. M.; Carmichael, N.; and Cavanagh, J. B. (1977). Ultrastructural changes in the nervous system of rabbits poisoned with methyl mercury. *Toxicol Appl Pharmacol* 39:249–261.

Jacobson, M. (1978). *Developmental Neurobiology,* pp. 58–60. New York: Plenum.

Johnston, M. V., and Coyle, J. T. (1980). Ontogeny of neurochemical markers for noradrenergic, GABAergic, and cholinergic neurons in neocortex lesioned with methylazoxymethanol acetate. *J Neurochem* 34:1429–1441.

Junghans, R. P. (1983). A review of toxicity of methyl mercury compounds with application to occupational exposure associated with laboratory uses. *Environ Res* 31:1–31.

Kabat, K.; Buterbaugh, G. G.; and Eccles, C. U. (1985). Methylazoxymethanol as a developmental model of neurotoxicity. *Neurobehav Toxicol Teratol* 7:519–525.

Kelman, B. J., and Sasser, L. B. (1977). Methylmercury movements across the perfused guinea pig placenta in late gestation. *Toxicol Appl Pharm* 39:119–127.

Khera, K. S. (1973). Teratogenic effects of methyl mercury in the cat: Note on the use of this species as a model for teratogenicity studies. *Teratology* 8:293–303.

Khera, K. S.; Iverson, F.; Hierlihy, L.; Tanner, R.; and Trivett, G. (1974). Toxicity of methyl mercury in neonatal cats. *Teratology* 10:69–76.

Khera, K. S., and Tabacova, S. A. (1973). Effects of methylmercuric chloride on the progeny of mice and rats treated before or during gestation. *Fd Cosmet Toxicol* 11:243–254.

Marsh, D. O.; Myers, G. J.; Clarkson, T. W.; Amin-Zaki, L.; Tikriti, S.; and Majeed, M. A. (1980). Fetal methylmercury poisoning: Clinical and toxicological data on 29 cases. *Ann Neurol* 7:348–353.

Matsumoto, E.; Koya, G.; and Takeuchi, T. (1964). Fetal Minamata disease: A neuropathological study of two cases of intrauterine intoxication by a methyl mercury compound. *J. Neuropathol Exp Neurolog* 24:563–574.

Menashi, M.; Ornoy, A.; and Yanai, J. (1982). Transplacental effects of methyl mercury chloride in mice with specific emphasis on audiogenic seizure response. *Dev Neurosci* 5:216–221.

Mirkin, B. L. (1976). *Perinatal Pharmacology and Therapeutics.* New York: Academic Press.

Mottet, N. K. (1974). Effects of chronic low-dose exposure of rat fetuses to methylmercury hydroxide. *Teratology* 10:173–190.

Murphy, J. M.; Meeker, R. B.; Porada, K. J.; and Nagy, Z. M. (1979). GABA-mediated behavioral inhibition during ontogeny in the mouse. *Psychopharmacology* 64:237–242.

Null, D. H.; Gartside, P. S.; and Wei, E. (1973). Methyl mercury accumulation in brains of pregnant, non-pregnant, and fetal rats. *Life Sci* 12(2):65–72.

O'Kusky, J., and McGeer, E. G. (1985). Methyl mercury poisoning of the developing nervous system in the rat: Decreased activity of glutamic acid decarboxylase in cerebral cortex and neostriatum. *Dev Brain Res* 21:299–306.

Olson, F. C., and Massaro, E. J. (1977). Pharmacodynamics of methyl mercury in the murine maternal/embryo: Fetal unit. *Toxicol Appl Pharmacol* 39:203–273.

Reuhl, K. R., and Chang, L. W. (1979). Effects of methylmercury on the development of the nervous system: A review. *Neurotoxicology* 1:21–55.

Reynolds, W. A., and Pitkin, R. M. (1975). Transplacental passage of methyl mercury and its uptake by primate fetal tissues. *Proc Soc Exp Biol Med* 148:523–526.

Robbins, M. S.; Hughes, J. A.; Sparber, S. B.; and Mannering, G. J. (1978). Delayed teratogenic effect of methyl mercury on hepatic cytochrome P-450-dependent monooxygenase systems of rats. *Life Sci* 22(4):287–293.

Rodier, P. M.; Aschner, M.; and Sager, P. R. (1984). Mitotic arrest in the developing CNS after prenatal exposure to methyl mercury. *Neurobehav Toxicol Teratol* 6:379–386.

Rodier, P. M.; Reynolds, S. S.; and Roberts, W. N. (1979). Behavioral consequences of interference with CNS development in the early fetal period. *Teratology* 19(3):327–336.

Sager, P. R.; Doherty, R. A.; and Rodier, P. M. (1982). Effects of methylmercury on developing mouse cerebellar cortex. *Exp Neurol* 77:179–193.

Schalock, R. L.; Brown, W. J.; Kark, R. A. P.; and Menon, N. K. (1981). Perinatal methylmercury intoxication: Behavioral effects in rats. *Dev Psychobiol* 14(3):213–219.

Schapiro, S. (1968). Some physiological, biochemical, and behavioral consequences of neonatal hormone administration: Cortisol and thyroxine. *Gen Comp Endocrinol* 10:214.

Shimai, S., and Satoh, H. (1985). Behavioral teratology of methyl mercury. *J Toxicol Sci* 10:199–216.

Sobotka, T. J.; Cook, M. P.; and Brodie, R. E. (1974). Effects of perinatal exposure to methyl mercury on functional brain development and neurochemistry. *Biolog Psychiatry* 8(3):307–320.

Spyker, J. M., and Smithberg, M. (1972). Effects of methylmercury on prenatal development in mice. *Teratology* 5:181–190.

Spyker, J. M.; Sparber, S. B.; and Goldberg, A. M. (1972). Subtle consequences of methylmercury exposure: Behavioral deviations in offspring of treated mothers. *Science* 177:621–623.

Stevens, M. W., and Harbison, R. D. (1974). Placental transfer of diphenylhydantoin: Effects of species, gestational age, and route of administration. *Teratology* 9:317–326.

Su, M., and Okita, G. T. (1976). Embryocidal and teratogenic effects of methylmercury in mice. *Toxicol App Pharmacol* 38:207–216.

Takeuchi, T., and Eto, K. (1977). Pathology and pathogenesis of Minamata disease. In *Minamata Disease: Methyl mercury poisoning in Minamata and Niigata, Japan,* edited by T. Tsubaki and K. Irukayama, pp. 103–141. Tokyo: Kodansha.

Takeuchi, T.; Eto, N.; and Eto, K. (1979). Neuropathology of childhood cases of methyl mercury poisoning: Minamata disease with prolonged symptoms, with particular reference to the decortication syndrome. *Neurotoxicology* 1:1–20.

Tanimura, T.; Emma, E.; and Kihara, T. (1980). Effects of combined treatment with methyl mercury and polychlorinated biphenyls (PCBs) on the development of mouse offspring. In T.V.N. Persaud, ed. *Advances in the Study of Birth Defects* vol. 4. *Neurol & Behavioural Teratology* pp. 163–198. MTP Press: Lancaster, England.

Taylor, L. L., and DiStefano, V. (1976). Effects of methyl mercury on brain biogenic amines in the developing rat pup. *Toxicol Appl Pharmacol* 38:489–497.

Thomas, D. J.; Fisher, H. L.; Hall, L. L.; and Mushak, P. (1982). Effects of age and sex on retention of mercury by methyl mercury treated rats. *Toxicol Appl Pharmacol* 62:445–454.

Wannag, A. (1976). The importance of organ blood mercury when comparing foetal and maternal rat organ distribution of mercury after methyl mercury exposure. *Acta Pharmacol Toxicol* 38:289–298.

Ware, R. A.; Chang, L. W.; and Burkholder, P. M. (1974). Ultra structural evidence for foetal liver injury induced by in utero exposure to small doses of methyl mercury. *Nature* 251:236–237.

Yang, M. G.; Krawford, K. S.; Gareia, J. D.; Wang, J. H. C.; and Lei, K. Y. (1972). Deposition of mercury in fetal and maternal brain. *Proc Soc Exp Med Biol* 141:1004–1007.

Zenick, H. (1974). Behavioral and biochemical consequences in methyl mercury chloride toxicity. *Pharmacol Biochem Behav* 2:709–713.

——— (1976). Evoked potential alterations in methyl mercury chloride toxicity. *Pharmacol Biochem Behav* 5:253–255.

NINE

The Alteration of Protein Synthesis by Methyl Mercury

David J. Thomas and Tore L. M. Syversen

Although the toxic effects of metallic and inorganic mercury have been recognized for centuries, identification of methyl mercury (MeHg) as a neurotoxin occurred only in the middle of the nineteenth century (for a historical review, see Goldwater 1972). Epidemiological studies have elucidated dose-response relationships between the body burden of methyl mercury and the frequency of various signs and symptoms of MeHg intoxication (Amin-Zaki et al. 1974; Clarkson et al. 1981), but the biochemical mechanisms underlying these toxic effects of MeHg in humans are not well understood. As a result, much effort has been devoted to studies of the distribution and fate of MeHg and of its neurotoxic effects in experimental animals.

In this chapter (which complements the recent review by Omata and Sugano [1985]), studies on the effects of methyl mercury on protein synthesis are reviewed and discussed in conjunction with a number of factors that are relevant to the effects of this toxin on protein synthesis in the central nervous system (CNS).

The data on the effects of methyl mercury on protein synthesis are considered both in terms of the mechanism of action and dose-effect relationships. Published reports on the effects of MeHg on protein synthesis in both intact animals and in vitro systems are reviewed, the designs of the studies are critically evaluated, special features of the procedures used to measure protein synthesis in vivo and in vitro are examined, and a number of issues concerning both the characteristics of the exposed organism and the systemic kinetics of methyl mercury which are relevant to assessing the role of altered protein synthesis in the toxicity of methyl mercury are discussed.

Special Characteristics of CNS Protein Synthesis

Protein synthesis in the central nervous system shares many common features with protein synthesis in other tissues. Among the various processes that may play a role in protein synthesis in the CNS are (1) uptake of amino acids at the blood-brain barrier (Rapoport 1976), (2) the transfer of amino acids between astrocytes, cells abutting endothelial cells of brain capillaries, and neurons (Samuels et al. 1983), (3) intracellular compartmentation of amino acids, (4) the extent and fidelity of DNA transcription to yield messenger RNA (mRNA), (5) the aggregation state of brain ribosomes, which is sensitive to a variety of metabolic insults (Westerlain 1972; Westerlain and Plum 1973;

Weiss et al. 1973), (6) the control of initiation, elongation, and termination of polypeptide chain synthesis (Moldave 1985), and (7) post-translational modification of proteins. Further, because the steady-state concentration of a protein is determined by the balance of synthetic and degradative processes, the role of proteases must be considered.

A further aspect of CNS protein synthesis that merits consideration is the concept of critical developmental periods. Such periods are intervals in development during which specific biochemical changes must occur in the organism if further growth and maturation are to be normal. The expression of particular biochemical processes at specific times in development is believed to be under the control of temporal genes that control the program of development (Paigen 1980). In the central nervous system, developmental changes in the expression of different poly $(A)^+$mRNAs have been demonstrated (Chaudhari and Hahn 1983). Such changes presumably reflect changes in the proteins synthesized in the CNS during growth and development. Further, a high percentage of the proteins synthesized in the CNS appear to be unique to that tissue (Sutcliffe et al. 1984). At an organismic level, the concept of critical developmental intervals for the CNS has been recognized. For instance, malnourishment during fetal or perinatal life has been shown to affect brain growth in experimental animals (Chase et al. 1969) and in children (Winick et al. 1970). Nutritional rehabilitation of deprived individuals after the critical period is not sufficient to reverse these neurodevelopmental effects (Winick and Noble 1966). Furthermore, exposure to such toxic agents as inorganic lead or triethyl tin during early life disrupts the normal developmental pattern for CNS myelination in the rat (Toews et al. 1980; Blaker et al. 1981). These effects are persistent; termination of toxin exposure and subsequent nutritional rehabilitation fail to reverse the deficit in myelination (Toews et al. 1983). These data indicate that alterations in CNS protein synthesis during critical developmental intervals can have long-lasting effects. Because methyl mercury readily enters the developing central nervous system (Null et al. 1973; King et al. 1976), particular emphasis in this chapter has been placed on the effects of MeHg on CNS protein synthesis during fetal and perinatal life.

Methyl Mercury and In Vivo CNS Protein Synthesis

Methodological Considerations

Certain factors may influence the capacity of experiments in intact animals to measure the rate of protein synthesis in specific tissues. Dunlop et al. (1977) and Dunn (1977) have reviewed the methodology for measuring protein synthesis in the central nervous system. The most significant factor may be delivery of labeled amino acids to the intracellular precursor pool that serves as the source of amino acids incorporated into newly synthesized protein. The regulation of amino acid delivery to precursor pools and the utilization of amino acids for protein synthesis are complex processes. For example, there is evidence that in isolated cells extracellular amino acids may be preferentially utilized for protein synthesis, thus sparing intracellular amino acid pools (Hider et al. 1969; Adamson et al. 1972; van Venrooij et al. 1972). Preferential utilization of amino acids from different pools may make it difficult to determine the exact experimental conditions under which protein synthesis is being measured.

In the central nervous system, the problem of labeling the precursor amino acid pool is complicated by the existence of several distinct compartments, including capillary endothelium, glial cells, and neurons. Determination of the amino acid content of the whole CNS will not necessarily indicate the extent of amino acid delivery to any of these individual compartments. Further, over the interval of any experiment it is possible that the radiolabeled amino acid contents of the precursor pool of any specific compartment may be increasing or decreasing. Because the specific activity of proteins synthesized depends on the specific activity of the precursor pool, temporal changes in the extent of precursor pool labeling can be the rate-limiting step in the radiolabeling of newly synthesized proteins.

Two strategies can be used to minimize the difficulties that occur in experiments where the labeling of the precursor amino acid pool is the rate-limiting step in labeling newly synthesized protein. First, the interval between administration of radiolabeled amino acid and termination of the experiment can be short (10–20 minutes). In this case, the labeling of the precursor pool would continue to increase throughout the experimental period, and the availability of radiolabeled precursor amino acid would not be rate-limiting. Second, the precursor pool can be flooded with large amounts of radiolabeled amino acids of low specific activity. This approach results in an expansion of precursor pool size, so that even in experiments of relatively long duration the extent of labeling of the precursor pool would not become rate-limiting.

Many in vivo studies have injected a limited amount of radiolabeled precursor and allowed incorporation into proteins to proceed for more than 1 hour (e.g., Cavanagh and Chen 1971; Brubaker et al. 1973; Richardson and Murphy 1974). Temporal changes in the labeling of the precursor amino acid pool were not determined in these studies. An indirect method to ensure that the labeling of the amino acid precursor pool was not the rate-limiting factor was used by Syversen (1977), who used a limited amount of radiolabeled precursor and a relatively short incubation time. Omata et al. (1978, 1980, 1981, 1982) have used the method of precursor flooding. Use of either method indicated that neuronal protein synthesis was reduced by exposure to methyl mercury. However, in any attempt to elucidate the dose-response relationship between MeHg exposure and reduced neuronal synthesis, these studies should be compared with great care.

Another component of the labeling of amino acid pools is the effect of methyl mercury on amino acid transport. Early work demonstrated that mercurials, including MeHg, affected the integrity and function of the blood-brain barrier (Steinwall 1961, 1968, 1969; Flodmark and Steinwall 1963; Steinwall and Olsson 1969; Steinwall and Snyder 1969; Chang and Hartmann 1972; Ware et al. 1974a). Recent work indicated that MeHg alters amino acid transport across the syncytiotrophoblast microvillus membrane of human placenta (Goodman et al. 1983). Alterations in the delivery of precursor amino acids to tissue by MeHg treatment may result in reduced availability of labeled amino acids for incorporation into newly synthesized proteins. Thus, a reduction in synthesis of labeled proteins in MeHg-treated animals could indicate either an effect of MeHg on protein synthesis or an alteration of the entry of labeled amino acids into the precursor pool.

Alteration of Protein Synthesis by Exposure to Methyl Mercury

In Utero and Perinatal Exposure   Protein synthesis during fetal and perinatal life differs both quantitatively and qualitatively from that found in the adult. For example, the protein synthetic capacity of the fetus is ultimately dependent on the integrity of the fetomaternal interface at which precursors for protein synthesis are transferred (Young 1979). Rapid accumulation of protein in the central nervous system during fetal life may be the result of low rates of protein degradation in the developing organism (Johnson 1985). Notably, the high rates of protein synthesis found in the CNS during the perinatal period have been shown to be sensitive to changes in the internal environment (e.g., altered thyroid function; Lindholm 1983).

Considerable epidemiological evidence indicates that the human fetus is particularly vulnerable to the toxic effects of methyl mercury. Congenital Minamata disease has been described in the offspring of women who consumed MeHg-contaminated seafood during pregnancy and who remained symptom-free (Takizawa 1979). Besides producing gross anatomical malformations (Murakami 1972), exposure to methyl mercury in utero also exerted a variety of effects on neurodevelopment (Amin-Zaki et al. 1974) that can be manifested years after cessation of exposure and occur in children with relatively low exposure to methyl mercury in utero (Marsh et al. 1977, 1979). Epidemiological data also suggest that children are particularly vulnerable to the lethal effects of MeHg (Greenwood 1985).

In experimental studies, the embryotoxicity of methyl mercury has been well documented. The transplacental toxicity of MeHg resulting from accumulation of methyl mercury in the fetal liver has been shown to produce biochemical and morphological changes (Ware et al. 1974b; Fowler and Woods 1977). The toxicity of methyl mercury to developing organisms may be related to the relative ease with which it crosses the placenta (Garrett et al.

1972; Mansour et al. 1973; Null et al. 1973; King et al. 1976). Studies with rat embryo explants indicated that exposure of the developing fetus to MeHg resulted in dysmorphogenic changes (Kitchin et al. 1984). Thus, fetal toxicity of MeHg was at least in part the result of a direct effect of the agent on the developing organism and not entirely mediated by alterations of the integrity of the fetomaternal interface. Exposure to MeHg in early postnatal life also affected development of the peripheral sympathetic nervous system, resulting in a disproportionate growth of the kidneys and heart in neonatal rats treated with methyl mercury (Bartolome et al. 1984).

Parallel studies in developing rodents have also demonstrated that in utero exposure to methyl mercury produces changes in postnatal development and behavior that are not associated with obvious signs of impairment at birth (Spyker et al. 1972; Hughes and Sparber 1978; Eccles and Annau 1982*a*, 1982*b*). A number of biochemical mechanisms may underlie these effects of MeHg exposure on the structure and function of the developing nervous system. Rodier (1983) has summarized the processes that may be especially subject to injury—neuron proliferation, glial production and myelination, neuron migration, elaboration of cell processes, and neurotransmitter turnover. Changes in protein synthesis could account for the vulnerability of each of these processes.

The relationship between maternal exposure to methyl mercury and fetal growth and development has been examined by Mottet and co-workers. Chronic exposure of pregnant Sprague-Dawley rats to MeHg starting at day 0 of gestation and continuing at 4-day intervals until day 21 was associated with increasing embryotoxicity as maternal liver Hg concentration increased (Mottet 1974). Notably, decreased fetal weight and increased Hg concentrations in fetal liver were also correlated with increased Hg concentration in the liver of the maternal rat. In a related study in which pregnant rats were continuously exposed to 25 parts per million (ppm) of MeHg in drinking water from day 1 to day 20 of gestation, Chen and associates (1979) found that MeHg exposure reduced fetal body weight and liver weight. Fetal liver DNA and protein concentrations were unaffected by treatment with methyl mercury. In the liver, kidneys, heart, and brain of MeHg-treated fetuses, incorporation of [^{3}H]-thymidine into DNA was reduced. These results suggested that a primary effect of in utero exposure to MeHg was to alter DNA replication; changes in protein synthesis might be secondary to this effect.

Farris and Smith (1975) examined the effects of methyl mercury on brain protein synthesis in utero. Pregnant rats received 1 mg MeHg subcutaneously (sc) on day 16 or day 17, or daily from day 16 through day 18, or daily from day 16 through day 19 of pregnancy. Controls received a subcutaneous injection of physiological saline on days 18 and 19 of gestation. At 48 hours of age, pups from MeHg-treated and control dams received intraperitoneal (ip) injections of [^{14}C]-leucine and were sacrificed after 30 minutes. A brain protein fraction was isolated and its [^{14}C] contents determined. Exposure to methyl mercury in utero did not affect CNS protein synthesis in early postnatal life.

Olson and Massaro (1978) examined the effects of in utero MeHg exposure on amino acid uptake, protein synthesis, and palate closure in fetal mice. Administration of 5 mg MeHg/kg sc to pregnant CFW mice at 12 days and 6 hours of gestation was associated with a delay in palate closure. At 24 hours after MeHg administration, total fetal protein was decreased 22 percent below controls, but DNA content did not differ between MeHg-treated fetuses and control fetuses. Maximal difference in fetal protein content (32 percent) occurred at 48 hours after treatment with methyl mercury. The rate of fetal protein synthesis was measured by injection of pregnant females with [^{3}H]-isoleucine 10–20 minutes prior to sacrifice at 3 hours after MeHg treatment. The rate of fetal protein synthesis was reduced about 5 percent. Up to 24 hours after treatment, the rate of fetal protein synthesis was reduced 22–26 percent in MeHg-treated fetuses, as compared with controls. The reduction in the rate of fetal protein synthesis was estimated to account for the observed reduction in the rate of accumulation of protein in the fetuses of MeHg-treated females. Notably, treatment with methyl mercury did not reduce placental blood flow or change fetal water space; however, at 2 hours after treatment, fetal uptake of cycloleucine and free amino acid concentrations in the fetus were both reduced. Therefore, the reduction of protein synthesis and accumulation in MeHg-treated fetal rats might be due to an MeHg-mediated reduction in the availability of precursor amino acids.

Joiner and Hupp (1979) investigated the effects of exposure to methyl mercury in early postnatal life on brain protein synthesis. In these studies, 1- to 21-day-old Sprague-Dawley rat pups received 8 mg CH$_3$HgCl (methyl mercury chloride) per kg ip. Twelve hours after treatment with methyl mercury, rats received an ip injection of [^{14}C]-leucine and were sacrificed 30 minutes later. Incorporation of radiolabel into protein was estimated as the amount of [^{14}C] precipitated in 9.1 percent trichloroacetic acid (TCA). Data were expressed as counts per minute per gram of brain. Methyl mercury treatment resulted in a significant increase in the incorporation of radiocarbon into protein in 5- and 15-day-old rats. At 17–21 days of age, MeHg treatment reduced incorporation of radiolabeled amino acid into brain protein significantly. The authors interpreted these data to suggest that MeHg exposure in early life resulted in a premature termination of cellular proliferation. Thus, exposure in early life to methyl mercury would interfere with brain growth and differentiation during a critical period in brain development.

The regional specificity of the effects of methyl mercury on protein and on nucleic acid metabolism has been examined in the central nervous system of neonatal rats (Slotkin et al. 1985). In these studies, Sprague-Dawley rat pups received 1.0 or 2.5 mg CH$_3$HgCl (MeHg hydroxide) per kg sc daily from the day after birth until weaning at 21 days of age. Control rat pups received daily sc injections of water. Treated and control pups were maintained with free access to lactating dams. Daily treatment with MeHg did not result in mortality, although there was a trend for reduced body weight in rats receiving the higher dosage level of MeHg. At 6, 10, 15, 20, 30, and 41 days of age, rats were sacrificed and the brain was dissected to yield midbrain and brain stem, cerebral cortex, and cerebellum. Aliquots of tissue homogenates were taken for protein analysis, and extracts of tissue homogenates were prepared for DNA and RNA analysis. Comparison between control and MeHg-treated animals used analysis of variance procedures.

In midbrain and brain stem, exposure to methyl mercury resulted in a significant decrease in DNA content, protein content, and tissue weight. RNA content of this brain region was unaffected by MeHg treatment. In the cerebral cortex, DNA contents were significantly increased and tissue weight was significantly decreased by MeHg treatments; protein and RNA contents were unaffected. In the cerebellum, MeHg treatment resulted in a significant increase in DNA and RNA content, but protein content and tissue weight were unchanged.

These results indicate that the effects of methyl mercury on cell growth and protein, DNA, and RNA metabolism depended not only on regional differences in the central nervous system but also on the developmental status of each region. For example, in the cerebellum, a late-maturing region, MeHg exposure resulted in increased DNA and RNA contents. This presumably represented compensatory cell divisions that replaced cells killed by exposure to methyl mercury. In regions that matured early, such as the midbrain and brain stem, similar increases in DNA and RNA contents were not seen after MeHg exposure. The decline in DNA and protein contents noted in brain regions of MeHg-treated rats probably reflected cell loss due to exposure to methyl mercury. The pattern of changes seen for the cerebral cortex also reflected the fact that its period of growth and development occurred after that of the midbrain and the brain stem.

Recent studies by Cheung and Verity (1985) carefully examined the effects of methyl mercury on individual steps in the translation of mRNA. In these studies, 10- to 20-day-old Sprague-Dawley rat pups received 8 mg MeHg/kg ip and were maintained with free access to lactating dams. At 20–24 hours after dosing, pups were killed and a 23,000 $\times$ g supernate (postmitochondrial supernate, PMS) was prepared from the brain. A pH 5 enzyme fraction was also prepared from the brains of MeHg-treated and control rats. Using PMS to direct a cell-free translation system, MeHg treatment was found to reduce the incorporation of [^{3}H]-leucine into protein by 39 percent, as compared with PMS from control rats. Because equal concentrations of RNA were found in the PMS prepared from the brains of control and MeHg-treated rats, this suggested that differences in incorporation were not due to differences in total RNA contents of PMS. Treatment with MeHg did not alter the free polyribosome sedimentation profile of PMS, compared with that found in control animals. Using [3H]-methionine, these investigators examined the initiation of translation in PMS prepared from untreated rat pups. Addition of 20 μM MeHg to the incubation medium increased the binding of [3H]-methionine to the 40S ribosomal unit. At 100 μM MeHg, a concentration that inhibits protein synthesis, the binding of methionine to the 40S complex persisted. This high concentration of methyl mercury also promoted binding of methionine to an 80S ribosome fraction. Addition of puromycin to this mixture reduced [3H] binding to the 80S fraction. This suggested that, even at high MeHg concentrations, 80S initiation complexes can synthesize the first peptide bond between methionine and puromycin. These data indicated that the initiation of peptide chain synthesis by brain PMS was relatively insensitive to inhibition by methyl mercury.

The effects of methyl mercury on peptide chain elongation were also evaluated by these investigators. For these studies, poly U-directed incorporation of phenylalanine into polyphenylalanine was examined in a system that is not dependent on normal reactions for chain initiation. It was found that poly U-directed phenylalanine incorporation was reduced about 22 percent using PMS prepared from brains of MeHg-treated rats. When endogenous mRNA was used to direct phenylalanine incorporation into protein, synthesis was reduced by about 35 percent. Peptidyl transferase activities of PMS were equal in fractions prepared from control or MeHg-treated rats.

The effect of methyl mercury on chain elongation was examined to determine whether tRNA aminoacylation was affected. Phenylalanyl-tRNA[Phe] synthetase activity was measured in the pH 5 enzyme fraction prepared from PMS from MeHg-treated or control rats. Treatment with methyl mercury resulted in a 22 percent reduction in the activity of this enzyme. In vitro addition of MeHg to PMS prepared from brains of control rats indicated that the IC_{50} for the effect of MeHg on this enzyme was about 8 μM. Correlation analysis indicated a positive association between the degree of inhibition of phenylalanine incorporation into protein and the inhibition of this enzyme activity. To test whether inhibitions of the enzymatic step leading to formation of phenylalanyl-tRNA[Phe] were sufficient to account for the reduction of phenylalanine incorporation into protein, this step was by-passed by addition of [3H]-phenylalanyl-tRNA[Phe] to an assay system containing PMS from brains of MeHg-treated or control rats. Under these conditions, poly U-directed phenylalanine incorporation was equal for PMS from control and MeHg-treated rats. However, if phenylalanine incorporation were directed by endogenous mRNA, use of PMS from MeHg-treated rats resulted in 27 percent less incorporation than did control PMS. This indicated that availability of other aminoacyl-tRNAs may be rate-limiting for translation in the PMS from MeHg-treated rats.

Taken together, these data argue that a primary lesion in the effect of methyl mercury on protein synthesis in the brain is the formation of aminoacyl-tRNAs. Inhibition of this process would lead to reduced rates of peptide chain elongation. Thus, protein synthesis could be inhibited in the absence of any effect of MeHg on peptide chain initiation or on peptide bond formation.

Exposure in Adult Life　The effects of methyl mercury treatment on protein metabolism in adult rats were examined by Brubaker et al. (1973). Adult male rats received 10 mg CH_3HgOH/kg sc daily for up to 7 days. Control rats received sc injections of vehicle only. The body weight of MeHg-treated rats declined over the course of treatment, but they displayed no other signs or symptoms of MeHg intoxication. Twenty minutes prior to sacrifice on day 2, 3, 6, or 8 of the study, rats received an intravenous injection of a mixture of $[^{14}C]$-labeled amino acids. The concentrations of protein and the amounts of radiolabeled protein in brain, liver, and kidneys were determined.

In the brain, there was no change in the protein concentration over the 8-day course of study. At all time points, however, incorporation of $[^{14}C]$ amino acids into protein was increased in the brains of MeHg-treated rats. The concentration of protein in liver declined over the experimental period, and the incorporation of radiolabeled amino acid increased at each time point. The concentration of protein in the kidney was increased, while the incorporation of amino acid into protein was inhibited.

These results were surprising in that an increase in protein synthesis was found in the liver and brain of MeHg-treated rats. These findings might relate to the time course of the study, as rats were sacrificed prior to the appearance of the signs and symptoms of MeHg intoxication. Further, these studies were not controlled for the inanitive effect of MeHg treatment. These factors have been examined more carefully in a number of more recent studies, which are reviewed below.

Because methyl mercury had been demonstrated to produce systemic effects such as weight loss and general debilitation, which might secondarily affect protein synthesis, an attempt was made to dissociate the specific neurotoxic effects of MeHg exposure from the systemic effects of chronic exposure to this agent by intracranial administration of MeHg (Richardson and Murphy 1974). Intracranial administration of methyl mercury at doses ranging from 10 to 100 μg 24 hours prior to sacrifice was accompanied by an increase in the rate of protein synthesis in brain homogenate. In vivo measurement of protein synthesis demonstrated an increased synthetic rate in both cerebrum and cerebellum of MeHg-treated rats. The stimulatory effect of MeHg on brain protein synthesis was transitory. By 3 days after intracranial administration, protein synthesis had returned to normal levels. Although the studies did not clearly separate systemic and neurotoxic effects of MeHg, they demonstrated that even in cases where relatively high mercury concentrations were attained in the central nervous system, protein synthesis was actually higher in MeHg-treated rats than in controls.

Farris and Smith (1975) examined the effects of methyl mercury exposure on CNS protein synthesis and the accumulation of MeHg in the brain. For these studies, adult female rats received sc injections of 5 mg MeHg and 10 mg L-cysteine, or 10 mg of L-cysteine alone, daily for 3 days. On the fourth day after the end of treatment, rats received intravenous injections of [^{14}C]-leucine. After 90 minutes, rats were decapitated, and brains were sectioned into hemispheres, midbrain, and occipital and cerebellar components. Brain protein was isolated, and the [^{14}C] contents of each brain region were expressed as a function of protein content. Although MeHg treatment increased the total amount of [^{14}C]-leucine per milligram of brain, it significantly decreased the amount of [^{14}C]-leucine incorporated per milligram of protein in all brain regions.

These investigators also determined the mercury concentration in the brains of adult rats exposed to methyl mercury. In females receiving 1 mg MeHg daily for 3 days, brain Hg concentration was 54 ± 4 μg per gram of tissue (mean $\pm$ SEM). It is notable that the concentration of mercury attained exceeded that associated with a variety of signs and symptoms of neurological dysfunction found in MeHg-treated animals (Suzuki 1969; Grant 1973; Magos and Butler 1976). Thus, data from this study probably cannot be used to define a lower limit of CNS methyl mercury concentration required to alter brain protein synthesis or to produce neurological dysfunction.

Omata et al. (1978) have used both in vivo and in vitro techniques to examine the effects of methyl mercury on protein synthesis. For studies of the effects on protein synthesis in vivo, adult female rats received 10 mg CH_3HgCl/kg sc daily for 7 days. Control rats received daily injections of the vehicle, sodium carbonate. On the seventh day after the last dose of MeHg or vehicle, rats received an ip injection of a mixture of [^{14}C]-labeled amino acids. Animals were sacrificed 30 minutes after dosing, and tissues were taken for mercury analysis and for determination of [^{14}C] incorporation into the acid-soluble and protein fractions. Treatment with methyl mercury reduced amino acid incorporation into the homogenate and the PMS fraction of brain, liver, and kidney. The amounts of labeled amino acid in the acid-soluble fraction of the PMS fraction of brain and kidney were not significantly different in MeHg-treated rats and control rats. However, the amount of [^{14}C] amino acid in the acid-soluble fraction of the liver PMS fraction was significantly increased. Thus, at least in brain and kidney, MeHg treatment did not alter the size of the free amino acid pool and thereby alter the availability of precursor amino acid required for protein synthesis. The significance of an increased free amino acid pool in livers of rats treated with methyl mercury may be considered in terms of the cachectic effect of the treatment. As noted by these investigators, MeHg treatment resulted in a steady decrease in body weight. On the seventh day after the end of treatment, the rats treated with methyl mercury had lost about 25 percent of their initial body weight. To test the effects of inanation on brain and liver protein synthesis, a parallel group of rats had restricted access to rat chow, so that they experienced a similar decrease in body weight over a 7-day period. The effects of food restriction on protein synthesis were measured using a cell-free system for [^{14}C]-L-leucine incorporation. When compared with control rats, food-restricted rats showed no reduction in brain protein synthesis, but liver protein synthesis was significantly reduced. Therefore, while the effects on liver protein synthesis found in MeHg-treated rats could be attributed to the reduction in food intake that accompanied methyl mercury intoxication, inanation alone did not reduce brain protein synthesis. This suggests that the effect on brain protein synthesis in MeHg-treated rats was due to a direct effect of MeHg on protein synthesis. This brings to mind the attempt of Richardson and Murphy (1974) to separate primary neurotoxic effects of MeHg from other, possibly secondary, systemic effects of the agent.

Food intake as a confounder in studies of the effects of methyl mercury on protein synthesis has been examined by Lapin and Carter (1982). Female rats received a single oral dose of 40 mg CH_3HgOH/kg, and controls received an oral dose of the vehicle alone. Control rats were divided into a group with free access to rat chow and a group pair-fed with MeHg-treated rats. Rats treated with methyl mercury manifested the characteristic signs and symptoms of MeHg intoxication on day 7 after exposure. Ad libitum, pair-fed, and MeHg-treated rats were sacrificed on day 1, 3, 7, or 13 of the study. Incorporation of labeled amino acids into protein was determined by ip injection of a [^{14}C]-labeled amino acid mixture 2 hours prior to sacrifice. Protein synthesis was measured as the amount of [^{14}C]-labeled amino acids that precipitated in 10 percent TCA per milligram of tissue. Data for pair-fed control and MeHg-treated rats were expressed as percentages of protein synthetic activity found in tissues of rats fed ad libitum. Analysis of variance procedures were used to compare results between groups.

Compared with controls fed ad libitum, treatment with methyl mercury increased [^{14}C] amino acid incorporation into whole-blood proteins at 1 and 3 days after dosing, while pair-fed control animals showed significantly less labeling than ad libitum fed MeHg-treated rats. In the liver, pair-fed animals showed greater inhibition of protein synthesis than did MeHg-treated rats. Pair-fed rats also showed consistent reduction in the labeling of proteins in the kidney, while MeHg treatment significantly reduced incorporation at day 7 and increased incorporation on day 13. Cerebellar protein synthesis was affected in both pair-fed and MeHg-treated rats. Notably, on days 7 and 13 after treatment, MeHg-treated rats showed significantly larger reductions in protein synthesis than did pair-fed rats.

These investigators also examined the role of amino acid uptake by tissues as a factor in the alteration of protein synthesis due to food restriction or treatment with methyl mercury. Using α-aminoisobutyric acid (AIB), a non-metabolized amino acid, as a tracer of tissue amino acid uptake, no differences were found between the concentration of AIB in the liver or cerebellum of pair-fed control and MeHg-treated rats. Compared with pair-fed rats, MeHg-treated rats had significantly higher AIB concentrations in blood and significantly lower concentrations in the kidney.

Taken together, these data indicate that some of the reported effects of methyl mercury on protein synthesis were clearly attributable to the inanation that accompanies MeHg intoxication. In particular, changes in liver protein synthesis seen in MeHg-treated rats have been found to be primarily attributable to reduced food intake, and not to a specific effect of MeHg. These investigators have also shown that MeHg treatment resulted in a reduction of protein synthesis in the central nervous system that was not accounted for by reduction in food intake. Use of AIB as a measure of tissue uptake of amino acids indicates that differences in liver and cerebellar protein synthesis between pair-fed and MeHg-treated rats were not due to differences in the uptake of precursor amino acids into the cell.

As described above, there are potential difficulties in measuring the rate of protein synthesis in intact animals. One approach (precursor flooding) has been used by Omata and co-workers (1980). In their studies, rats were sacrificed at relatively short intervals after injection of large amounts of radiolabeled precursor amino acid. Male Wistar rats received either sodium carbonate (control) or 10 mg CH_3HgCl/kg sc (treated) for 7 days. Following the approach used in an earlier study (Omata et al. 1978), rats sacrificed on day 10 after the beginning of treatment were considered to be in the latent period of MeHg poisoning and those sacrificed on day 15 were considered to be symptomatic. Rats were sacrificed 30 minutes after receiving ip injections of 1.5 mmoles of [^{14}C]-labeled-L-valine per 100 grams of body weight. Tissue homogenates were prepared, and proteins were precipitated with sulfosalicylic acid. Treatment with MeHg did not affect the concentration of valine soluble in sulfosalicylic acid in either the cerebral cortex or the cerebellum. Thus, there was equivalent labeling of precursor amino acid pools in control and MeHg-treated animals.

On day 10 after the beginning of treatment, rats treated with methyl mercury displayed less labeling of proteins in the pons, hypothalamus, striatum, midbrain, hippocampus, cerebral and cerebellar cortex, and spinal cord than did control rats. Notably, reductions in the rate of protein synthesis in regions of the brain of MeHg-treated rats were greater during the latent period (day 10) than during the symptomatic period (day 15). The rise in protein synthesis during the symptomatic period may represent a compensatory response to injury. Recent studies on the effects of MeHg on RNA synthesis in the dorsal root ganglia of rats indicated that, during the asymptomatic period, RNA synthesis was unaffected, suggesting that alterations in protein synthesis in this tissue were not due to changes in RNA metabolism (Nagumo et al. 1985).

Further understanding of the mechanism by which methyl mercury alters protein synthesis has come from the work of Omata et al. (1981). These investigators also examined the adrenal function in the stimulation of hepatic protein and RNA synthesis by MeHg. Adult female Sprague-Dawley rats were bilaterally adrenalectomized 5–6 days prior to use and maintained with access to 0.9 percent sodium chloride. Treated rats received 0.5–50.0 mg MeHg/kg sc, and controls received the vehicle—sodium carbonate. Protein synthesis in vivo was measured 30 minutes after ip injection of [^{14}C]-leucine. In the intact animal, treatment with 50 mg MeHg/kg resulted in increased incorporation of [^{14}C] into liver homogenate and a large increase in the incorporation of radiolabel into serum proteins. To assess the role of endocrine factors in the effect of MeHg on hepatic protein synthesis, studies of in vitro protein synthesis using the cell-free system described by Omata et al. (1978) were undertaken. Administration of 10–50 mg MeHg/kg resulted in significant increases in the amino acid incorporation in the cell-free system when the liver was used as the source of PMS. The use of brain PMS from MeHg-treated animals did not stimulate amino acid incorporation in the cell-free system.

In order to determine the mechanism by which methyl mercury might increase hepatic protein synthesis, the effect of MeHg on the activity of RNA polymerases in liver nuclei was investigated (Omata et al. 1981). Treatment of donor rats with 20–50 mg MeHg/kg increased Mg^{2+}-dependent RNA polymerase activity but had a small effect on Mn^{2+}-dependent polymerase activity. These investigators postulated that the stimulatory effect of MeHg on hepatic protein and RNA synthesis was due to a stimulation of corticosterone secretion from the adrenal glands. To test this hypothesis, adrenalectomized rats were treated with MeHg. At the 10 mg MeHg/kg dosage level, adrenalectomized animals did not manifest an increase in hepatic RNA or protein synthesis, but at the 20 mg MeHg/kg dosage level, effects on both protein synthesis and polymerase activity were found. These findings suggested that some of the effects of MeHg on protein and RNA metabolism were mediated by a change in corticosterone secretion from the adrenals. At high-dosage levels, however, these glucocorticoid-mediated effects were superseded by other effects of exposure to methyl mercury. Burton and Meikle (1980) showed that MeHg exposure affected adrenal function in the rat. Acute or chronic MeHg exposure increased adrenal gland weight but did not affect serum corticosterone concentrations. However, when subjected to ether stress or treated with adrenocorticotropic hormone, MeHg-treated rats showed a smaller rise in serum corticosterone concentrations than did rats receiving the vehicle alone. Burton and Meikle concluded that MeHg treatment produced a defect in steroidogenesis that reduced the ability of the animal to respond to stress. The relationship between this effect of MeHg and the effects on hepatic protein synthesis observed by Omata et al. (1981) requires further investigation.

Sauve and Nicholls (1981) examined the effect of methyl mercury exposure on protein synthesis in the liver, particularly the production and secretion of plasma proteins by this organ. Because the effect of MeHg on liver protein synthesis might be due to an effect of MeHg on the pituitary, both intact and hypophysectomized adult male rats were used. Animals received 10 mg CH_3HgOH/kg or vehicle (distilled water) sc daily for 3 days. At 24 hours after the third injection and 12–60 minutes before sacrifice, rats received 5 μCi of $[^{14}C]$-leucine ip. Serum was prepared for analyses of the concentrations of free leucine and of serum proteins, and liver homogenate was prepared for measurement of free leucine and of newly synthesized proteins. Treatment with methyl mercury did not alter the specific activity of leucine in the serum or liver homogenate. However, MeHg treatment significantly increased the specific activity of leucine in serum proteins and in proteins of the liver homogenate. In MeHg-treated rats, there was a significant increase in the specific activity of microsomal proteins, but no increase in cytosolic proteins. This finding was consistent with an increase in the synthesis of secreted proteins and was associated with a marked increase in the labeling of two serum proteins of 43,000 and 63,000 daltons molecular mass.

Studies of protein synthesis in vitro using 105,000 × g supernate and ribosomes prepared from the livers of control or MeHg-treated rats demonstrated that use of either fraction from the liver of MeHg-treated rats was associated with an increase in the incorporation of radioleucine into protein. Assays of poly U-directed synthesis of polyphenylalanine were performed using postmicrosomal supernate from the liver of control rats or rats treated with methyl mercury. More polyphenylalanine was synthesized when the postmicrosomal supernate was obtained from the livers of MeHg-treated rats. Further studies using a pH 5 supernate fraction prepared from the postmicrosomal fraction suggested that there were higher levels of elongation factors 1 and 2 in the cytosols of livers of MeHg-treated rats than in control rats. Parallel studies using hypophysectomized rats treated with the vehicle or MeHg indicated that ablation of the pituitary had no influence on the effect of MeHg on protein synthesis in the liver.

In summary, these results indicated that the effects of methyl mercury on hepatic protein synthesis was a direct effect and not related to an effect on endocrine status. The increase in plasma protein synthesis that accompanied MeHg exposure suggested that exposure to this agent may provoke an acute phase reaction similar to that found after exposure to a number of toxins (Kushner 1982). This aspect of cellular response to MeHg exposure requires further investigation.

Methyl Mercury and CNS Protein Synthesis In Vitro

Studies with Tissue Slices

Yoshino et al. (1966*a*) observed that the mercury concentration in the central nervous system of rats treated with methyl mercury rose rapidly; however, exposed animals were initially symptom-free, with evidence of CNS dysfunction appearing only 6–10 days after MeHg treatment. Notably, mercury concentrations in the CNS were as high during the latent (or symptom-free) period as during the period when signs of CNS dysfunction were manifested. Thus, these investigators undertook studies of protein synthesis in the CNS during the latent and symptomatic periods following MeHg exposure (Yoshino et al. 1966*b*).

In these studies, male Wistar rats received 7.5 mg MeHg thioacetamide per 100 grams of body weight ip. MeHg-treated rats developed signs of MeHg poisoning (ataxia and abnormal posture) 5 or more days after treatment. For these studies, rats were divided into controls (not treated with MeHg), rats in the latent period, and rats with MeHg-induced neurological symptoms. Animals were killed by decapitation, and three or four cortical slices about 0.35 mm thick were prepared from each hemisphere. Six slices were pooled for measurement of the rate of [U-^{14}C]-leucine incorporation into protein. Slices were incubated at 37° C for 2 hours in modified Krebs-Ringer phosphate buffer containing radioleucine. After addition of 0.4 ml of 30% TCA, contents of the Warburg flask were homogenized in 8 ml of 5% TCA. The precipitate was washed twice with 10% TCA and heated to 90° C for 15 minutes. Following delipidation, precipitates were radioassayed.

Incorporation of radioleucine into protein by brain cortex slices was reduced whether the donor rat was in the latent period or was symptomatic. The relative reduction was greater when the donor was symptomatic (42 percent vs. 57 percent of control values), and the reduction in protein synthesis during the latent period appeared to be a sensitive indicator of impending CNS injury. For comparison, later studies by Cavanagh and Chen (1971) showed that protein synthesis was decreased in the peripheral nervous system of the rat prior to histological evidence of neuronal injury. Thus, a decline in protein synthesis may precede the appearance of neuronal injury. This temporal separation of a primary biochemical lesion (reduced protein synthesis) from evidence of injury (morphological or functional changes) may reflect in part the fact that protein synthesis in neurons occurs primarily in the cell body and that newly synthesized proteins are transported by axoplasmic flow to distant sites in the cells. Therefore, injury may not be manifested until the supply of proteins to peripheral sites in the neuron has declined. Because thioacetamide modifies the distribution of inorganic mercury in rats (Trojanowska et al. 1971), these results may not be directly comparable to studies with other MeHg compounds.

Verity et al. (1977) have compared the effects of methyl mercury treatment on protein synthesis in tissue slices prepared from the cerebrum and the cerebellum. For these studies, female Sprague-Dawley rats (100–150 g) received 10 mg CH_3HgCl/kg by mouth daily for 6 to 8 days. Slices prepared from cerebra and cerebella of rats at different time points during methyl mercury treatment were incubated with [^{14}C]-leucine at 37° C. Reactions were terminated by removal and blotting of tissue slices, and slices were homogenized in 50% TCA. Data on [^{14}C]-leucine incorporation in slices prepared from MeHg-treated rats were compared with the incorporation of the labeled amino acid in slices prepared from age-matched controls. At 10 days after the beginning of MeHg treatment, cerebellar slices from MeHg-treated rats incorporated about 50 percent as much leucine as did slices from control rats, and cerebral slices incorporated about 80 percent of the amount incorporated by controls. This reduction in protein synthesis persisted for up to 21 days after the beginning of MeHg exposure and was always greater in cerebellar slices than in cerebral slices. Notably, these effects of MeHg on protein synthesis in cerebral and cerebellar slices appeared to be independent of the inanative effect of MeHg treatment. Parallel studies of leucine incorporation into tissue slices prepared from cerebra and cerebella of pair-fed animals indicated that weight loss alone did not consistently reduce radiolabeling of proteins.

These investigators also examined the effects of MeHg exposure in vitro on protein synthesis in cerebral slices. Half-maximal inhibition of [^{14}C]-leucine incorporation into protein was found at an MeHg concentration of about 7.5 μM.

Studies on Isolated Cells

Neuronal Cell Types   The effects of methyl mercury on protein synthesis have also been examined by use of isolated cells. Two aspects of this approach merit consideration. First, techniques are available for the bulk isolation of specific cell types (Nagata and Tsukada 1978). In studies of the effects of MeHg on protein synthesis in the central nervous system, the ability to examine the effects of MeHg on a particular cell type can be useful. Second, isolated cell systems may avoid difficulties in the delivery of radiolabeled amino acids to the target cells. Whereas, in intact animals, specific barriers exist to regulate amino acid uptake into the CNS, in isolated cell preparations such barriers are removed. Theoretically, labeling of precursor-free amino acid pools within isolated cells should be easily accomplished, facilitating direct measurement of protein synthetic rates.

The use of cells isolated from the central nervous system in the measurement of the effects of methyl mercury on protein synthesis was first reported by Syversen (1977). This investigation combined exposure in vivo to MeHg and a radiolabeled amino acid with isolation of specific cell types from the cerebrum and cerebellum. In these studies, male rats received 10 mg MeHg (as CH_3HgCl) per kg ip. On 1–10 days after treatment, rats received a subcutaneous injection of $[^{14}C]$-leucine. Rats were sacrificed 30 minutes later and neurons were isolated from the cerebrum, and granule and Purkinje cells were isolated from the cerebellum. A 30-minute period for in vivo incorporation of radioleucine into protein was chosen because incorporation was found to be linear for at least 50 minutes. Thus, at 30 minutes, the availability of precursor amino acid was not rate-limiting, and protein synthesis was itself the rate-limiting process.

Rates of protein synthesis were determined in MeHg-treated and control rats 1, 2, 3, 5, 7, and 10 days after exposure to methyl mercury or the vehicle. Results for MeHg-treated rats were expressed as percentages of those obtained for control rats. At 1, 2, 3, and 5 days after dosing, cerebral neurons from MeHg-treated rats displayed rates of protein synthesis that were 10–20 percent below those found in controls. On day 7 the protein synthetic rate for cerebral neurons isolated from MeHg-treated donors rebounded and exceeded that found in the controls by about 10 percent. On day 10, synthetic rates for cerebral neurons were the same in MeHg-treated and control animals. For Purkinje cells from MeHg-treated rats, a similar pattern of initial depression and subsequent rebound in protein synthetic rates was found. On days 1, 2, 3, and 5 after dosing, rates were decreased 5–20 percent; on days 7 and 10, rates were increased between 10 and 20 percent above those found in controls. In contrast, the rate of protein synthesis in granule cells was consistently reduced by MeHg treatment. At 1 day after dosing, the rate in MeHg-treated rats was reduced about 30 percent. Between days 2 and 10, the rates were consistently reduced to about 80 percent of those found in control rats.

These findings have interesting correlations with the distribution and clearance of methyl mercury. In parallel studies, Syversen (1977) also measured the concentrations of mercury per milligram of protein in the three cell types isolated from the brains of MeHg-treated rats. Among these cell types, the highest peak concentration of Hg (about 20 mg Hg per mg of protein) was attained in cerebral neurons on day 3 after treatment. In contrast, peak Hg concentrations (about 16–17 mg Hg per mg of protein) were attained in both cerebellar granule and Purkinje cells on day 2 after treatment. These results were notable in that granule cells, which demonstrated the most severe and persistent reduction in protein synthesis, did not attain a higher Hg concentration or retain Hg more avidly than did cells that showed reversible alterations in the rate of protein synthesis. Morphological studies have indicated that granule cells show early and selective injury following MeHg exposure (Herman et al. 1973; Syversen et al. 1981). For comparison, in myelinating cultures of newborn mouse cerebella, MeHg exposure also produced more severe injury in granule cells than in Purkinje cells (Kim 1971). Thus, granule cells were apparently more sensitive to MeHg-induced injury displaying persistent alterations in morphology and protein synthesis at levels of Hg exposure that did not produce structural or functional alterations in other cell types. Similar studies of RNA and protein synthesis in cerebral neurons and cerebellar Purkinje and granule cells of MeHg-treated rats demonstrated that decreases in [^{3}H]-uridine incorporation into RNA occurred prior to decreases in [^{14}C]-leucine incorporation into protein. Effects on RNA synthesis were more persistent in cerebellar granule cells than in the other cell types (Syversen 1982*a*).

Effects on protein and RNA synthesis in isolated cerebral and cerebellar cells have been demonstrated following a single injection of 10 mg MeHg/kg (Syversen 1977, 1982*a*). This level of MeHg exposure did not produce weight loss or any of the other typical signs and symptoms of MeHg intoxication. Peak Hg concentrations attained in either cerebrum or cerebellum were less than 2 μg Hg/g of tissue. The temporal separation of the effects of MeHg on RNA and protein synthesis suggested that changes in RNA metabolism were required prior to any change in protein synthesis.

To examine the effects of chronic exposure to methyl mercury on protein synthesis in isolated neurons, Syversen (1982*b*) administered 1 mg or 5 mg MeHg/kg by mouth daily for up to 45 days. Control rats received daily oral doses of the vehicle. No effect on body weight was found in rats receiving up to 45 doses of 1 mg MeHg/kg. Rats receiving 5 mg MeHg/kg daily showed a reduced rate of increase in body weight after 20 daily doses. After 23–28 daily doses, these rats displayed hind-limb crossing, a characteristic sign of MeHg intoxication (Klein et al. 1972). For up to 31 days of MeHg dosing, cerebral and cerebellar MeHg concentrations were highly correlated with the cumulative MeHg dose. Following the in vivo labeling of brain protein as described above, rats were sacrificed and cerebral neurons and cerebellar granule and Purkinje cells were isolated. As in the study of the effects of acute MeHg exposure on protein synthesis, cerebellar granule cells were found to be the most sensitive to the inhibitory effect of MeHg. At a cerebellar Hg concentration of 0.78 μg/g, granule cells from MeHg-treated rats displayed a 34 percent reduction in the specific activity of protein, compared with control animals. Following longer dosing regimens or a higher dosing rate, similar reductions in protein synthesis were found in Purkinje cells at a cerebellar Hg concentration of 3–6 μg/g.

The effect of in vitro exposure to methyl mercury on protein synthesis by isolated cerebellar cells has been examined by Sarafian et al. (1984). For these studies, a population consisting predominantly of granule cells and interneurons was prepared from cerebella of Sprague-Dawley rat pups (7–15 days old). Freshly isolated cells were suspended in Krebs-Ringer buffer and exposed to MeHg at concentrations up to 40 μM. Protein synthesis was measured by the incorporation of [^{3}H]-phenylalanine into material precipitated at a final TCA concentration of 6.7 percent. This pellet was washed with 2 ml of 10% TCA and solubilized for radioassay. To determine whether the effects of MeHg on protein synthesis were due to changes in adenine nucleotide metabolism, the AMP, ADP, and ATP contents of cells exposed to MeHg were determined. Cellular integrity was determined by the leakage of lactate dehydrogenase (LDH) into the incubation media and by determination of intracellular K^+ and Na^+ concentrations.

Increasing concentrations of methyl mercury, up to 40 μM, decreased incorporation of phenylalanine into newly synthesized protein. The estimated IC_{50} for the effect of MeHg on protein synthesis was about 15 μM. The reduction of protein synthesis by MeHg exposure was apparently not due to changes in the uptake of precursor amino acid, because up to 40 μM MeHg did not alter intracellular concentration of [^{3}H]-phenylalanine. LDH leakage was also not increased by MeHg exposure. Cellular ATP contents and cellular energy charge (the ratio of adenine di- and tri-phosphorylated nucleotides to total cellular adenine nucleotides) were found to be less sensitive to MeHg than polyphenylalanine synthesis was. Exposure to the estimated IC_{50} (15 μM) for the effects of MeHg on protein synthesis produced less than a 20 percent reduction in ATP contents and no change in cellular energy charge. Although exposure to 20 μM MeHg decreased cellular K^+ concentrations, use of a high concentration of KCl in the incubation medium did not reverse the inhibition of protein produced by MeHg. Taken together, these results suggested that the effects of MeHg on protein synthesis were due to effects on translation of mRNA. Uptake of precursor amino acid, cellular energy status, and membrane integrity appeared to be resistant to the effects of MeHg indicating that altered protein synthesis was not secondary to effects of MeHg on these processes.

In more recent work, Sarafian and Verity (1985) have examined both RNA and protein synthesis by isolated cerebellar cells that were exposed to MeHg either in vivo or in vitro. In studies of the effects of MeHg exposure in vitro, donors were 2- to 21-day-old Sprague-Dawley rat pups. For studies of the effects of MeHg exposure in vivo, 6- to 13-day-old Sprague-Dawley rat pups received 45 nmols MeHg/g body weight ip 20–24 hours prior to sacrifice; controls received ip injections of distilled water. Protein synthesis was measured as incorporation of [^{3}H]-phenylalanine in TCA-precipitable material, and RNA synthesis was measured as incorporation of [^{3}H]-uridine into the TCA-insoluble pellet. In studies of the effects of MeHg exposure in vitro, RNA synthesis was found to be more sensitive to the inhibitory effects of MeHg than protein synthesis, especially at low MeHg concentrations. For example, at 5 μM MeHg, RNA synthesis was 60 percent of its control value, and protein synthesis was 80 percent of its control value. However, this difference in sensitivity was lost as MeHg concentration increased. At 10 μM MeHg, both RNA and protein synthesis were both about 40 percent of their control values. MeHg exposure in vitro did not increase [^{3}H]-uridine uptake.

Following exposure in vivo to methyl mercury, RNA synthesis was reduced to 77 percent of that found in cerebellar cells from control animals, but protein synthesis was 92 percent of its control value. Using PMS prepared from the brain of these MeHg-treated rats, it was found that protein synthesis directed by endogenous mRNA or by added poly U was decreased to about 70 percent of that found in control rats.

These results concerning the effects of methyl mercury exposure in vivo and in vitro on isolated cerebellar cells indicated that RNA synthesis was more sensitive than protein synthesis to the toxic effects of this agent. For both processes, it was suggested that alterations of synthetic rates were not due to changes in precursor availability, but rather to direct effects of MeHg on the machinery of RNA or protein synthesis. The ability of MeHg to disrupt RNA synthesis may be particularly significant in the production of effects following chronic exposure to this toxin during growth and development of the central nervous system.

Non-neuronal Cell Types   Studies of the effects of methyl mercury protein synthesis have also been profitably pursued in non-neuronal cells. Such studies are useful not only for direct comparison with results obtained in neuronal cells, but also because many of the cell lines used in these studies are better characterized than cells derived from the central nervous system. Important data concerning both mechanisms of toxicity and dose-effect relationships have been obtained in these studies.

Nakazawa et al. (1975) examined the effects of acute exposure in vitro of mouse L5178Y leukemic cells to methyl mercury, phenyl mercuric acetate (PMA), or $HgCl_2$. Cells were exposed to various concentrations of the mercurials for 60 minutes at $37°$ C in the presence of $[^3H]$-thymidine or $[^3H]$-uridine. At the end of exposure, cells were pelleted, lysed with sodium dodecyl sulfate and lysate collected on filter paper. Filters were washed with TCA and ethanol, dried, and radioassayed. For inhibition of DNA synthesis, the approximate IC_{50} for MeHg was 1 μM, for divalent Hg was 6 μM, and for PMA was 4 μM. These investigators found that increasing MeHg concentrations over the range of 1–10 μM was associated with increasing single strand scission of DNA. Further studies showed that the rate of DNA chain elongation was reduced in the presence of 1 μM MeHg. These results suggested that MeHg exerted a direct effect on DNA replication and that the effect of MeHg on DNA metabolism was not due to an effect on the availability of precursor nucleotides.

Further dose-effect studies were reported by Gruenwedel and Cruikshank (1979), who investigated the effects of methyl mercury on DNA, RNA, and protein synthesis in HeLa S3 cells. In these studies, cells were exposed to various concentrations of MeHg for 12 hours prior to addition of the labeled precursors ($[^3H]$-thymidine, $[^3H]$-uridine, or $[^3H]$-leucine). After a 30-minute labeling period, cells were harvested and lysed and material precipitable in 5% TCA was collected on Millipore filters. Dried filters were radioassayed to determine the amount of tritium incorporated into DNA, RNA, or protein. For DNA synthesis, there was no inhibition at an MeHg concentration of 1 μM; at 10 μM, however, inhibition approached 100 percent. Similar results were found for RNA synthesis. By comparison, protein synthesis was less sensitive to the effects of MeHg than either DNA or RNA synthesis. Complete inhibition of protein synthesis was attained at an MeHg concentration of about 35 μM. Notably, DNA, RNA, and protein synthesis were all more sensitive indicators of cellular injury than was cell viability, and for each synthetic parameter measured the dose-effect relationship was extremely steep.

Further studies by these investigators (Gruenwedel et al. 1981) examined the relationship between cellular methyl mercury accumulation and DNA and protein synthesis. In these studies, [^{3}H]-thymidine or [^{3}H]-leucine incorporation into DNA or protein in HeLa S3 cells was expressed as a function of the amount of MeHg bound to cells (moles of MeHg per cell). The estimated IC_{50} for MeHg inhibition of DNA synthesis was 35.5×10^{-16} moles per cell; and for protein synthesis it was 63.1×10^{-16} moles per cell. As found in earlier studies, dose-effect relationships were quite steep. These investigators suggested that MeHg interfered with DNA synthesis by specific binding to the basic N(3) and N(1) of thymidine and guanosine, which disrupted H-bonding and base-stacking in the DNA molecule.

Other studies of the mechanistic basis of the effect of methyl mercury on cellular metabolism have been reported. Frenkel and Randles (1982) measured DNA and RNA synthesis in nuclei isolated from HeLa cells and in intact HeLa cells. For DNA synthesis in intact cells, the IC_{50} was estimated at 20 μM; in nuclei, the IC_{50} was 8 μM. For RNA synthesis in intact cells, the IC_{50} was about 35 μM. In contrast, addition of MeHg to isolated nuclei increased RNA synthesis. This stimulation of RNA synthesis was due to stimulation of α-amanitin-sensitive RNA polymerase (RNA polymerase II) by MeHg. Other studies indicated that MeHg inhibited initiation of RNA chain synthesis by RNA polymerase and chain elongation by polymerases I and II. Exposure of calf thymus DNA to MeHg concentrations greater than 1 mM results in increased transcription of the DNA template by RNA polymerase II (Frenkel et al. 1985). This increase may be due to an MeHg-induced increase in the number or affinity of polymerase binding sites.

Comparative studies of the effects of methyl mercury and inorganic mercury on protein synthesis have been reported. Nakada et al. (1980) examined protein synthesis in mouse glioma cells, in Yoshida ascites sarcoma cells, and in rabbit reticulocytes exposed to these agents. Protein synthesis was measured by incorporation of [^{3}H]-leucine into the acid-insoluble fraction of intact cells and by use of a PMS-directed cell-free system. In the sarcoma cell line, MeHg was a more potent inhibitor of protein synthesis than was inorganic Hg. In rabbit reticulocytes and mouse glioma cells, the agents were about equally potent inhibitors of protein synthesis. This difference in relative potency may reflect differences in the ability of MeHg and inorganic Hg to cross cell membranes. For example, at equimolar concentrations of the two mercurials in the incubation medium, mouse glioma cells attained a higher burden of MeHg than of inorganic Hg. Thus, the cell membrane may play a critical role in controlling the entry of this toxin into cells and in its subsequent effect on protein synthesis.

These studies in non-neuronal cells have permitted a partial characterization of relationships between methyl mercury accumulation and effects on DNA, RNA, and protein synthesis. Mechanistic studies have contributed to our understanding of the processes by which MeHg perturbs DNA and RNA synthesis. To date, less is known about the mechanism by which MeHg affects protein synthesis in isolated cells.

Studies with Cell-Free Systems

The effects of methyl mercury on protein synthesis in cell-free systems have also been investigated. The cell-free system allows evaluation of the direct effects of MeHg on the synthetic process without some of the potential difficulties that accompany studies of protein synthesis in intact organisms or in isolated cells. Further, by reconstitution studies, it is also possible to use the cell-free system to determine the site of action of methyl mercury.

Sugano et al. (1975) determined the effects of MeHg, inorganic Hg, and Cd on cell-free protein synthesis using the liver and brain from adult male rats. Livers were homogenized, and the homogenate was centrifuged at 12,000 × g to prepare PMS. The PMS was layered over 0.55 M sucrose in HEPES buffer and centrifuged at 100,000 × g for 2 hours. The supernate was designated as the cytosolic fraction, and the pellet as the microsomal fraction. Cell-free amino acid incorporating systems consisted of the cellular fractions incubated with various concentrations of MeHg, Hg, or Cd and [^{14}C]-leucine for 30 minutes at 37° C. Reactions were terminated by addition of 5% TCA; following heating to 95° C for 15 minutes, precipitates were collected on Millipore filters and radioassayed.

Methyl mercury decreased [^{14}C]-leucine incorporation into cell-free systems that contained either the microsomal or the polysomal fraction from liver or brain. For the microsomal fraction from either tissue, the IC$_{50}$ for incorporation of [^{14}C]-leucine into protein was between 0.25 and 0.50 mM. Complete inhibition of protein synthesis by the microsomal fraction was found at an MeHg concentration of 0.5 mM. For the brain polysomal fraction used in the cell-free amino acid incorporation system, complete inhibition of [^{14}C] incorporation into protein occurred at an MeHg concentration of 0.25 mM. About 70 percent inhibition of protein synthesis occurred in the liver polysomal fraction at an MeHg concentration of 0.25 mM; inhibition was complete at an MeHg concentration of 0.5 mM. Notably for both liver and brain and for both the microsomal and polysomal fractions, Cd and Hg were each about 10 times more potent (on a molar basis) than MeHg as inhibitors of protein synthesis in the cell-free system. Because the polysomal-cytosol system was found to be more sensitive to metal-induced reduction in protein synthesis than the microsomal-cytosol system, the effects of methyl mercury and inorganic mercury on polysome structure were examined. Incubation of polysomes and cytosol derived from brain or liver with MeHg resulted in disaggregation of polysomes to yield monosomes and disomes. Brain polysomes appeared more sensitive than liver polysomes to the disaggregative effects of MeHg. Brain polysomes were present primarily as monosomes and disomes at an MeHg concentration of 0.25 mM, while liver polysomes fully dissociated to monosomes and disomes at an MeHg concentration of 0.5 mM. Inorganic mercury was found to be more potent than methyl mercury in disaggregating polysomes. Dissociation of polysomes to yield monosomes and disomes was attained for brain polysomes at 0.025 mM Hg and for liver polysomes at 0.05 mM Hg. Notably, the concentrations of methyl mercury or inorganic mercury that dissociated brain or liver polysomes were equal to those that fully inhibited protein synthesis in the cell-free amino acid incorporating system. The disaggregation of polysomes in mouse kidney following mercuric chloride treatment has been reported (Pezerovic et al. 1981).

The relationship between polysome disaggregation and exposure to MeHg or divalent Hg was further investigated by determining the effects of these metals on cytosolic RNase (ribonuclease) activity (Sugano et al. 1975). Both metals were found to increase RNase activity. Their effects on this activity could be prevented by concurrent addition of β-mercaptoethanol to the incubation mixture. These results were consistent with a metal-dependent inactivation of a cytosolic RNase inhibitor. To test this hypothesis, either β-mercaptoethanol or *L*-cysteine was added to a cell-free amino acid incorporating system containing the PMS fraction from liver and brain and various concentrations of MeHg or Hg. At a concentration of 1 mM, MeHg inhibited protein synthesis by brain PMS by about 73 percent. In the presence of 1 mM MeHg, addition of 5 mM β-mercaptoethanol or 5 mM *L*-cysteine resulted in 28 percent and 10 percent reductions respectively in brain-PMS-directed protein synthesis. Similarly, addition of β-mercaptoethanol reduced the degree of inhibition of protein synthesis directed by liver PMS that was produced by addition of MeHg or Hg to the cell-free amino acid incorporating system. Thus, it was concluded that MeHg and Hg can affect protein synthesis by altering polysome stability. This effect may be attributable to the ability of MeHg and Hg to inactivate a cytosolic RNase inhibitor. The resulting increase in RNase activity may result in a breakdown of polysomes and a reduction in protein synthesis.

In a study utilizing MeHg-treated rats as donors for the preparation of liver and brain PMS and cytosol, Omata et al. (1978) investigated the effects of chronic methyl mercury treatment on protein synthesis in a cell-free system. Adult female rats received daily subcutaneous injections of 10 mg $CH_3HgCl/$ kg. Controls received daily injections of the vehicle—10 mM $NaCO_3$. Rats received up to 7 daily injections of methyl mercury. Animals were sacrificed on days 3, 5, 8, 10,11, and 14 of the study. PMS was prepared from the liver and brain of MeHg- and vehicle-treated rats. Incorporation of $[^{14}C]$-leucine into 5% TCA-precipitable material was measured using liver or brain PMS in a cell-free system.

The effects of methyl mercury on cell-free protein synthesis by liver or brain PMS can be presented in terms of the progression of signs and symptoms of MeHg intoxication in the rat. In the study described in the following paragraph, a latent period (days 7–11) and a symptomatic period (days 13 and 14) for MeHg poisoning were defined by these investigators.

Brain-PMS-directed cell-free protein synthesis was slightly increased in MeHg-treated rats for the first 7 days of the study period. During both the latent period and the symptomatic period, however, treatment with methyl mercury resulted in a progressive decline in cell-free protein synthesis directed by brain PMS. By day 14, incorporation directed by brain PMS of MeHg-treated rats was 56 percent of that found in vehicle-treated animals. In contrast, MeHg treatment markedly increased protein synthesis by liver PMS between days 3 and 11 of the study to between 150 and 250 percent of control values. On day 14, when rats were symptomatic, cell-free protein synthesis using liver PMS had declined to 56 percent of the control activity. To further characterize the site of action of MeHg on protein synthesis in the brain, PMS from MeHg-treated or vehicle-treated rats was centrifuged at 100,000 × g to yield cytosol and a microsomal pellet. Recombination of these fractions from MeHg-treated or control rats indicated that the reduction of protein synthesis by PMS was about equally inhibited when either microsomes or cytosol from an MeHg-treated rat was used. Thus, the contribution of both fractions to brain protein synthesis appeared to be affected similarly by in vivo exposure to methyl mercury.

The effects of methyl mercury and inorganic mercury on protein synthesis by brain PMS have been compared (Syversen 1981). In this study, brain PMS prepared from adult male rats was chromatographed on Sephadex G-25 gel to yield a high molecular weight fraction, which was then added to a cell-free amino acid incorporating system. The IC_{50} for protein synthesis for Hg was 2.5 mM, and for MeHg it was mM. Two inhibitors of protein synthesis, puromycin and cycloheximide, were each added at a 100 mM concentration to the cell-free system, and the combined effects of MeHg and these agents on protein synthesis were determined. It was found that addition of cycloheximide did not change the shape of the inhibition curve or the IC_{50} for protein synthesis. Addition of puromycin to the incubation medium changed the shape of the inhibition curve and also shifted the IC_{50} for MeHg to about 1 mM. This finding suggested an interaction between the effects of MeHg and puromycin in the alteration of protein synthesis. Notably, puromycin has been reported to promote polysome disaggregation and premature release of the polypeptide, and MeHg had earlier been shown to promote polysome disaggregation in liver and brain (Sugano et al. 1975). In intact animals, disorganization of neuronal ribosomes has been reported to be an early sign of MeHg intoxication (Jacobs et al. 1977). Thus, MeHg may act in a manner analogous to puromycin and alter protein synthesis by polysomal disaggregation or by affecting peptide release from the ribosome.

Cheung and Verity (1983) have compared the effects of in vivo and in vitro exposure to methyl mercury on brain cell-free protein synthesis. For these studies, 10- to 25-day-old neonatal rats received single ip injections of MeHg chloride or of distilled water. Treated and control rats were sacrificed 18–20 hours after dosing, and PMS, ribosomes, and a pH 5 enzyme fraction were prepared. The extent of protein synthesis directed by PMS or ribosomes was determined using a cell-free amino acid incorporating system. Relative to control rats, PMS prepared from neonates receiving 30–40 nM MeHg/g body weight showed up to a 60 percent inhibition of amino acid incorporation. At MeHg doses below 30 nM/g, PMS-directed protein synthesis was not affected. Addition of MeHg directly to the PMS-directed cell-free system resulted in a biphasic effect on protein synthesis. Addition of up to 40 mM MeHg to the incubation medium increased protein synthesis to about 150–200 percent of control values. At higher MeHg concentrations, protein synthesis was inhibited. The estimated IC_{50} for MeHg in this system was about 60 mM. As previously reported by Sugano et al. (1975), these effects of MeHg added in vitro on PMS-directed protein synthesis were antagonized by addition of sulfhydryl compounds. However, addition of sulfhydryl compounds to cell-free systems containing PMS prepared from the brains of MeHg-treated rats did not restore amino acid incorporating capacity to control values. In fact, addition of these agents to the PMS-directed systems led to a further decrease in protein synthetic activity. Thus, the interaction between sulfhydryls and MeHg, and the effect of MeHg on protein synthesis, depended on whether MeHg exposure occurred in the intact animal or in vitro.

Cheung and Verity (1983) also examined the effects of methyl mercury administration on ribosomal protein synthesis. For these studies, the two components of the system—ribosomes and the pH 5 enzyme preparation—were obtained from MeHg-treated or control neonatal rats. By combining ribosomes and pH 5 enzymes from MeHg-treated and control rats, these investigators showed that the inhibitory effect of MeHg on protein synthesis was due to perturbation of the activity of the pH 5 enzyme fraction and not to an effect in the ribosomal fraction. Exposure of PMS in vitro to a low concentration of MeHg (20 mM) resulted in a stimulation of cell-free protein synthetic activity. This perturbation of activity was also found to be attributable to an effect of MeHg on the pH 5 enzyme fraction. These investigators suggested that the effects of MeHg on protein synthesis might stem from the existence of an endogenous regulator of protein synthesis that is sensitive to methyl mercury. This regulator is postulated to be in the pH 5 enzyme fraction. It is hypothesized that the rate of protein synthesis in vivo is determined by the functional activities of the ribosomal fraction and the pH 5 enzymes, which are modulated by the action of the postulated regulator. Low concentrations of MeHg reduce the effective concentrations of the regulator and thus stimulate protein synthesis. At higher MeHg concentrations, however, the capacity of the regulator to bind MeHg is exceeded, and MeHg then binds to other components of the pH 5 enzyme mixture. This binding alters the ability of these components to participate in protein synthesis. The net result of the reduction of endogenous regulator activity by MeHg and the interaction of MeHg with other components of the pH 5 enzyme mixture is to reduce protein synthesis.

The Use of Synaptosomal Preparations

Synaptosomal preparations have also been used to examine the neurotoxic effects of methyl mercury. These membrane-bounded vesicles are prepared from the synaptic region of neurons and as such are relatively homogeneous, both structurally and functionally. This lack of heterogeneity may permit more definitive studies of the effects of MeHg on cellular function.

Verity et al. (1975) examined the effects of MeHg on respiration in synaptosomes exposed to MeHg in vivo or in vitro. For in vivo exposure, adult male or female Sprague-Dawley rats received daily intragastric doses of 10 mg MeHg/kg. Rats were sacrificed for the preparation of synaptosomes during either the latent phase (6–10 days after beginning of MeHg treatment) or the neurotoxic phase (more than 10 days after beginning of treatment). Respiratory control, state 3, state 4, and 2,4-dinitrophenol(DNP)-stimulated respiration were measured using succinate, glutamate, or pyruvate plus malate as substrates. During the latent phase, none of these variables was affected; but during the neurotoxic phase, respiratory control was reduced significantly for each substrate. Cerebellar synaptosomes displayed a larger inhibition of DNP-stimulated respiration using glutamate during either the latent phase or the neurotoxic phase.

For in vitro studies, synaptosomes were prepared from brains of untreated rats and exposed to various concentrations of MeHg in the incubation medium. At MeHg concentrations of 5–10 μM, the respiratory control index (the ratio of the respiratory rate in the presence of ADP to the rate after phosphorylation) declined when glutamate or succinate, or malate plus pyruvate, was used as a substrate. State 4 respiratory rate was increased by increasing MeHg concentrations from 5 to 15 μM. At higher concentrations, state 4, state 3, and DNP-stimulated respiration rates were reduced. Because oxidative phosphorylation and coupled respiration in synaptosomes depend on mitochondrial Mg^{2+}-dependent-ATPase, the effect of MeHg on activity of this enzyme was determined. No inhibition of Mg^{2+}-dependent-ATPase activity was noted at MeHg concentrations up to 20 μM. Thus, the inhibitory effects on respiration seen at MeHg concentrations less than 20 μM could not be attributed to an effect on this enzyme activity. The effect of MeHg on terminal electron transfer was examined by determining its effect on cytochrome-*c*-oxidase activity. For these studies, the enzyme was examined not only in its native form but also following activation, by freeze-thawing in liquid nitrogen. In its activated form, the approximate IC_{50} for MeHg was 2 μM; for the native enzyme, however, the estimated IC_{50} would be greater than 50 μM. The differential effect of MeHg on native and activated enzyme probably reflects a permeability barrier affecting access of MeHg to an enzyme that is bound to the inner mitochondrial membrane. Thus, the effects of MeHg upon respiration cannot be directly attributed to its effect on cytochrome-*c*-oxidase activity. The stimulation of the state 4 respiratory rate by MeHg was postulated to be attributable to an MeHg-dependent increase in the permeation of K^+ ions across the membrane.

The effect of methyl mercury exposure in vivo or in vitro on synaptosomal protein synthesis was investigated by Verity et al. (1977). For studies of exposure in vivo, female Sprague-Dawley rats received 10 mg CH_3HgCl/kg by mouth daily for 6–8 days. Rats were sacrificed both during the asymptomatic phase (10 days after beginning of treatment) and the symptomatic phase (20–22 days after the beginning of treatment), and synaptosomes were prepared from cerebrum and cerebellum as described by Verity et al. (1975). During the asymptomatic period, MeHg treatment did not alter incorporation of [^{14}C]-leucine into synaptosomal proteins in either cerebral or cerebellar preparations. During the symptomatic period, however, MeHg treatment resulted in a 40–60 percent decrease in leucine incorporation by synaptosomes prepared from cerebrum or cerebellum. Using synaptosomes prepared from the cerebral cortex of untreated rats, inhibition of synaptosomal protein synthesis by MeHg was shown to be noncompetitive. These investigators also examined the uptake of [^{14}C]-leucine into synaptosomes exposed to MeHg in vitro. At an MeHg concentration of 12 μM, no alteration in leucine uptake was found. This finding suggested that alteration of synaptosomal protein synthesis by MeHg exposure was not due to changes in amino acid availability. Similarly, no relationship was found between Na^+/K^+-ATPase activity and MeHg-induced alterations in synaptosomal protein synthesis. Addition of sulfhydryl group reagents (cysteine and glutathione) to synaptosomal preparations protected protein synthesis against the inhibitory effects of MeHg. Both the mitochondrial and extramitochondrial components of synaptosomal protein synthesis were found to be affected by MeHg exposure in vitro.

These studies were extended to examine the effects of MeHg upon synaptosomal integrity and capacity for protein synthesis (Cheung and Verity 1981). In synaptosomes, both a prokaryotic ribosome-dependent system and a eukaryotic ribosomal-like system are available for protein synthesis. Because these systems are sensitive to chloramphenicol or cycloheximide, respectively, it is possible to examine them separately. Further, it is possible to enumerate the factors that permit optimal synthesis in the synaptosome. These criteria are an osmotically intact, membrane-limited structure, coupled mitochondrial respiration and oxidative phosphorylation, maintenance of an Na^+-K^+ gradient across the membrane, capacity for amino acid uptake, and intact intrasynaptosomal ribosomes. Because these factors can be identified, it is possible to examine the effects of MeHg on each of them.

For these studies, synaptosomes were prepared from either 12- to 18-day-old neonatal or adult female Sprague-Dawley rats. Synaptosomes were prepared from brain cortices by means of a discontinuous Ficoll-sucrose gradient procedure. Synaptosomal protein synthesis was assayed by incubating synaptosomes in a medium containing 10 μCi [^{3}H]-leucine/ml. Proteins were precipitated at a final TCA concentration of 8 percent. Exposure to 25 μM MeHg reduced the amount of protein synthesized per milligram of synaptosomal protein by 27 percent for neonates and 53 percent for adults. At an MeHg concentration of 50 μM, protein synthesis by neonatal synaptosomes was inhibited 67 percent and, by adult synaptosomes, 91 percent. The mechanisms by which MeHg might exert these effects on protein synthesis were examined. The osmotic integrity of synaptosomes was assessed by measuring the release of the cytosolic enzyme, lactate dehydrogenase (LDH), into the incubation medium. Up to 50 μM MeHg did not increase the LDH release by neonatal synaptosomes, suggesting that the agent did not disrupt the synaptosomes. Addition of up to 100 μM MeHg to the incubation medium also failed to change synaptosomal volume as measured by the distribution of [^{3}H]-water and [^{14}C]-dextran. However, exposure to up to 100 μM MeHg was associated with a decrease in the K^+ contents and an increase in the Na^+ contents of synaptosomes.

Because protein synthesis by the microsomal fractions from neonatal rat brain was known to be K^+- and ATP-dependent, chloramphenicol-resistant, and cycloheximide-sensitive, these investigators postulated that MeHg may exert its effect on protein synthesis by disrupting the microsomal-dependent portion of synaptosomal protein synthesis. Further investigation indicated that exposure of synaptosomes to MeHg led to a dose-dependent reduction in synaptosomal ATP contents (approximate IC_{50} for MeHg of 35 μM). Integrating these data, it can be suggested that MeHg exerted its effects upon synaptosomal protein synthesis by increasing the efflux of K^+. This increased efflux may be related to the decline in the K^+ contents of intraterminal mitochondria and a decline in mitochondrial oxidation, resulting in a reduction in synaptosomal ATP levels. In parallel, a decline in synaptosomal K^+ contents led to reduced rates of ribosomal translation. Thus, these interactions of MeHg reduced the K^+- and ATP-dependent synthesis of proteins by synaptosomal microsomes.

Conclusions

This chapter has examined the literature on the effects of methyl mercury on protein synthesis. Although MeHg is considered primarily a neurotoxin, this review also includes studies of the effects of MeHg upon protein synthesis in non-neuronal cells and in tissues besides the nervous system. The objectives of this chapter can be summarized as a series of questions that have served as guides evaluating the data reviewed herein. (1) What are the mechanisms by which protein synthesis is affected by MeHg? (2) What is the dose-effect relationship between MeHg exposure and effects on protein synthesis? (3) How can these data be used to assess the hazard associated with exposure to methyl mercury?

Mechanistic Studies

Studies of the mechanisms by which methyl mercury affects protein synthesis have been pursued not only in intact animals but also in a variety of tissue slices, in isolated cells and organelles, and in cell-free amino acid incorporation systems. Each of these preparations offers advantages and limitations. Thus, while studies in intact animals have been important in characterizing the time course of the effects of MeHg on protein synthesis, there are distinct limitations for studies of protein synthesis in such complex systems. Nevertheless, the results of studies in intact animals indicate the areas in which research using better defined systems might be conducted.

Of particular interest are studies of the differential effects of methyl mercury on protein synthesis in the liver and the brain. Beginning with the work of Sugano et al. (1975), different effects of MeHg on protein synthesis in the liver and the brain have been reported. Further studies (Omata et al. 1978, 1981) demonstrated that MeHg disaggregated CNS polysomes at concentrations lower than those required to disaggregate liver polysomes. This effect was attributed to inactivation of a putative cytosolic RNase inhibitor by MeHg, which resulted in the destabilization of polysomes. Stimulation by MeHg of protein synthesis in vitro using liver PMS has been related to increased Mg^{2+}-dependent RNA polymerase activity following MeHg exposure (Omata et al. 1981). A similar role of MeHg in the inactivation of an endogenous cytosolic inhibitor of protein synthesis has been suggested by Cheung and Verity (1983). Inactivation of an inhibitor by MeHg might account for stimulation of protein synthesis noted after MeHg exposure. Stimulation of protein synthesis by MeHg may also be related to an MeHg-induced increase in peptide elongation factors 1 and 2. Recent studies have examined the effects of MeHg on peptide chain initiation and elongation (Cheung and Verity 1985). A high concentration of MeHg (100 μM) added in vitro to neonatal rat brain PMS did not interfere with methionine binding to polyribosomes, and synthesis of peptide bonds was unaffected. Exposure to methyl mercury affected peptide chain elongation, probably because of an inhibition of tRNA synthetase activity. Alteration of the rate of protein synthesis following MeHg exposure may also be due to the inanative effects of this agent. Other research has shown that hepatic protein synthesis was sensitive to changes in food intake, while CNS protein synthesis was relatively unchanged by alterations in food intake (Omata et al. 1978; Lapin and Carter 1982).

The relative sensitivity of protein, DNA, and RNA synthesis to the effects of methyl mercury were compared. Following exposure in vivo to MeHg, cerebellar granule and Purkinje cells and cerebral neurons all displayed decreased RNA and protein synthesis. The effects on RNA synthesis may precede changes in protein synthesis in these cells (Syversen 1982a). Studies with isolated cerebellar cells also indicated that RNA synthesis may be more sensitive than protein synthesis to the toxic effect of MeHg (Sarafian et al. 1984; Sarafian and Verity 1985). MeHg exposure also reduced thymidine incorporation into DNA, increased DNA single-strand scission, and reduced the rate of DNA chain elongation (Nakazawa et al. 1975). In contrast, RNA synthesis may have been increased by MeHg exposure, possibly by activation of RNA polymerase II (Frenkel and Randles 1982) or by an increase in the number or affinity of RNA polymerase II binding sites on DNA (Frenkel et al. 1985). In HeLa S3 cells, both DNA and RNA synthesis were more sensitive than protein synthesis to the inhibitory effects of MeHg. The relationship between the relative sensitivities of protein, DNA, and RNA synthesis to modulation by MeHg exposure requires further study.

Another approach to understanding the mechanism by which methyl mercury alters CNS protein synthesis was pursued by Verity and associates. Using synaptosomal preparations to determine the effects of MeHg on metabolic status and protein synthesis, these investigators showed that MeHg exposure altered synaptosomal membrane permeability (Verity et al. 1975). As a consequence of this change, synaptosomal K^+ contents decreased, and Mg^{2+}-ATPase activity declined and microsomal protein synthesis decreased. Thus, an effect of MeHg on membrane permeability may account ultimately for the alteration of protein synthesis following MeHg exposure.

These investigators also demonstrated that alterations of synaptosomal protein synthesis by methyl mercury were not related to changes in precursor amino acid availability and could be reversed by adding the sulfhydryl-containing reagents—cysteine and glutathione (Verity et al. 1977). The former point was of interest in that it indicated that the effect of MeHg did not depend on altered availability of precursor amino acids but was a direct effect on the synthetic process. The modulation of the effects of MeHg by glutathione is of interest because glutathione is a major soluble binding ligand for MeHg in the CNS (Thomas and Smith 1979*b*). Modulation of MeHg availability by its binding to glutathione may play a role in the neurotoxicity of this agent. Further studies (Cheung and Verity 1981) indicated that MeHg exposure increased the efflux of K^+ from the synaptosome and thus altered ATP production. Decline in protein synthesis in the synaptosome may relate to these changes in K^+ fluxes and energy metabolism.

In summary, available data suggest that methyl mercury has a number of effects on protein synthesis, which not only vary among tissues, cells, or organelles examined but probably also change as a function of MeHg concentration and the interval between exposure and analysis. The particular vulnerability of CNS protein synthesis to alteration by MeHg may relate to the sensitivity of CNS polysomes to disaggregation by MeHg. However, the molecular basis for this effect remains uncharacterized.

Dose-Effect Relationships

The dose-dependence for biological effects of an agent is a fundamental concept in toxicology. Determination of the relationship between toxin distribution and biological effect is commonly an early step in evaluating the hazard of exposure for any agent. In studies of the toxic effects of MeHg, much effort has been expended in an attempt to relate the concentration of MeHg in biological indicator media, such as hair or blood, to the intake of MeHg or to its deleterious effects (e.g., Sherlock et al. 1982; Kershaw et al. 1980; Turner et al. 1980). Studies in experimental animals have also examined the relationship between exposure to MeHg, accumulation of MeHg in tissues, and the development of signs and symptoms of MeHg intoxication. Similarly, the extent of CNS injury following MeHg exposure was shown to be a function of integrated exposure of the CNS to this toxin (Magos et al. 1978). These general topics have recently been reviewed by Piotrowski and Inskip (1981).

In terms of neurotoxic effects of methyl mercury, the work by Suzuki (1969) and Grant (1973) indicated that signs of MeHg intoxication appeared in mice, rats, cats, and squirrel monkeys when brain Hg concentrations rose to between 10 and 30 μg Hg/g of tissue. Early work by Sugano et al. (1975) demonstrated a reduction of brain protein synthesis in the rat when brain Hg concentration was about 30 $\mu g/g$ of tissue. It is worth noting that the relatively narrow range of brain Hg concentrations associated with the development of neurotoxicity contrasted markedly with the very wide range of blood Hg concentrations attained in various species during MeHg exposure. In particular, rats attained much higher concentrations of MeHg in blood than did other species. This accumulation of Hg in blood was attributable to the high capacity of the rat erythrocyte for MeHg (Norseth and Clarkson 1970). Despite this difference, rats displayed signs and symptoms of MeHg intoxication at brain Hg concentrations approximately the same as those producing effects in other species.

Other data from isolated cells indicate that MeHg exposure affects protein, DNA, and RNA synthesis. For HeLa S3 cells, DNA synthesis appeared to be more sensitive to inhibition by MeHg than protein synthesis was (Gruenwedel and Cruikshank 1979). The IC_{50} for protein synthesis was about 7 μg Hg/ml of medium and, for DNA synthesis, about 2 $\mu g/ml$. Similar studies in which Hg concentration was expressed as mole of Hg per cell indicated that the IC_{50} for protein synthesis was about twice that for DNA synthesis (Gruenwedel et al. 1981). Data from studies with L5178Y leukemic cells indicated that the IC_{50} for DNA synthesis was very low (2 ng/ml) (Nakazawa et al. 1975). In contrast, other studies with HeLa S3 cells indicated a much higher IC_{50} for DNA synthesis (7 $\mu g/ml$). Differences in IC_{50} estimates among different studies probably reflect differences in experimental design or in the sensitivity of cell lines used. It is likely that, in general, DNA synthesis is more sensitive to the inhibitory effects of MeHg than is protein synthesis.

Studies with isolated cells from the central nervous system have also provided useful data on the sensitivity of protein synthesis to methyl mercury. Syversen (1977) showed that the previously characterized difference of cerebral neurons and cerebellar Purkinje and granule cells to the toxic effects of MeHg was accompanied by differences in protein synthesis. Thus, granule cells, which manifest morphological change earliest during MeHg exposure, were found to display the largest and most prolonged reduction in protein synthesis. However, the difference in sensitivity was not related to obvious differences in the kinetic profile for MeHg accumulation and loss from the various cell types. All cell types attained roughly equal Hg concentrations and showed similar patterns of MeHg loss. These data suggested that kinetic differences in Hg uptake and loss did not explain differences in cellular sensitivity. There must be qualitative differences in the response of the different cell types to MeHg. Studies with cells isolated from rats chronically exposed to MeHg indicated that protein synthesis can be inhibited at Hg concentrations as low as 0.78 $\mu g/g$ in granule cells and between 3 and 6 $\mu g/g$ in Purkinje cells and cerebral neurons (Syversen 1982b). These concentrations were considerably below those that produced effects on protein synthesis in other studies in intact animals discussed above. Because injury to the central nervous system was a product of the integrated exposure of the CNS to MeHg (Magos et al. 1978), long-term exposure to relatively low levels of MeHg may affect protein synthesis in the CNS. Further studies of the effects of chronic MeHg exposure on CNS protein synthesis are required.

Studies with cell-free systems have contributed significantly to understanding of the mechanisms of the effects of methyl mercury on CNS protein synthesis. However, it is difficult to extrapolate results from these studies to the concentrations attained in the central nervous system in intact animals. In general, these studies have employed rather high concentrations of MeHg. For example, Cheung and Verity (1983) determined the IC_{50} for protein synthesis of about 12 mg/ml of incubation media, and Syversen (1981) estimated the IC_{50} for protein synthesis to be 1.4 mg/ml. One notable finding in these studies with cell-free systems is that of Sugano et al. (1975), indicating that the concentration of MeHg that disaggregated brain polysomes into monosomes was about half that required to disaggregate liver polysomes. This suggested a tissue-dependent difference in liver and brain, which might account for the greater vulnerability of the CNS to the toxic effects of this agent. Studies on the effects of MeHg on peptide chain initiation and elongation have demonstrated that MeHg exposure altered elongation (Cheung and Verity 1985). This effect was thought to be due to inhibition of tRNA synthetase by MeHg. The estimated IC_{50} for this effect was 8 μM (1.6 $\mu g/ml$).

Comparative Sensitivity of Developing and Mature Organisms

The vulnerability of developing organisms to the effects of MeHg is of special interest. Studies on children exposed in utero to MeHg have demonstrated that MeHg can be a teratogen (Murakami 1972) and can affect neurodevelopment (Amin-Zaki et al. 1974; Clarkson et al. 1981; Greenwood 1985). In experimental studies, these effects of MeHg exposure in utero on neurodevelopment have been further characterized. In particular, the ability of in utero exposure to relatively low levels of MeHg to produce alterations in behavior at maturity is striking (Spyker et al. 1972; Hughes and Sparber 1978; Eccles and Annau 1982*a*, 1982*b*).

The relationship between these effects of methyl mercury on neurodevelopment and behavior and on protein synthesis is not known. Exposure to MeHg was not found to alter protein synthesis in fetal rats (Chen et al. 1979) or in early postnatal life (Farris and Smith 1975). In the mouse, exposure in utero to MeHg reduced protein accumulation in the fetus (Olson and Massaro 1978). This effect may result from decreased availability of precursor amino acids in the fetus exposed to MeHg. Studies of the effect of MeHg exposure on rats during early postnatal life indicated that MeHg increased protein synthesis in young animals (5–15 days old) but inhibited it in older (17–21 days old) rats (Joiner and Hupp 1979). Slotkin et al. (1985) recently showed that the effects of postnatal exposure to MeHg upon protein synthesis in the

CNS are dependent not only upon the brain region examined but also on the developmental status of the regions at the time of investigation. Recent studies by Verity and co-workers (Cheung and Verity 1983, 1985; Sarafian et al. 1984; Sarafian and Verity 1985) on the mechanism by which MeHg alters protein synthesis in vivo or in vitro have employed neonatal rats. These studies indicate that MeHg affected protein synthesis in the CNS by reducing the rate of tRNA aminoacylation.

While these studies have contributed to our understanding of the effects of methyl mercury on protein synthesis in the developing central nervous system, they have not, as a whole, addressed the question of the comparative sensitivity of protein synthesis in the developing and mature CNS to the effects of this toxin. However, it can be surmised that protein synthesis in the developing CNS is at least as sensitive as that in the mature CNS to the effects of MeHg. The issue of the sensitivity of protein synthesis in the developing CNS to MeHg is complicated by the fact that developing rodents avidly retain both MeHg (Doherty et al. 1977; Thomas et al. 1982) and inorganic Hg (Jugo 1976; Thomas and Smith 1979a). For example, rats treated with either MeHg or inorganic Hg at 7 days of age excrete these metals very slowly until about 15–18 days of age, when there is the abrupt onset of a more rapid clearance process. During this interval, the integrated exposure of tissues to MeHg or its metabolite, inorganic Hg, will be quite high. If the magnitude of CNS injury by MeHg reflects the integrated exposure to this agent (Magos et al. 1978), the effects of MeHg on protein synthesis in the developing organism may be influenced by avid retention of MeHg by the neonate. Other studies suggest that following MeHg exposure the fetal CNS attains higher Hg concentrations than does the maternal CNS (Null et al. 1973; King et al. 1976). However, the Hg concentration attained in the CNS of 7-day-old rats treated with 1 μm of MeHg/kg subcutaneously was not higher than that found in adult rats treated at the same dosage level (D. J. Thomas, H. L. Fisher, L. L. Hall, and P. Mushak, unpublished observation). Taken together, these data indicate that kinetic factors, particularly developmental changes in distribution and retention of methyl mercury, must be carefully evaluated in a study of the dose-dependency of the effects of this agent on protein synthesis in the developing central nervous system.

Acknowledgments

We thank Dr. Saburo Omata, Department of Biochemistry, Niigata University, for providing an extensive bibliography of recent Japanese papers on effects of methyl mercury on protein synthesis. In addition, one of us (D.J.T.) received partial support from the Center for Alternatives to Animal Testing, School of Hygiene and Public Health, Johns Hopkins University.

References

Adamson, L. F.; Herington, A. C.; and Bornstein, J. (1972). Evidence for selection by the membrane transport system of intracellular and extracellular amino acids for protein synthesis. *Biochem Biophys Acta* 282:352–365.

Amin-Zaki, L.; Elhassani, S.; Majeed, M. A.; Clarkson, T. W.; Doherty, R. A.; and Greenwood, M. R. (1974). Intra-uterine methylmercury poisoning in Iraq. *Pediatrics* 54:587–595.

Bartolome, J.; Trepanier, P. A.; Chait, E. A.; Barnes, G. A.; Lerea, L.; Whitmore, W. L.; Weigel, S. J.; and Slotkin, T. A. (1984). Neonatal methyl mercury poisoning in the rat: Effects on development of the peripheral sympathetic nervous system. Neuronal participation in methyl mercury induced cardiac and renal overgrowth. *Neurotoxicol* 5:45–54.

Blaker, W. D.; Krigman, M. R.; Thomas, D. J.; Mushak, P.; and Morell, P. (1981). Effects of triethyltin on myelination in the developing rat. *J Neurochem* 36:44–52.

Brubaker, P. E.; Herman, S. P.; Lucier, G. W.; Alexander, L. T.; and Long, M. D. (1973). DNA, RNA, and protein synthesis in brain, liver, and kidneys of asymptomatic methylmercury treated rats. *Exp Mol Pathol* 18:263–280.

Burton, G. V., and Meikle, A. W. (1980). Acute and chronic methyl mercury poisoning impairs rat adrenal and testicular function. *J Toxicol Environ Health* 6:597–606.

Cavanagh, J. B., and Chen, F. C. K. (1971). Amino acid incorporation in protein during the "silent phase" before organo-mercury and *p*-bromophenyl-acetylurea neuropathy in the rat. *Acta Neuropathol* 19:216–224.

Chang, L. W., and Hartmann, H. (1972). Blood-brain barrier dysfunction in experimental mercury poisoning. *Acta Neuropathol* 20:122–128.

Chase, H. P.; Lindsley, W. F. B. Jr.; and O'Brien, D. (1969). Undernutrition and cerebellar development. *Nature* 221:554–555.

Chaudhari, N., and Hahn, W. E. (1983). Genetic expression in the developing brain. *Science* 220:924–928.

Chen, W. J.; Body, R. L.; and Mottet, N. K. (1979). Some effects of continuous low-dose congenital exposure to methylmercury on organ growth in the rat fetus. *Teratol* 20:31–36.

Cheung, M. K., and Verity, M. A. (1981). Methylmercury inhibition of synaptosomal protein synthesis: Role of mitochondrial dysfunction. *Environ Res* 24:286–298.

——— (1983). Experimental methylmercury neurotoxicity: Similar in vivo and in vitro perturbation of brain cell-free protein synthesis. *Exp Mol Pathol* 38:230–242.

——— (1985). Experimental methylmercury neurotoxicity: Locus of mercurial inhibition of brain protein synthesis in vivo and in vitro. *J Neurochem* 44:1799–1808.

Clarkson, T. W.; Cox, C.; Marsh, D. O.; Myers, G. J.; Al Tikriti, S. K.; Amin-Zaki, L.; and Dabbagh, A. R. (1981). Dose-response relationships for adults and prenatal exposures to methylmercury. In *Measurement of Risks,* edited by G. G. Berg and H. D. Maillie, pp. 111–130. New York: Plenum.

Doherty, R. A.; Gates, A. H.; and Landry, T. D. (1977). Methyl mercury excretion: Developmental changes in mouse and man. *Pediatr Res* 11:416.

Dunlop, D.; Lajtha, A.; and Toth, J. (1977). Measuring brain protein metabolism in young and adult rats. In *Mechanism, Regulation, and Special Functions of Protein Synthesis in the Brain*, edited by S. Roberts, A. Lajtha, and W. H. Gipsen, pp. 79–96. Amsterdam: Elsevier-North Holland.

Dunn, A. J. (1977). Measurement of the rate of brain protein synthesis. In *Mechanisms, Regulation, and Special Function of Protein Synthesis in the Brain*, edited by S. Roberts, pp. 97–105. Amsterdam: Elsevier-North Holland.

Eccles, C. U., and Annau, Z. (1982a). Prenatal methylmercury exposure, I: Alterations in neonatal activity. *Neurobehav Toxicol Teratol* 4:371–376.

——— (1982b). Prenatal methylmercury poisoning, II: Alterations in learning and psychotropic drug sensitivity in adult offspring. *Neurobehav Toxicol Teratol* 4:377–382.

Farris, F. F., and Smith, J. C. (1975). In vivo incorporation of ^{14}C-leucine into brain protein of methylmercury treated rats. *Bull Environ Contam Toxicol* 13:451–455.

Flodmark, S., and Steinwall, O. (1963). Differential effects on certain blood-brain barrier phenomena and on the EEG produced by means of intracerebrally applied mercuric dichloride. *Acta Physiol Scand* 57:446–453.

Fowler, B. A., and Woods, J. S. (1977). The transplacental toxicity of methyl mercury to fetal rat liver mitochondria: Morphometric and biochemical studies. *Lab Invest* 36:122–130.

Frenkel, G. D.; Cain, R.; and Chao, E. S.-E. (1985). Exposure of DNA to methyl mercury results in an increase in the rate of its transcription by RNA polymerase, II. *Biochem Biophys Res Commun* 127:849–856.

Frenkel, G. D., and Randles, K. (1982). Specific stimulation of α-amanitin-sensitive RNA synthesis in isolated HeLa nuclei by methyl mercury. *J Biol Chem* 257:6275–6279.

Garrett, N. E.; Garrett, R. J. B.; and Archdeacon, J. W. (1972). Placental transmission of mercury to the fetal rat. *Toxicol Appl Pharmacol* 22:649.

Goldwater, L. J. (1972). *Mercury: A History of Quicksilver.* Baltimore: York Press.

Goodman, D. R.; Fant, M. E.; and Harbison, R. D. (1983). Perturbation of aminoisobutyric acid transport in human placental membranes: Direct effects by $HgCl_2$, CH_3HgCl, and $CdCl_2$. *Teratogenesis Carcinog Mutagen* 3:89–100.

Grant, C. A. (1973). Pathology of experimental methyl mercury intoxication: Some problems of exposure and response. In *Mercury, Mercurials, and Mercaptans*, edited by M. W. Miller and T. W. Clarkson, pp. 294–312. Springfield, Ill.: Charles C Thomas.

Greenwood, M. R. (1985). Methyl mercury poisoning in Iraq: An epidemiological study of the 1971–1972 outbreak. *J Appl Toxicol* 5:148–159.

Gruenwedel, D. W., and Cruikshank, M. W. (1979). Effect of methyl mercury (II) on the synthesis of deoxyribonucleic acid, ribonucleic acid, and protein in HeLa S3 cells. *Biochem Pharmacol* 28:651–655.

Gruenwedel, D. W.; Glaser, J. F.; and Cruikshank, M. W. (1981). Binding of methyl mercury (II) by HeLa S3 suspension-culture cells: Intracellular methyl mercury levels and their effects on DNA replication and protein synthesis. *Chem Biol Interact* 36:259–274.

Herman, S. P.; Klein, R.; Talley, F. A.; and Krigman, M. R. (1973). An ultrastructural study of methyl mercury induced primary sensory neuropathy in the rat. *Lab Invest* 28:104–118.

Hider, R. C.; Fern, E. B.; and London, D. R. (1969). Relationship between intracellular amino acids and protein synthesis in the extensor digitorum longus muscle of rats. *Biochem J* 114:171–178.

Hughes, J. A., and Sparber, S. B. (1978). *d*-Amphetamine unmasks potential consequences of exposure to methylmercury in utero: Methods for studying behavioral teratogenesis. *Pharmacol Biochem Behav* 8:365–375.

Jacobs, J. M.; Carmichael, N.; and Cavanagh, J. B. (1977). Ultrastructural changes in the nervous system of rabbits poisoned with methyl mercury. *Toxicol Appl Pharmacol* 39:249–261.

Johnson, J. D. (1985). Protein turnover in brain of the rat fetus. *J Neurochem* 44:260–264.

Joiner, F. E., and Hupp, E. W. (1979). Developmental and methyl mercury effects on brain protein synthesis. *Arch Environ Contam Toxicol* 8:465–470.

Jugo, S. (1976). Retention and distribution of $^{203}HgCl_2$ in suckling and adult rats. *Health Phys* 30:240–241.

Kershaw, T. G.; Dhahir, P. M.; and Clarkson, T. W. (1980). The relationship between blood levels and dose of methylmercury in man. *Arch Environ Health* 35:28–36.

Kim, S. U. (1971). Neurotoxic effects of alkyl mercury compound on myelinating cultures of mouse cerebellum. *Exp Neurol* 32:237–246.

King, R. B.; Robkin, M. A.; and Shepherd, T. H. (1976). Distribution of ^{203}Hg in pregnant and fetal rats. *Teratol* 13:275–280.

Kitchin, K. T.; Ebron, M. T.; and Svendsgaard, D. (1984). In vitro study of embryotoxic and dysmorphogenic effects of mercuric chloride in the rat. *Fd Chem Toxicol* 22:31–37.

Klein, R.; Herman, S.; Brubaker, P. E.; Lucier, G. W.; and Krigman, M. R. (1972). A model of acute methyl mercury intoxication in rats. *Arch Pathol* 93:408–418.

Kushner, I. (1982). The phenomenon of the acute phase response. *Ann NY Acad Sci* 389:39–48.

Lapin, C. A., and Carter, D. E. (1982). The role of food consumption and amino acid uptake in the action of methylmercury on protein synthesis. *J Toxicol Environ Health* 10:689–698.

Lindholm, D. B. (1983). Age-dependent inhibition of neuronal protein synthesis by hypothyroidism in the developing rat brain cortex. *Biochem Biophys Res Commun* 109:805–812.

Magos L., and Butler, W. H. (1976). The kinetics of methyl mercury administered repeatedly to rats. *Arch Toxicol* 35:25–39.

Magos, L.; Peristianis, G. C.; and Snowden, R. T. (1978). Post exposure preventive treatment of methylmercury intoxication in rats with dimercaptosuccinic acid. *Toxicol Appl Pharmacol* 45:463–475.

Mansour, M. M.; Dyer, N. C.; Hoffman, L. H.; Schulert, A. R.; and Brill, A. B. (1973). Maternal-fetal transfer of organic and inorganic mercury via placenta and milk. *Environ Res* 6:479–484.

Marsh, D. O.; Myers, G. J.; Clarkson, T. W.; Amin-Zaki, L.; and Tikriti, S. (1977). Fetal methylmercury poisoning: New data on clinical and toxicological aspects. *Trans Am Neurol Assoc* 102:1–3.

Marsh, D. O.; Myers, G. J.; Clarkson, T. W.; Amin-Zaki, L.; Tikriti, S.; Majeed, M.; and Dabbagh, A. R. (1979). Dose-response relationships for human fetal exposure to methylmercury. *Abstract for International Congress of Neurotoxicology, Varese, Italy,* September 27–30.

Moldave, K. (1985). Eukaryotic protein synthesis. *Ann Rev Biochem* 54:1109–1149.

Mottet, N. K. (1974). Effects of chronic low-dose exposure of rat fetuses to methylmercury hydroxide. *Teratol* 10:173–190.

Murakami, U. (1972). The effect of organic mercury on intrauterine life. In *Drugs and Fetal Development,* edited by M. A. Klingberg, A. Abramovici, and J. Chemke, pp. 309–336. New York: Plenum.

Nagata, Y., and Tsukada, Y. (1978). Bulk separation of neuronal cell bodies and glial cells from mammalian brain and some of their biochemical properties. In *Reviews of Neuroscience,* vol. 3, edited by S. Ehrenpreis and I. Kopin, pp. 195–221. New York: Raven Press.

Nagumo, S.; Omata, S.; and Sagano, H. (1985). Alteration of RNA synthesis in dorsal root ganglia of methylmercury-treated rats. *Arch Toxicol* 56:236–241.

Nakada, S.; Nomoto, A.; and Imura, N. (1980). Effect of methylmercury and inorganic mercury on protein synthesis in mammalian cells. *Ecotoxicol Environ Safety* 4:184–190.

Nakazawa, N.; Makino, F.; and Okada, S. (1975). Acute effects of mercuric compounds on cultured mammalian cells. *Biochem Pharmacol* 24:489–493.

Norseth, T., and Clarkson, T. W. (1970). Studies in the biotransformation of [203]Hg-labeled methylmercury chloride in the rat. *Arch Environ Health* 21:717–727.

Null, D. U.; Gartside, P. S.; and Wei, E. (1973). Methylmercury accumulation in brains of pregnant, nonpregnant, and fetal rats. *Life Sci* 12:65–72.

Olson, F. C., and Massaro, E. J. (1978). Effects of methyl mercury on murine fetal amino acid uptake, protein synthesis, and palate closure. *Teratol* 16:187–194.

Omata, S.; Horrigome, T.; Momose, Y.; Kambayashi, M.; Mochizuki, M.; and Sugano, H. (1980). Effect of methylmercury chloride on the in vivo rate of protein synthesis in the brain of the rat: Examination with the injection of a large quantity of [^{14}C]-valine. *Toxicol Appl Pharmacol* 56:207–215.

Omata, S.; Momose, Y.; Ueki, H.; and Sugano, H. (1982). In vivo effect of methylmercury on protein synthesis in peripheral nervous tissues of the rat. *Arch Toxicol* 49:203–214.

Omata, S.; Sakimura, K.; Tsubaki, H.; and Sugano, H. (1978). In vivo effect of methylmercury on protein synthesis in brain and liver of the rat. *Toxicol Appl Pharmacol* 44:367–378.

Omata, S., and Sugano, H. (1985). Methyl mercury: Effects on protein synthesis in nervous tissue. In *Neurotoxicology,* edited by K. Blum and L. Manzo, pp. 369–383. New York: Marcel Dekker.

Omata, S.; Tsubaki, H.; Sakimura, K.; Sato, M.; Yoshimura, R.; Hirakawa, E.; and Sugano, H. (1981). Stimulation of protein and RNA synthesis by methylmercury chloride in the liver of intact and adrenalectomized rats. *Arch Toxicol* 47:113–123.

Paigen, K. (1980). Temporal genes and other developmental regulators in mammals. In *The Molecular Genetics of Development,* edited by T. Leighton and W. F. Loomis, Jr., pp. 419–470. New York: Academic Press.

Pezerovic, D.; Narancsik, P.; and Gamulin, S. (1981). Effects of mercury bichloride on mouse kidney polyribosome structure and function. *Arch Toxicol* 48:167–172.

Piotrowski, J. K., and Inskip, M. J. (1981). *Health Effects of Methyl Mercury,* Monitoring and Assessment Research Centre, Report 24. London: Chelsea College, University of London.

Rapoport, S. I. (1976). *Blood-Brain Barrier in Physiology and Medicine.* New York: Raven Press.

Richardson, R. J., and Murphy, S. D. (1974). Neurotoxicity produced by intracranial administration of methylmercury in rats. *Toxicol Appl Pharmacol* 29:289–300.

Rodier, P. M. (1983). Critical processes in CNS development and the pathogenesis of early injuries. In *Reproductive and Developmental Toxicity of Metals,* edited by T. W. Clarkson, G. F. Nordberg, and P. R. Sager, pp. 455–473. New York: Plenum.

Rozalski, M., and Wierzbicki, R. (1983). Effects of mercuric chloride on cultured rat fibroblasts: Survival, protein biosynthesis, and binding of mercury to chromatin. *Biochem Pharmacol* 32:2124–2126.

Samuels, S.; Fish, I.; Schwartz, S. A.; and Hochgeschwender, U. (1983). Age related changes in blood-to-brain amino acid transport and incorporation into brain protein. *Neurochem Res* 8:167–177.

Sarafian, T. A.; Cheung, M. K.; and Verity, M. A. (1984). In vitro methyl mercury inhibition of protein synthesis in neonatal cerebellar perikarya. *Neuropathol Appl Neurobiol* 10:85–100.

Sarafian, T. A., and Verity, M. A. (1985). Inhibition of RNA and protein synthesis in isolated cerebellar cells by in vitro and in vivo methyl mercury. *Neurochem Pathol* 3:27–39.

Sauve, G. J., and Nicholls, D. M. (1981). Liver protein synthesis during the acute response to methyl mercury administration. *Int J Biochem* 13:981–990.

Sherlock, J. C.; Lindsay, D. G.; Hislop, J. E.; Evans, W. H.; and Collier, T. R. (1982). Duplication diet study on mercury intake by fish consumers in the United Kingdom. *Arch Environ Health* 37:271–278.

Slotkin, T. A.; Pachman, S.; Kavlock, R. J.; and Bartolome, J. (1985). Effects of neonatal methylmercury exposure on development of nucleic acids and protein in rat brain: Regional specificity. *Brain Res Bul* 14:397–400.

Spyker, J. M.; Sparber, S. B.; and Goldberg, A. M. (1972). Subtle consequences of methylmercury exposure: Behavioral deviations in offspring of treated mothers. *Science* 177:621–623.

Steinwall, O. (1961). Transport mechanism in certain blood-brain barrier phenomena: A hypothesis. *Acta Psychiatr Neurol Scand* 36(Supp. 150):314–318.

——— (1968). Transport inhibition phenomena in unilateral chemical injury of blood-brain barrier. In *Brain Barrier Systems: Progress in Brain Research,* vol. 29, edited by A. Lajtha and D. H. Ford, pp. 357–365. Amsterdam: Elsevier.

——— (1969). Brain uptake of Se[75]-selenomethionine after damage to blood-brain barrier by mercuric ions. *Acta Neurol Scand* 45:362–368.

Steinwall, O., and Olsson, Y. (1969). Impairment of the blood-brain barrier in mercury poisoning. *Acta Neurol Scand* 45:352–361.

Steinwall, O., and Snyder, S. H. (1969). Brain uptake of C[14]-cycloleucine after damage to blood-brain barrier by mercuric ions. *Acta Neurol Scand* 45:369–375.

Sugano, H.; Omata, S.; and Tsubaki, H. (1975). Methylmercury inhibition of protein synthesis in brain tissues, I: Effects of methylmercury and heavy metals on cell-free protein synthesis in rat brain and liver. In *Studies on the Health Effects of Alkylmercury in Japan,* edited by T. Tsubaki, pp. 129–135. Tokyo: Environment Agency.

Sutcliffe, J. G.; Milner, R. J.; Gottesfeld, J. M.; and Reynolds, W. (1984). Control of neuronal gene expression. *Science* 225:1308–1318.

Suzuki, T. (1969). Neurological symptoms from concentrations of mercury in the brain. In *Chemical Fallout,* edited by M. W. Miller and G. G. Berg, pp. 245–257. Springfield, Ill.: Charles C Thomas.

Syversen, T. L. M. (1977). Effects of methylmercury on in vivo protein synthesis in isolated cerebral and cerebellar neurons. *Neuropathol Appl Neurobiol* 3:225–236.

——— (1981). Effects of methylmercury on protein synthesis in vitro. *Acta Pharmacol Toxicol* 49:422–426.

——— (1982a). Changes in protein and RNA synthesis in rat brain neurons after a single dose of methylmercury. *Toxicol Lett* 10:31–34.

——— (1982b). Effects of repeated dosing of methyl mercury in vivo protein synthesis in isolated neurons. *Acta Pharmacol Toxicol* 50:391–397.

Syversen, T. L. M.; Totland, G.; and Flood, P. R. (1981). Early morphological changes in rat cerebellum caused by a single dose of methylmercury. *Arch Toxicol* 47:101–111.

Takizawa, Y. (1979). Epidemiology of mercury poisoning. In *The Biogeochemistry of Mercury in the Environment,* edited by J. Nriagu, pp. 325–365. Amsterdam: Elsevier/North Holland.

Thomas, D. J.; Fisher, H. L.; Hall, L. L.; and Mushak, P. (1982). Effects of age and sex on retention of mercury by methyl mercury-treated rats. *Toxicol Appl Pharmacol* 62:445–454.

Thomas, D. J., and Smith, J. C. (1979a). Distribution and excretion of mercuric chloride in neonatal rats. *Toxicol Appl Pharmacol* 48:43–47.

——— (1979b). Partial characterization of a low-molecular weight methylmercury complex in rat cerebrum. *Toxicol Appl Pharmacol* 47:547–556.

Toews, A. D.; Blaker, W. D.; Thomas, D. J.; Gaynor, J. J.; Krigman, M. R.; Mushak, P.; and Morell, P. (1983). Myelin deficits produced by early postnatal exposure to inorganic lead or triethyltin are persistent. *J Neurochem* 41:814–822.

Toews, A. D.; Krigman, M. R.; Thomas, D. J.; and Morell, P. (1980). Effects of inorganic lead exposure on myelination in the rat. *Neurochem Res* 5:605–616.

Trojanowska, B.; Piotrowski, J. K.; and Szendsikowski, S. (1971). The influence of thioacetamide on the excretion of mercury in rats. *Toxicol Appl Pharmacol* 18:374–386.

Turner, M. D.; Marsh, D. O.; Smith, J. G.; Inglis, J. B.; Clarkson, T. W.; Rubio, C. E.; Chiriboga, J.; and Chiriboga, C. C. (1980). Methylmercury in populations consuming large quantities of marine fish. *Arch Environ Health* 35:367–378.

van Venrooij, W. J.; Poort, C.; Kramer, M. F.; and Jansen, M. T. (1972). Relationship between extracellular amino acids and protein synthesis in vitro in the rat pancreas. *Eur J Biochem* 30:427–433.

Verity, M. A.; Brown, W. J.; and Cheung, M. (1975). Organic mercurial encephalopathy: In vivo and in vitro effects of methyl mercury on synaptosomal respiration. *J Neurochem* 25:759–766.

Verity, M. A.; Brown, W. J.; Cheung, M.; and Czer, G. (1977). Methyl mercury inhibition of synaptosome and brain slice protein synthesis: In vivo and in vitro studies. *J Neurochem* 29:673–669.

Ware, R. A.; Chang, L. W.; and Burkholder, P. M. (1974*a*). An ultrastructural study on the blood-brain barrier dysfunction following mercury intoxication. *Acta Neuropathol* 30:211–214.

———— (1974*b*). Ultrastructural evidence for foetal liver injury induced by in utero exposure to small doses of methyl mercury. *Nature* 251:236–237.

Weiss, B. F.; Wurtman, R. J.; and Munro, H. N. (1973). Disaggregation of brain polysomes by *L*-5-hydroxytryptophan: Mediation by serotonin. *Life Sci* 13:411–416.

Westerlain, C. G. (1972). Breakdown of brain polysomes in status epilepticus. *Brain Res* 39:278–284.

Westerlain, C. G., and Plum, F. (1973). Vulnerability of developing rat brain to electroconvulsive seizures. *Arch Neurol* 29:39–45.

Winick, M., and Noble, A. (1966). Cellular responses in rats during malnutrition at various ages. *J Nutr* 89:300–306.

Winick, M.; Rosso, P.; and Waterlow, J. (1970). Cellular growth of cerebrum, cerebellum, and brainstem in normal and marasmic children. *Exp Neurol* 26:393–400.

Yoshino, Y.; Mozai, T.; and Nakao, K. (1966*a*). Distribution of mercury in the brain and its subcellular units in experimental organic mercury poisoning. *J Neurochem* 13:397–406.

———— (1966*b*). Biochemical changes in the brains of rats poisoned with an alkylmercury compound, with special references to the inhibition of protein synthesis in brain cortex slices. *J Neurochem* 13:1223–1230.

Young, M. (1979). Transfer of amino acids. In *Placental Transfer,* edited by G. Chamberlain and A. Wilkinson, pp. 142–158. Baltimore: University Park Press.

TEN

The Neurochemical Effects of Methyl Mercury in the Brain

Hannu Komulainen and Jouko Tuomisto

Methyl mercury is one of the most potent neurotoxins of any compound tested in neurobehavioral tests so far (Pryor et al. 1983). The involvement of the central nervous system (CNS) in intoxication is well known. Accordingly, the symptoms of human poisoning include, for example, tremor, ataxia, and mental disturbances (Kojima and Fujita 1973; Gerstner and Huff 1977). In animals, concomitant with the behavioral changes induced by methyl mercury, several biochemical parameters are altered in the brain (Salvaterra et al. 1973; Chang et al. 1973). In the same dose range, neurochemical alterations have also been observed. It is tempting to speculate that these neurochemical changes in the brain are related to the altered behavior, mental disturbances, and other subtle symptoms of poisoning.

In this chapter we summarize and review the neurochemical data obtained so far for methyl mercury in the mammalian brain. In spite of several human catastrophes and the seriousness of environmental contamination by methyl mercury, neurochemical studies on the brain are sparse. In particular, the consequences of prenatal exposure to methyl mercury have seldom been studied, although this period of life is most sensitive to methyl mercury (Amin-Zaki et al. 1974; Marsh et al. 1980; for review, see Reuhl and Chang 1979). Hence, the present data do not cover all aspects of neurotransmission to allow one to predict the most sensitive steps in central neurotransmission to methyl mercury toxicity and correlate the changes with specific symptoms of poisoning.

In several studies, direct effects of methyl mercury on neurochemical parameters have been assessed in vitro. Interpreting the results from these experiments is difficult, however, because experimental conditions drastically affect the results obtained. The effect of methyl mercury in vitro depends on the total protein and tissue content of an assay system (Macfarlane 1981; Omata et al. 1982; Tuomisto and Komulainen 1983a). When the amount of tissue increases, the potency of methyl mercury decreases. Therefore, in vitro results on one parameter cannot be compared directly with another without relating them to the tissue preparation used. However, in vitro experiments reveal whether the enzyme or process is sensitive to methyl mercury at all and help to explain the mechanisms of action in the whole brain.

Cholinergic Neurotransmission

Methyl mercury inhibits several stages of cholinergic neurotransmission in brain tissue in vitro: choline uptake (Kobayashi et al. 1979; Bondy et al. 1979; Araki et al. 1981), choline acetyltransferase (ChAT) (Tunnicliff and Wood 1973; Kobayashi et al. 1979; Omata et al. 1982), muscarinic (Eldefrawi et al. 1977; Von Burg et al. 1980; Abd-Elfattah and Shamoo 1981), and nicotinic receptor binding (Eldefrawi et al. 1977). Brain acetylcholine esterase (AChE), the enzyme terminating the effect of acetylcholine (ACh) in the synaptic cleft, is not sensitive to methyl mercury in vitro (Omata et al. 1982; Tunnicliff and Wood 1973; Hösli and Hösli 1974; Kobayashi et al. 1979). Acetylcholine synthesis is inhibited by methyl mercury at concentrations that do not cause release of endogenous ACh from the same brain slices (Kobayashi et al. 1979). Hence, the synthesis of ACh appears to be a very sensitive stage in vitro, and the most important mechanism is evidently the inhibition of ChAT. Decreased neuronal choline uptake, the rate-limiting step in ACh synthesis, may also contribute to the inhibition of ACh synthesis in vitro.

Methyl mercury has a suppressive effect on some stages of cholinergic neurotransmission also in vivo (Table 10.1). The doses able to produce significant alterations in the cholinergic parameters of the mature brain are already high enough to induce typical peripheral symptoms (hind-limb paresis) in animals. At these same doses, neurochemical changes in the dorsal root ganglion are even more profound than in the central nervous system (Araki et al. 1981; Omata et al. 1982). However, the neurochemical alterations in the brain are more immediate than those in the peripheral nervous system.

After long-term administration of methyl mercury to adult rats, the activity of ChAT is slightly but uniformly decreased (Dwivedi et al. 1980; Tsuzuki 1981; Omata et al. 1982). The decrease is not clearly dose-dependent and is not augmented as the treatment progresses. As a result of this inhibition, the ACh synthesis rate and regional ACh levels are slightly decreased (Hrdina et al. 1976; Kobayashi et al. 1980). The decrease of ACh levels is transient, disappearing after cessation of methyl mercury administration (Hrdina et al. 1976). The inhibition of ChAT activity appears to be the critical effect, because neither choline uptake (Araki et al. 1981) nor AChE (Sobotka et al. 1974; Hrdina et al. 1976; Omata et al. 1982) is as sensitive to methyl mercury in vivo. However, the exact mechanism of the inhibition of the activity of ChAT is not known. On the basis of the in vitro data, a direct inhibitory effect on the enzyme is possible.

The few published studies from prenatal exposure of animals to methyl mercury indicate no delayed effects on cholinergic neurons. The activity of ChAT in mouse brain (Spyker et al. 1972) as well as that of AChE in rat brain, even after moderately toxic doses (Sobotka et al. 1974), are normal in

Table 10.1 Effect of methyl mercury on brain cholinergic neurotransmission

Parameter	Type of Exposure and Dose (mg/kg)	Species	Brain Region	Result	Reference
Choline uptake	Subacute (adult), 10	Rat	Cortex	No change	Araki et al. 1981
ChAT	Acute (prenatal), 8	Mouse	Whole brain	No change	Spyker et al. 1972
	Subacute (adult), 10, 50 µg/ml	Rat	Whole brain	17–67% decrease	Dwivedi et al. 1980
	Subacute (adult), 10	Rat	Whole brain	25–30% decrease	Omata et al. 1982
	Chronic (adult), 4	Rat	Cerebellum	32% decrease	Tsuzuki 1981
ACh synthesis rate	Subacute (adult), 5	Mouse	Cortex, striatum, cerebellum	Decrease	Kobayashi et al. 1980
ACh levels	Subacute (adult), 5	Mouse	Cortex, striatum	Decrease	Kobayashi et al. 1980
			Cerebellum	No change	
AChE	Chronic (adult), 0.4, 4.0	Rat	Cortex	23–24% decrease	Hrdina et al. 1976
	Acute (prenatal), 8	Mouse	Whole brain	No change	Spyker et al. 1972
	Subacute (prenatal), 0.1, 0.5, 2.5	Rat	Telencephalon, midbrain–diencephalon, pons–medulla, cerebellum	No change	Sobotka et al. 1974
	Subacute (adult), 10	Rat	Whole brain	No change	Omata et al. 1982
	Chronic (adult), 0.4, 4.0	Rat	Cortex	No change	Hrdina et al. 1976
	Chronic (adult), 4	Rat	Cerebellum	29% decrease	Tsuzuki 1981

adulthood. At present there are no published data on the effects of methyl mercury on brain ACh receptors in vivo, so the most sensitive stage of cholinergic neurotransmission in vivo cannot be deduced as yet. The symptoms caused by methyl mercury in adult mice (hypothermia, decreased spontaneous motor activity) can be induced by an inhibitor of choline uptake or ChAT in vivo (Kobayashi et al. 1981). This supports the concept of hypofunction of cholinergic neurotransmission in methyl mercury intoxication.

Catecholaminergic Transmission

Methyl mercury inhibits in vitro enzymes responsible for the metabolism of catecholamines and their precursors. Tyrosine hydroxylase (TH), DOPA decarboxylase, monoamine oxidase (MAO), and catechol-O-methyltransferase (COMT) are inhibited in mouse brain homogenate by high concentrations of methyl mercury (Tunnicliff and Wood 1973), whereas AChE remains intact. In addition, methyl mercury inhibits dopamine (DA) (Bondy et al. 1979; Komulainen and Tuomisto 1981) and noradrenaline (NA) uptake (Komulainen and Tuomisto 1981) into synaptosomes at micromolar concentrations in vitro. Concomitantly, it induces spontaneous release of these catecholamines from synaptosomes (Komulainen and Tuomisto 1981). The stimulation of dopamine release from synaptosomes is more profound than that of noradrenaline.

In striatal tissue, methyl mercury also potently inhibits antagonist binding to D_2-receptors (Bondy and Agrawal 1980; our unpublished results). The binding affinity is decreased, while receptor numbers remain unchanged (our unpublished results). Little is known about the effects of methyl mercury on later postsynaptic events of catecholaminergic transmission in vitro. In rat neuroblastoma cultures, neither the basal nor the NA-stimulated activity of adenylate cyclase is affected by methyl mercury at concentrations that otherwise are toxic (Spuhler and Prasad 1980). In contrast, the prostaglandin E_1-stimulated adenylate cyclase is inhibited both in glial cells (Spuhler and Prasad 1980) and in platelets (Macfarlane 1981).

The effect of methyl mercury on catecholaminergic pathways in vivo depends on the age of animals and accordingly on the developmental stage of the nervous system. A continuous administration of methyl mercury from day 1 of life to day 21, covering the postnatal developmental spurt of the nervous system, causes a permanent defect in both dopaminergic and noradrenergic neurons (Bartolome et al. 1982). Within the course of administration of methyl mercury (when its concentration in the brain is supposedly high) DA uptake into synaptosomes is inhibited. On the basis of the in vitro data, this may be a direct inhibitory effect of methyl mercury on uptake. Concurrently with decreased DA uptake, both DA and NA turnover are increased, and NA levels are elevated. TH activity and vesicular uptake of NA are unchanged.

After cessation of methyl mercury administration DA uptake, as well as NA uptake, remains permanently increased, at least up to 60 days of life. The damage is dose-dependent and occurs at a dose (2.5 mg/kg) that does not significantly decrease body or brain weight during development. It is not yet known why dopaminergic and noradrenergic neurons become hyperactive, and the extent to which these neurochemical changes are related to observed postnatal hyperactivity (Eccles and Annau 1982*a*) and learning deficits (Zenick 1974; Hughes et al. 1975; Hughes and Annau 1976; Eccles and Annau 1982*b*) in rats.

In adult rats, dopaminergic neurons may be more sensitive to methyl mercury than noradrenergic or serotonergic neurons. The whole-brain DA synthesis rate is already impaired when those of NA or 5-hydroxytryptamine (5-HT) are unaffected (Sharma et al. 1982). It is decreased already at doses that do not cause symptoms of peripheral toxicity or detectable changes in steady-state levels of DA or DOPAC in the brain. The activity of TH, the rate-limiting step in DA synthesis, is not decreased at these doses as measured ex vivo. On the contrary, it is either increased (Omata et al. 1982) or unchanged (Tsuzuki 1982). TH associated with dopaminergic and noradrenergic neurons is, however, regulated differently, and the measured total activity of the enzyme does not necessarily reveal subtle changes in each type of neuron.

The steady-state levels of dopamine are altered only after a chronic high-dose administration (Table 10.2). Increased DA levels have been reported with concomitant decreases in its metabolites, DOPAC and HVA (Tsuzuki 1982). These changes may be explained by the inhibition of monoamine oxidase, the main degradative enzyme of DA in the brain. Both monoamine oxidase and catechol-O-methyltransferase are inhibited in the cerebellum, while dopamine-beta-hydroxylase activity is not altered (Tsuzuki 1981).

Neither striatal DA uptake (our unpublished results) nor D_2-receptor binding (Agrawal et al. 1981; Corda et al. 1981) is influenced by acute administration of methyl mercury to adult rats.

The levels of NA (Table 10.3) are increased concomitantly with DA in chronic high-dose administration to adult rats (Hrdina et al. 1976; Tsuzuki 1982). There is, however, substantial regional variation in NA concentrations. The brain stem seems to be particularly vulnerable. At lower doses and after shorter exposures, the changes in NA levels are inconsistent. It is interesting to note that there appears to be a diurnal rhythm in the methyl mercury induced alterations in regional NA levels (Sudo and Arito 1982). The changes are detectable in the morning but disappear at night, suggesting some deficiency in the adaptation of the neuronal pathways to diurnal variation.

There are no data on the effects of methyl mercury on noradrenergic receptors in the brain. The concentration of cyclic AMP does not change in

Table 10.2 Effect of methyl mercury on brain dopaminergic neurotransmission

Parameter	Type of Exposure and Dose (mg/kg)	Species	Brain Region	Result	Reference
Tyrosine levels	Subacute (adult), 1, 3, 10	Rat	Whole brain	13% decrease	Sharma et al. 1982
Tyrosine hydroxylase	Acute (postnatal), 5	Rat	Whole brain	No change	Taylor and DiStefano 1976
	Chronic (postnatal), 1, 2.5, 5	Rat	Whole brain	No change	Bartolome et al. 1982
	Subacute (adult), 10	Rat	Whole brain	50–20% increase	Omata et al. 1982
	Chronic (adult), 4	Rat	Cerebellum	No change	Tsuzuki 1981
Dopamine levels	Subacute (prenatal), 0.1, 0.5, 2.5	Rat	Telencephalon, midbrain-diencephalon	No change	Sobotka et al. 1974
	Acute (postnatal), 5	Rat	Whole brain	15% decrease	Taylor and DiStefano 1976
	Chronic (postnatal), 1, 2.5, 5	Rat	Whole brain	No change	Bartolome et al. 1982
	Subacute (adult), 1, 3, 10	Rat	Whole brain	No change	Sharma et al. 1982
	Chronic (adult), 4	Rat	Striatum, brain stem, pons-medulla, hypothalamus	21–33% increase	Tsuzuki 1982
Synthesis rate	Subacute (adult), 1, 3, 10	Rat	Whole brain	27–54% decrease	Sharma et al. 1982
Turnover	Chronic (postnatal), 1, 2.5, 5	Rat	Whole brain	20% increase	Bartolome et al. 1982
DOPAC	Subacute (adult), 1, 3, 10	Rat	Whole brain	No change	Sharma et al. 1982
	Chronic (adult), 4	Rat	Striatum, brain stem, pons-medulla, hypothalamus	20–33% decrease	Tsuzuki 1982
HVA	Chronic (adult), 4	Rat	Striatum, brain stem, pons-medulla, hypothalamus	3–21% decrease	Tsuzuki 1982
MAO	Acute (postnatal), 5	Rat	Whole brain	15% decrease, 17% increase	Taylor and DiStefano 1976
	Subacute (adult), 10	Rat	Whole brain	10–20% increase	Omata et al. 1982
COMT	Chronic (adult), 4	Rat	Cerebellum	31% decrease	Tsuzuki 1981
	Chronic (adult), 4	Rat	Cerebellum	25% decrease	Tsuzuki 1981
Uptake	Chronic (postnatal), 1, 2.5, 5	Rat	Whole brain	58–30% decrease, 40–70% increase	Bartolome et al. 1982
	Acute (adult), 10	Rat	Striatum	No change	Komulainen and Tuomisto (unpublished)
Receptor binding	Acute (adult), 14	Rat	Striatum	No change	Agrawal et al. 1981
	Acute (adult), 10	Rat	Cortex, caudate nucleus	No change	Corda et al. 1981
cAMP	Acute (adult), 10	Rat	Cerebellum	No change	Corda et al. 1981
cGMP	Acute (adult), 10	Rat	Cerebellum	50% decrease	Corda et al. 1981

177

Table 10.3 Effect of methyl mercury on brain noradrenergic neurotransmission

Parameter	Type of Exposure and Dose (mg/kg)	Species	Brain Region	Result	Reference
Dopamine-β-hydroxylase	Chronic (adult), 4	Rat	Cerebellum	No change	Tsuzuki 1981
Synthesis rate	Subacute (adult), 1, 3, 10	Rat	Whole brain	No change	Sharma et al. 1982
Turnover	Chronic (postnatal), 1, 2.5, 5	Rat	Whole brain	25–50% increase	Bartolome et al. 1982
Noradrenaline levels	Subacute (prenatal), 0.1, 0.5, 2.5	Rat	Midbrain-diencephalon Telencephalon, pons-medulla	25% decrease No change	Sobotka et al. 1974
	Acute (postnatal), 5	Rat	Whole brain	15% decrease	Taylor and DiStefano 1976
	Chronic (postnatal), 1, 2.5, 5	Rat	Whole brain	10–20% increase	Bartolome et al. 1982
	Acute (adult), 15	Rat	Diencephalon-midbrain, pons-medulla Cerebral hemispheres	Increase Decrease	Sudo and Arito 1982
	Subacute (adult), 1, 3, 10	Rat	Whole brain	No change	Sharma et al. 1982
	Chronic (adult), 0.4, 4.0	Rat	Brain stem	38–19% increase	Hrdina et al. 1976
	Chronic (adult), 4	Rat	Striatum, brain stem Pons-medulla, hypothalamus	23–25% increase No change	Tsuzuki 1982
Uptake	Chronic (postnatal), 1, 2.5, 5	Rat	Whole brain	20–100% increase	Bartolome et al. 1982
Vesicular uptake	Chronic (postnatal), 1, 2.5, 5	Rat	Whole brain	No change	Bartolome et al. 1982

178

the cerebellum after a single dose (10 mg/kg), while cyclic GMP (cGMP) decreases by 50 percent (Corda et al. 1981). Whether this is a direct effect of methyl mercury or an adaptive change is not known, but the decrease is one of the earliest neurochemical changes reported so far in the brain.

Serotonergic Transmission

Direct effects of methyl mercury have been demonstrated only on a few stages of serotonergic transmission. Methyl mercury inhibits uptake of 5-hydroxytryptamine (5-HT) into hypothalamic synaptosomes at micromolar concentrations and also stimulates its spontaneous release (Komulainen and Tuomisto 1981). It potently inhibits 5-HT uptake and releases 5-HT also in blood platelets (Macfarlane 1981; Tuomisto and Komulainen 1983*a*), a suggested peripheral model of serotonergic neurons for 5-HT uptake studies. At the same micromolar range of concentrations, it inhibits imipramine binding in platelet membranes (Tuomisto and Komulainen 1983*b*), suggesting a blockade of 5-HT uptake carrier.

As measured by 5-HT levels, serotonergic neurons (Table 10.4) would appear to be more vulnerable during neonatal administration than catecholaminergic neurons. A dose-dependent decrease in 5-HT levels lasting to adulthood has been observed in the rat midbrain-diencephalon area after prenatal administration, while DA and NA do not show consistent regional changes (Sobotka et al. 1974). Postnatally, a biphasic change in the concentrations of 5-HT and 5-HIAA takes place (Taylor and DiStefano 1976). There is first a decrease in their levels in the presence of high levels of methyl mercury in the brain, and later a long-lasting increase (at least up to day 50 of life). Serotonergic neurons differ biochemically from catecholaminergic neurons at least in two aspects, which may explain their apparently higher susceptibility. The availability of tryptophan, the precursor of 5-HT, from blood is suggested to contribute directly to 5-HT turnover (Green and Grahame-Smith 1975). Second, tryptophan hydroxylase, the rate-limiting step in 5-HT synthesis, does not obey sensitive feedback inhibition by 5-HT permitting 5-HT levels to be elevated in nerve endings. Hence, the decrease in 5-HT is likely to be due to the simultaneous decrease in tryptophan levels and tryptophan hydroxylase activity (Taylor and DiStefano 1976). The permanent increase of 5-HT and 5-HIAA reflects a more indirect adaptive change in the activity of serotonergic pathways.

In the mature brain, chronic administration of methyl mercury decreases 5-HT regionally (Hrdina et al. 1976; Tsuzuki 1982), and this effect is reversible (Hrdina et al. 1976). The doses required for these changes are high enough to induce peripheral neurotoxicity. There also appears to be a delayed circadian variation in regional response of serotonergic neurons to methyl mercury (Sudo and Arito 1982). 5-HT and 5-HIAA tend to be decreased at

Table 10.4 Effect of methyl mercury on brain serotonergic neurotransmission

Parameter	Type of Exposure and Dose (mg/kg)	Species	Brain Region	Result	Reference
Tryptophan levels	Acute (postnatal), 5	Rat	Whole brain	20% decrease	Taylor and DiStefano 1976
	Acute (adult), 15	Rat	Diencephalon-midbrain, pons-medulla, cerebral hemispheres	Decrease	Sudo and Arito 1982
Tryptophan hydroxylase	Subacute (adult), 1, 3, 10	Rat	Whole brain	No change	Sharma et al. 1982
	Acute (postnatal), 5	Rat	Whole brain	26% decrease	Taylor and DiStefano 1976
	Chronic (adult), 4	Rat	Cerebellum	46% decrease	Tsuzuki 1981
5-HT turnover	Subacute (adult), 1, 3, 10	Rat	Whole brain	No change	Sharma et al. 1982
5-HT levels	Subacute (prenatal), 0.1, 0.5, 2.5	Rat	Midbrain-diencephalon	30% decrease	Sobotka et al. 1974
			Telencephalon, pons-medulla	No change	
	Acute (postnatal), 5	Rat	Whole brain	20% decrease, 20% increase	Taylor and DiStefano 1976
	Acute (adult), 15	Rat	Diencephalon-midbrain	Increase	Sudo and Arito 1982
			Pons-medulla, cerebral hemispheres	No change	
	Subacute (adult), 1, 3, 10	Rat	Whole brain	No change	Sharma et al. 1982
	Chronic (adult), 4	Rat	Striatum, hypothalamus, brain stem	20–28% decrease	Tsuzuki 1982
			Pons-medulla	No change	
5-HIAA	Chronic (adult), 0.4, 4.0	Rat	Brain stem	24% decrease	Hrdina et al. 1976
	Subacute (prenatal), 0.1, 0.5, 2.5	Rat	Telencephalon, midbrain-diencephalon, pons-medulla	No change	Sobotka et al. 1974
	Acute (postnatal), 5	Rat	Whole brain	20% decrease, 20% increase	Taylor and DiStefano 1976
	Acute (adult), 5	Rat	Diencephalon-midbrain	Decrease	Sudo and Arito 1982
			Pons-medulla, cerebral hemispheres	No change	
5-HT uptake	Subacute (adult), 1, 3, 10	Rat	Whole brain	No change	Sharma et al. 1982
	Acute (adult), 10	Rat	Hypothalamus	No change	Komulainen and Tuomisto (unpublished)

180

night when brain tryptophan levels are also decreased. Uptake of 5-HT into hypothalamic synaptosomes is unaffected after a single dose (10 mg/kg) of methyl mercury to adult rats (our unpublished results).

GABA and Amino Acids

Methyl mercury inhibits the uptake of GABA (gamma-aminobutyric acid), glycine, and glutamate by brain tissue preparations in vitro (Bondy et al. 1979; Araki et al. 1981). In addition, their release is slightly stimulated (Bondy et al. 1979), and ligand binding to glycine and benzodiazepine receptors is inhibited in vitro (Bondy and Agrawal 1980). However, respective dopaminergic parameters are clearly more vulnerable in these conditions.

In the light of the present data (Table 10.5), GABAergic transmission in the rat brain is not so sensitive to methyl mercury as monoaminergic or cholinergic transmission. This is in agreement with the symptoms of poisoning; methyl mercury is not particularly convulsive (Adler and Adler 1977). At ultimately lethal doses, GABA levels are, however, increased, and those of glycine, aspartate, and glutamate are decreased (Hoskins and Hupp 1978). In contrast, GABA metabolism in the dorsal root ganglion is seriously affected when changes in the brain are slight (Araki et al. 1981).

Benzodiazepine receptor binding sites increase in the rat brain regions after a single dose of 10 mg/kg (Corda et al. 1981). The receptors display a long-lasting supersensitivity. Because GABA content and binding are not concurrently changed, the defect is not in the GABA-regulated site of the receptor.

Contribution of Pharmacokinetics to Neurochemical Effects

As observed above, the in vitro results do not correlate well with neurochemical changes in vivo. Several steps of neurotransmission are inhibited in vitro but not in vivo. However, the concentrations of methyl mercury in the brain achieve the range of 10–100 μM in these studies. Hence, pharmacokinetic factors are important determinants in the neurochemical toxicity. Especially, the distribution in the brain must be critical. It has been observed in vitro that a certain threshold concentration must be reached before methyl mercury is toxic (Gruenwedel and Friend 1980). Binding of methyl mercury to multiple proteins decreases the effective fraction acting on critical sites. In addition, the effect depends on the total cumulated dose rather than on the exposure time, suggesting a similar threshold (Berthoud et al. 1976; MacDonald and Harbison 1977). There is some evidence that methyl mercury accumulates first in glial cells and only later enters neurons (Berlin et al. 1975; Sakai 1974). This might partly explain why neuronal processes are spared in spite of the apparently high concentration of methyl mercury in the brain.

Table 10.5 Effect of methyl mercury on brain GABAergic and amino-acid related transmission

Parameter	Type of Exposure and Dose (mg/kg)	Species	Brain Region	Result	Reference
GAD	Chronic (adult), 4	Rat	Cerebellum	No change	Tsuzuki 1981
GABA levels	Acute (adult), 10	Rat	Cortex, cerebellum, caudate nucleus	No change	Corda et al. 1981
	Subacute (adult), 34	Rat	Cerebellum, brain stem, cerebral hemisphere	No change	Hoskins and Hupp 1978
	Subacute (adult), 6–20	Monkey	Cerebellum, brain stem, cerebral hemisphere	Increase	Hoskins and Hupp 1978
	Chronic (adult), 4	Rat	Hypothalamus, pons-medulla, brain stem, striatum	No change	Tsuzuki 1982
GABA uptake	Subacute (adult), 10	Rat	Cortex	No change	Araki et al. 1981
			Cerebellum	17% decrease	
GABA receptors	Acute (adult), 10	Rat	Cortex, cerebellum, caudate nucleus	No change	Corda et al. 1981
Glycine and glutamate levels	Subacute (adult), 34	Rat	Cerebellum, brain stem, cerebral hemisphere	No change	Hoskins and Hupp 1978
	Subacute (adult), 6–20	Monkey	Cerebellum, brain stem, cerebral hemisphere	Decrease	Hoskins and Hupp 1978
Benzodiazepine receptors	Acute (adult), 10	Rat	Cortex, cerebellum, striatum, and retina	27–60% increase	Corda et al. 1981

Possible Mechanisms of Neurochemical Effects

The neurochemical effects cited above have been detected at the same range of doses that usually also causes histopathological damage in the brain and overt peripheral toxicity. Thus neurochemical alterations represent to some extent biochemical implications of this morphological damage and neuronal loss. Interpretation of these neurochemical changes is difficult because they must be partly indirect. Decreased activity of one pathway (e.g., dopaminergic) may increase the activity of the second (e.g., cholinergic) or increase its own presynaptic activity by feedback mechanisms (dopaminergic). Neuronal loss leads to hypofunction in damaged pathways, but the observed increases in synthesis and turnover rates and in receptor densities represent adaptation to altered neuronal activity.

In the light of the present data, there are several mechanisms that affect neurons more or less directly. Because methyl mercury binds avidly to SH-groups (Vallee and Ulmer 1972), every process where these are essential would be expected to be disturbed at some concentrations. The inhibition of neuronal protein synthesis (Yoshino 1966; Verity et al. 1977; Omata et al. 1978; Syversen 1982) may contribute significantly to the effects observed. Decreased protein synthesis, together with inhibited axonal transport (Abe et al. 1975), would lead to an apparent decrease in enzyme activity (such as choline acetyltransferase) in nerve terminals. Especially, it must delay and impair the maturation of the developing brain. The depression of the mitochondrial glycolytic pathway, oxidative phosphorylation, and tissue respiration (Chang et al. 1973; Fox et al. 1975; Verity et al. 1975; Bull and Lutkenhoff 1975) may disturb energy-requiring processes. By affecting mitochondria (O'Kusky 1983), methyl mercury may also impair intracellular calcium homeostasis. Mitochondria are important regulators of the free intracellular calcium concentration (Åkerman and Nicholls 1983). Increased free cytoplasmic calcium could explain the rapid stimulative effect of methyl mercury on the release of neurotransmitters in vitro.

Finally, certain unspecific factors must be excluded as contributing factors. Prenatal and postnatal undernutrition, as such, causes neurochemical changes by delaying and impairing brain development (for review, see Michaelson 1980). The cholinergic system is generally suppressed. Turnover in serotonergic neurons is increased, but catecholaminergic neurons are variably affected. Because methyl mercury decreases the weight gain of pups and their brains at higher doses (Bartolome et al. 1982), the extent to which the postnatal changes in monoaminergic parameters are due to specific effects or to unspecific effects remains unclear.

Conclusion

Methyl mercury is a potent inhibitor of several stages of brain chemical neurotransmission in vitro. After administration to animals, however, it is less often inhibitory. This suggests that pharmacokinetics, particularly distribution and binding in the brain, is an important regulatory factor of its toxicity. The data accumulated so far do not cover all aspects of neurotransmission to permit conclusions to be drawn on the most sensitive neuronal pathways or the exact sites and mechanisms of action. In addition to gaps in information, methodological inconsistencies and differences between studies make it difficult to form the final concept of the critical neurochemical mechanisms of action of methyl mercury. However, certain trends can already be observed. In the mature brain, methyl mercury appears to have a slight suppressive effect on cholinergic and serotonergic parameters. The effect on catecholaminergic neurons is more variable and depends on the total dose. One of the earliest signs is the supersensitivity of benzodiazepine receptors, and future studies are likely to reveal more such changes to explain the symptoms of poisoning. In general, however, the doses required for these changes are high enough to induce morphological changes in the brain and peripheral neurotoxicity. Hence, it remains to be shown whether methyl mercury disturbs neurotransmission independently from histopathological damage. As yet, the study has been too crude to reveal subtle changes in small, critically important brain areas.

It is already clear that the developing brain is more vulnerable to methyl mercury than the mature brain. Permanent disturbances, at least in serotonergic, dopaminergic, and noradrenergic neurons, can be detected in later life after neonatal methyl mercury administration to animals. Hence, the behavioral and learning deficits are not unexpected, although their neurochemical basis cannot yet be explained.

References

Abd-Elfattah, A.-S. A., and Shamoo, A. E. (1981). Regeneration of a functionally active rat brain muscarinic receptor by *d*-penicillamine after inhibition with methylmercury and mercuric chloride. *Mol Pharmacol* 20:492–497.

Abe T.; Haga, T.; and Kurokawa, M. (1975). Blockage of axoplasmic transport and depolymerization of reassembled microtubules by methyl mercury. *Brain Res* 86:504–508.

Adler, M. W., and Adler, C. H. (1977). Toxicity of heavy metals and relationship to seizure thresholds. *Clin Pharmacol* 22:774–779.

Agrawal, A. K.; Seth, P. K.; Squibb, R. E.; Tilson, H. A.; Uphouse, L. L.; and Bondy, S. C. (1981). Neurotransmitter receptors in brain regions of acrylamide treated rats, I: Effects of a single exposure to acrylamide. *Pharmacol Biochem Behav* 14:527–531.

Akerman, K. E. O., and Nicholls, D. G. (1983). Physiological and bioenergetic aspects of mitochondrial calcium transport. *Rev Physiol Biochem Pharmacol* 95:149–201.

Amin-Zaki, L.; Elhassani, S.; Majeed, M. A.; Clarkson, T. W.; Doherty, R. A.; and Greenwood, M. (1974). Intra-uterine methyl mercury poisoning in Iraq. *Pediatrics* 54:587–595.

Araki, K.; Wakabayashi, M.; Sakimura, K.; Kushiya, E.; Ozawa, H.; Kunamoto, T.; and Takahashi, Y. (1981). Decreased uptake of GABA by dorsal ganglia in methylmercury-treated rats. *Neurotoxicology* 2:557–566.

Bartolome, J.; Trepanier, P.; Chait, E. A.; Seidler, F. J.; Deskin, R.; and Slotkin, T. A. (1982). Neonatal methylmercury poisoning in the rat: Effects on development of central catecholamine neurotransmitter systems. *Toxicol Appl Pharmacol* 65:92–99.

Berlin, M.; Blomstrand, C.; Grant, C. A.; Hamberger, A.; and Trofast, J. (1975). Tritiated methylmercury in the brain of squirrel monkeys. *Arch Environ Health* 30:591–597.

Berthoud, H. R.; Garman, R. H.; and Weiss, B. (1976). Food intake, body weight, and brain histopathology in mice following chronic methylmercury treatment. *Toxicol Appl Pharmacol* 36:19–30.

Bondy, S. C., and Agrawal, A. K. (1980). The inhibition of cerebral high affinity receptor sites by lead and mercury compounds. *Arch Toxicol* 46:249–256.

Bondy, S. C.; Anderson, C. L.; Harrington, M. E.; and Prasad, K. N. (1979). The effects of organic and inorganic lead and mercury on neurotransmitter high affinity transport and release mechanisms. *Environ Res* 19:102–111.

Bull, R. J., and Lutkenhoff, S. D. (1975). Changes in the metabolic responses of brain tissue to stimulation, in vitro, produced by in vivo administration of methyl mercury. *Neuropharmacol* 14:351–359.

Chang, L. W.; Ware, R. A.; and Desnoyers, P. A. (1973). A histochemical study on some enzyme changes in the kidney, liver, and brain after chronic mercury intoxication in the rat. *Food Cosmet Toxicol* 11:283–286.

Corda, M. G.; Concas, A.; Rossetti, Z.; Guarneri, P.; Corongiu, F. P.; and Biggio, G. (1981). Methyl mercury enhances [^{3}H] diazepam binding in different areas of the brain. *Brain Res* 229:264–269.

Dwivedi, C.; Raghunathan, R.; Joshi, B. C.; and Foster, H. W. (1980). Effect of mercury compounds on cholinacetyl transferase. *Res Commun Chem Pathol Pharmacol* 30:381–384.

Eccles, C. U., and Annau, Z. (1982a). Prenatal methyl mercury exposure, I: Alterations in neonatal activity. *Neurobehav Toxicol Teratol* 4:371–376.

——— (1982b). Prenatal methyl mercury exposure, II: Alterations in learning and psychotropic drug sensitivity in adult offspring. *Neurobehav Toxicol Teratol* 4:377–382.

Eldefrawi, M. E.; Mansour, N. A.; and Eldefrawi, A. T. (1977). Interactions of acetylcholine receptors with organic mercury compounds. *Adv Exp Med Biol* 84:449–463.

Fox, J. H.; Patel-Mandlik, K.; and Cohen, M. M. (1975). Comparative effects of organic and inorganic mercury on brain slice respiration and metabolism. *J Neurochem* 24:757–762.

Gerstner, H. B., and Huff, J. E. (1977). Clinical toxicology of mercury. *J Toxicol Environ Health* 2:491–526.

Green, A. R., and Grahame-Smith, D. G. (1975). 5-Hydroxytryptamine and other indoles in the central nervous system. In *Handbook of Psychopharmacology*, Vol. 3: *Biochemistry of Biogenic Amines*, edited by L. L. Iversen, S. D. Iversen, and S. H. Snyder, pp. 169–245. New York: Plenum Press.

Gruenwedel, D. W., and Friend, D. (1980). Long-term effects of methyl mercury (II) on the viability of HeLa S3 cells. *Bull Environ Contam Toxicol* 25:441–447.

Hoskins, B. B., and Hupp, E. W. (1978). Methylmercury effects in rat, hamster, and squirrel monkey. *Environ Res* 15:5–19.

Hösli, E., and Hösli, L. (1974). The effects of methyl mercury on morphological and histochemical properties of human and rat spinal cord and cerebellum in tissue culture. *Experientia* 30:1300–1304.

Hrdina, P. D.; Peters, D. A. V.; and Singhal, R. L. (1976). Effects of chronic exposure to cadmium, lead, and mercury on brain biogenic amines in the rat. *Res Commun Chem Pathol Pharmacol* 15:483–493.

Hughes, J. A., and Annau, Z. (1976). Postnatal behavioral effects in mice after prenatal exposure to methyl mercury. *Pharmacol Biochem Behav* 4:385–391.

Hughes, R.; Belser, R.; and Brett, C. W. (1975). Behavioral impairment produced by exposure to subclinical amounts of methylmercury chloride. *Environ Res* 10:54–58.

Kobayashi, H.; Yuyama, A.; Matsusaka, N.; Takeno, K.; and Yanagiya, I. (1979). Effects of methyl mercury chloride on various cholinergic parameters in vitro. *J Toxicol Sci* 4:351–362.

——— (1980). Effect of methylmercury on brain acetylcholine concentration and turnover in mice. *Toxicol Appl Pharmacol* 54:1–8.

——— (1981). Neuropharmacological effect of methylmercury in mice with special reference to the central cholinergic system. *Japan J Pharmacol* 31:711–718.

Kojima, K., and Fujita, M. (1973). Summary of recent studies in Japan on methyl mercury poisoning. *Toxicol* 1:43–62.

Komulainen, H., and Tuomisto, J. (1981). Interference of methyl mercury with monoamine uptake and release in rat brain synaptosomes. *Acta Pharmacol Toxicol* 48:214–222.

MacDonald, J. S., and Harbison, R. D. (1977). Methyl mercury-induced encephalopathy in mice. *Toxicol Appl Pharmacol* 39:195–205.

Macfarlane, D. E. (1981). The effects of methyl mercury on platelets: Induction of aggregation and release via activation of the prostaglandin synthesis pathway. *Mol Pharmacol* 19:470–476.

Marsh, D. O.; Myers, G. J.; Clarkson, T. W.; Amin-Zaki, L.; Tikriti, S.; and Majeed, M. A. (1980). Fetal methylmercury poisoning: Clinical and toxicological data on 29 cases. *Ann Neurol* 7:348–353.

Michaelson, A. (1980). An appraisal of rodent studies on the behavioral toxicity of lead: The role of nutritional status. In *Lead Toxicity*, edited by L. Singhal and J. A. Thomas, pp. 301–365. Baltimore: Urban and Schwarzenberg.

O'Kusky, J. (1983). Methylmercury poisoning of the developing nervous system: Morphological changes in neuronal mitochondria. *Acta Neuropathol* 61:116–122.

Omata, S.; Hirakawa, E.; Daimon, Y.; Uchiyama, M.; Nakashita, H.; Horigome, T.; Sugano, I.; and Sugano, H. (1982). Methylmercury-induced changes in the activities of neurotransmitter enzymes in nervous tissues of the rat. *Arch Toxicol* 51:285–294.

Omata, S.; Sakimura, K.; Tsubaki, H.; and Sugano, H. (1978). In vivo effect of methylmercury on protein synthesis in brain and liver of the rat. *Toxicol Appl Pharmacol* 44:367–378.

Pryor, G. T.; Uyeno, E. T.; Tilson, H. A.; and Mitchell, C. L. (1983). Assessment of chemicals using a battery of neurobehavioral tests: A comparative study. *Neurobehav Toxicol Teratol* 5:91–117.

Reuhl, K. R., and Chang, L. W. (1979). Effects of methylmercury on the development of the nervous system: A review. *Neurotoxicol* 1:21–55.

Sakai, K. (1974). Time-dependent distribution of [203]Hg-methylmercuric chloride in tissues and cells of rats. *Japan J Exp Med* 45:63–77.

Salvaterra, P.; Lown, B.; Morganti, J.; and Massaro, E. J. (1973). Alterations in neurochemical and behavioural parameters in the mouse induced by low doses of methyl mercury. *Acta Pharmacol Toxicol* 33:177–190.

Sharma, R. P.; Aldous, C. N.; and Farr, C. H. (1982). Methylmercury induced alterations in brain amine synthesis in rats. *Toxicol Lett* 13:195–201.

Sobotka, T. J.; Cook, M. P.; and Brodie, R. E. (1974). Effects of perinatal exposure to methyl mercury on functional brain development and neurochemistry. *Biol Psychiatr* 8:307–320.

Spuhler, K., and Prasad, K. N. (1980). Inhibition by methylmercuric chloride of prostaglandin E_1-sensitive adenylate cyclase activity in glioma but not in neuroblastoma cells in culture. *Biochem Pharmacol* 29:201–203.

Spyker, J. M.; Sparber, S. B.; and Goldberg, A. M. (1972). Subtle consequences of methylmercury exposure: Behavioral deviations in offspring of treated mothers. *Science* 18:621–623.

Sudo, A., and Arito, H. (1982). Neurochemical correlates of sleep disorder of rats administered with methylmercury chloride. *Ind Health* 20:67–70.

Syversen, T. L. M. (1982). Changes in protein and RNA synthesis in rat brain neurons after a single dose of methylmercury. *Toxicol Lett* 10:31–34.

Taylor, L. L., and DiStefano, V. (1976). Effects of methylmercury on brain biogenic amines in the developing rat pup. *Toxicol Appl Pharmacol* 38:489–497.

Tsuzuki, Y. (1981). Effects of chronic methylmercury exposure on activities of neurotransmitter enzymes in rat cerebellum. *Toxicol Appl Pharmacol* 60:379–381.

———— (1982). Effect of methylmercury on different neurotransmitter systems in rat brain. *Toxicol Lett* 13:159–162.

Tunnicliff, G., and Wood, J. D. (1973). The inhibition of mouse brain neurotransmitter enzymes by mercury compounds and a comparison with the effects of hyperbaric oxygen. *Comp Gen Pharmacol* 4:101–105.

Tuomisto, J., and Komulainen, H. (1983a). Release and inhibition of uptake of 5-hydroxytryptamine in blood platelets in vitro by copper and methyl mercury. *Acta Pharmacol Toxicol* 52:292–297.

———— (1983b). Uptake inhibiting metals do not inhibit 5-HT binding to platelet membranes. *Toxicol Lett* 18(Suppl. 1):103.

Vallee, B. T., and Ulmer, D. D. (1972). Biochemical effects of mercury, cadmium, and lead. *Ann Rev Biochem* 41:91–128.

Verity, M. A.; Brown, W. J.; and Cheung, M. (1975). Organic mercurial encephalopathy: In vivo and in vitro effects of methyl mercury on synaptosomal respiration. *J Neurochem* 25:759–766.

Verity, M. A.; Brown, W. J.; Cheung, M.; and Czar, G. (1977). Methyl mercury inhibition of synaptosome and brain slice protein synthesis: In vivo and in vitro studies. *J Neurochem* 29:673–679.

Von Burg, R.; Northington, F. K.; and Shamoo, A. (1980). Methylmercury inhibition of rat brain muscarinic receptors. *Toxicol Appl Pharmacol* 53:283–292.

Yoshino, Y.; Mozai, T.; and Nakao, K. (1966). Biochemical changes in the brain in rats poisoned with an alkylmercury compound, with special reference to the inhibition of protein synthesis in brain cortex slices. *J Neurochem* 13:1223–1230.

Zenick, H. (1974). Behavioral and biochemical consequences in methyl mercury chloride toxicity. *Pharmacol Biochem Behav* 2:709–713.

ELEVEN

Neurophysiological Effects of Mercurials

William D. Atchison

In contrast to the neuropathology of methyl mercury poisoning, the functional effects of methyl mercury on electrical impulse conduction by nerve and muscle membranes and chemical transmission at synapses have not been studied as extensively. The fundamental properties of information transfer within the nervous system—impulse conduction and chemical transmission across synapses—are both vitally dependent on electrochemical flux of cations such as Na^+, K^+, and Ca^{2+}. There is abundant evidence in the literature that abnormal mono- and polyvalent cations, such as Li^+, Mg^{2+}, Co^{2+}, Mn^{2+}, and La^{3+}, can alter the nature of these cationic conductances (del Castillo and Engbaek 1954; Baker et al. 1971; Heuser and Miledi 1971; Kajimoto and Kirpekar 1972; Weakly 1973; Balnave and Gage 1973; Branisteanu and Volle 1975). Thus, it should come as no surprise that mercury in both organic and inorganic forms would also affect these processes. Indeed, given the propensity of mercury in general, and organomercurials in particular, to interact with functional groups in biological membranes (such as sulfhydryls and amino groups), it would be surprising if functional damage to the nervous system were not observed. One may well ask what relevance these functional changes following acute exposure to mercury have to the histopathological findings in patients poisoned by chronic exposure to methyl mercury. The answer, of course, is that in many cases there may be no direct relationship, but that these functional changes may signal early cellular effects of methyl mercury that have not progressed in the whole organism to the extent of observable pathology. Moreover, effects of mercurials on the processes responsible for synaptic transmission—processes that are highly Ca^{2+}-dependent—may be representative of other effects of methyl mercury on the nervous system. Thus, studies of acute and semi-acute exposure of in vitro systems to organic and inorganic mercurials may permit us to predict more generally the nature of their neurotoxicity.

This chapter reviews the clinical effects as well as the results of studies that have dealt with functional changes in neurotransmission wrought by methyl mercury as studied by neurophysiological techniques. A variety of experimental systems using both vertebrates, including mammals, and invertebrates have been used in these studies.

Clinical Studies

There are few reports of clinical studies of electromyographic measurements in individuals intoxicated with methyl mercury. Those that do exist deal with the outbreak of subchronic mercurialism in Iraq in the 1970s (Bakir et al. 1973). Studies of conduction velocity of sensory nerve action potentials and mixed nerve action potentials in 19 patients, all victims of this episode of poisoning and all exhibiting a variety of signs of neurological dysfunction, indicated no differences from control values in either conduction velocity or amplitude (Le Quesne et al. 1974). In a second electromyographic study of 14 randomly selected patients 7 months after their hospitalization for mercury poisoning, no effects on motor or sensory conduction velocity, sensory threshold, or latency were observed (Von Burg and Rustam 1974). No fibrillations or fasciculations—signs of denervation—were observed. An unusual observation made during the course of this latter study was that 2 of the 14 patients exhibited a decremental response of the evoked muscle action potential recorded from the *abductor pollicis brevis* following median nerve stimulation (Rustam et al. 1975). During stimulation at 4–10 Hz, muscle action potentials decreased from 30 to 33 percent of the initial amplitude. Administration of the reversible acetylcholinesterase inhibitor neostigmine methylsulfate (0.5 mg) prevented the decrease in amplitude of the muscle action potential. Initiation of neostigmine therapy led to a marked improvement in muscular strength, an effect reversed almost immediately by replacement of neostigmine with placebo. The decrement in muscle action potential amplitude during repetitive nerve stimulation, and its amelioration by neostigmine, suggested a myasthenia gravis–like syndrome to the authors. Because the normal incidence of this disease is on the order of 0.005 percent (Keynes 1969), and because neither of the patients had a history of muscle weakness prior to ingestion of methyl mercury, the authors concluded that neuromuscular defects may be associated with methyl mercury poisoning. The mechanism underlying this apparent block of neuromuscular transmission by methyl mercury (MeHg) is unknown.

Experimental Studies

In contrast to the paucity of clinical information regarding neurophysiological effects of methyl mercury, there are a number of reports that indicate that inorganic and organic mercurials alter neurotransmission in experimental animals. In isolated nerve-skeletal muscle preparations from the rat (diaphragm) and frog (sartorius), acute bath application of micromolar concentrations of mercuric chloride and methyl mercuric chloride produced a time-dependent block of twitches evoked by electrical stimulation of the motor nerve (Von Burg and Landry 1976; Juang 1976a) (Figure 11.1). Responses evoked by direct electrical stimulation of the muscle were either unaffected or

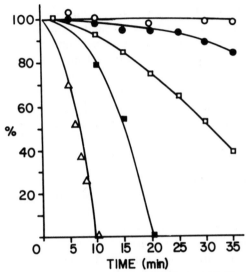

Figure 11.1. Time course of contraction inhibition at the indicated bath concentrations of methyl mercury. ($\bigcirc$, 1; $\bullet$, 10; $\square$, 15; $\blacksquare$, 20; $\triangle$, 29 μM MeHg. Y axis = % of premercury control.) (Reprinted, by permission, from Von Burg and Landry 1976, p. 549.)

depressed to a much lesser extent, indicating that the depressant effect of mercurials could be attributed either to effects on conduction of the nerve action potential or to effects on synaptic transmission, or both. Reports regarding the reversibility of these effects conflict. Von Burg and Landry (1976) reported that after washing the preparations four to five times with a mercury-free solution over a period of 20 minutes, twitch height recovered from complete block to 10–30 percent of premercury-control tension. Juang (1976a), on the other hand, reported that if methyl mercury was washed out of the preparation prior to complete block of twitch, block continued to progress 30 minutes after washing with mercury-free solutions. Efforts to reverse methyl mercury induced block with choline, *L*-cysteine, or *d*-penicillamine (10^{-5}–10^{-3}M) were unsuccessful (Von Burg and Landry 1976). When muscle contractility measurements were made in situ—from rats poisoned either acutely (10 mg/kg/day subcutaneously [sc] for 7 days) or subchronically (2 mg/kg/day sc for 5 days/wk for 3–4 wk) with methyl mercury (Somjen et al. 1973)—gastrocnemius twitch tension was also diminished, compared with food-deprived controls. Twitch tension was reduced to 75 percent of control values, while tetanic tension was 78 percent of control. The frequency at which a fused tetanus was first observed (fusion frequency) was not altered in methyl mercury intoxicated rats, nor was maximal tetanic tension elicited during a 10-second train at 75 or 100 Hz subject to fatigue. Responses to direct electrical stimulation of the gastrocnemius-soleus were not measured, so it is impossible to determine whether these effects were the result of direct effects of methyl mercury on skeletal muscle, as opposed to effects on either nerve impulse conduction or neuromuscular transmission. However, these results are important in that they signify that effects of methyl mercury on skeletal muscle contractility occur not only with direct bath application but also at periods of 2–10 days following systemic application of the toxicant. These studies have provided the basis for further experimentation on effects of mercurials on synaptic transmission.

Effects of Mercurials on Synaptic Transmission

Preferential effects of inorganic and organic mercurials on twitches evoked by motor nerve stimulation, compared with effects evoked by direct skeletal muscle stimulation, are indicative of effects on either synaptic transmission, conductance of nerve action potentials into the axon terminal, or both. In recent years, a number of investigators have focused on the direct effects of inorganic and organic mercurials on synaptic and, in particular, neuromuscular transmission. Release of transmitter at chemical synapses occurs in two forms (see Katz 1969). The first, in response to stimulation of the presynaptic neuron, is assumed to result in the synchronous discharge of multiple packets or quanta of transmitter and gives rise to a graded polarization (either depolarization or hyperpolarization, depending on the ionic conductances involved) of the postsynaptic cell, known respectively as an excitatory postsynaptic potential or an inhibitory postsynaptic potential. The second form occurs spontaneously, and presumably consists of random discharge of single quanta of transmitter, although this is still open to some debate. The postsynaptic responses to these random discharges are known as miniature postsynaptic potentials. The process of chemical neurotransmission can be simplified into two steps: (1) processes associated directly with the synthesis and release of neurotransmitter, which occur in the presynaptic nerve terminal (presynaptic processes), and (2) processes associated with the binding of transmitter to its receptor sites in the postsynaptic membrane, with subsequent opening of ionic conductance channels leading to the postsynaptic polarization (postsynaptic processes). Effects at either presynaptic or postsynaptic sites would be expected to alter neurotransmission and hence depress the final result, which at the neuromuscular junction is the muscle twitch. Consequently, to obtain further information on the nature of potential effects on neurotransmission, both processes must be studied independently.

The first study of the effects of mercury on synaptic transmission was reported by Kostial and Landeka (1975). Using the intact perfused superior cervical ganglion of the cat treated with eserine to block acetylcholinesterase, the release of acetylcholine (ACh) at rest and following 5 minutes of preganglionic stimulation was measured before and at various times after perfusion with mercuric chloride ($HgCl_2$). Before treatment with mercury, no ACh was measured in the ganglion perfusate at rest, while approximately 40 ng were obtained following stimulation. Administration of 100 μM $HgCl_2$ initially decreased the amount of the ACh released during stimulation to 75 percent of that in nonmercury-exposed ganglia. However, resting release was increased to approximately 15 ng. Following an initial return to normal Lockes solution, stimulus-evoked release apparently returned to normal levels, but resting release remained elevated. Subsequent exposure to 100 μM $HgCl_2$ for 5 minutes 10 minutes later decreased both resting and stimulus-evoked ACh release. Following this second exposure to mercury, subsequent return to normal Lockes solution could not reverse the effect. The authors were unable to distinguish experimentally between ACh released spontaneously during nerve stimulation and that evoked by nerve stimulation. For this reason, and because the depression of stimulus-evoked release was irreversible after more than one exposure to $HgCl_2$, Kostial and Landeka reasoned that the increase in ACh following stimulation during the first washout phase may have represented a long-lasting increase in spontaneous release, while stimulus-evoked release was in fact depressed. Thus, the initial observations on effects of mercurials on synaptic transmission were (1) an irreversible decrease in nerve-evoked neurotransmitter release and (2) a biphasic, irreversible stimulation followed by depression of spontaneous neurotransmitter release.

More recent studies utilizing conventional intracellular microelectrode recording techniques have clarified the effects of mercurials on synaptic transmission. These techniques make it possible to differentiate between responses due to synchronous nerve-evoked release of neurotransmitter (excitatory postsynaptic potentials [EPSPs] or end-plate potentials [EPPs]) and those occurring asynchronously at rest or during nerve stimulation (miniature EPSPs [MEPSPs] or miniature EPPs [MEPPs]).

Effects on Synchronous Nerve-Evoked Release of Transmitter

In studies of ganglionic transmission at the guinea pig superior cervical ganglia (Juang and Yonemura 1975) and of neuromuscular transmission in the frog sartorius (Manalis and Cooper 1975; Juang 1976*b;* Cooper and Manalis 1983) and rat (Atchison and Narahashi 1982; Atchison et al. 1984; Atchison et al. 1986; Traxinger and Atchison 1987*a*) and mouse diaphragm (Atchison et al. 1984), the primary effect of mercurials is to decrease nerve-evoked release of acetylcholine. End-plate block of preparations in which neuromuscular transmission is blocked with *d*-tubocurarine is characterized by a steady decline in mean EPP amplitude (Figure 11.2), while in magnesium-paralyzed preparations it is characterized by a decline in mean EPP amplitude and an increase in the number of failures of transmission in response to a nerve stimulus (Atchison and Narahashi 1982; Atchison et al. 1984). In contrast, in preparations in which contractions are blocked by

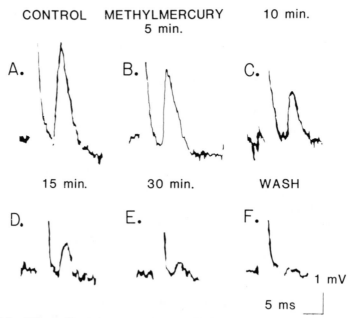

CONTROL   METHYLMERCURY   10 min.
5 min.

A.   B.   C.

15 min.   30 min.   WASH

D.   E.   F.

1 mV

5 ms

Figure 11.2. Effects of methyl mercury (20 μM) on EPP amplitude at the rat neuromuscular junction. EPPs were elicited at 0.5 Hz before application of methyl mercury (A), during application of methyl mercury (B–D), and during washout of methyl mercury (E). Skeletal muscle contractions were blocked with *d*-tubocurarine (1 μM).

cutting the myofibers near the main intramuscular branch of the motor nerve, transmission block induced by MeHg is characterized by sudden failure of the EPP to be generated in response to nerve stimulation. Under these conditions, block occurs in approximately 8 to 9 minutes (Traxinger and Atchison 1987*a*). At the time of EPP block, MEPPs of normal amplitude and duration still occur (Atchison and Narahashi 1982). In every instance where it was tested, block of nerve-evoked transmitter release by inorganic or organic mercury could not be reversed by washing the preparation with mercury-free solutions (Atchison and Narahashi 1982; Atchison et al. 1986; Atchison and Traxinger 1986; Traxinger and Atchison 1987*a*). However, more recent studies (Atchison and Traxinger 1986; Traxinger and Atchison 1987*b*) indicate that under some conditions at least a temporary reversal of MeHg-induced block of neuromuscular transmission can be induced.

The effect of inorganic and methyl mercury on nerve-evoked transmitter release is time- and concentration-dependent (Figure 11.3)—the higher the concentration, the shorter the time required to produce an effect. At low concentrations of mercurials (0.1–10.0 μM), complete block of the EPP was not seen for 60 minutes or more (Manalis and Cooper 1975; Juang 1976*b*); a concentration of 100 μM methyl mercury produced a virtually complete block of nerve-evoked postsynaptic responses between 5 and 15 minutes

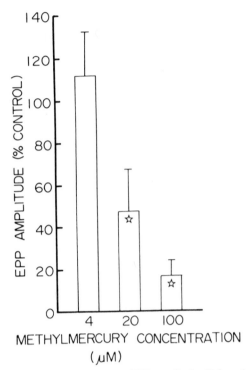

Figure 11.3. Effects of methyl mercury on EPP amplitude. Values (mean ± SEM of 4–8 determinations) are expressed as a percentage of pretreatment values. The EPP was recorded in solutions containing high Mg^{2+} and low Ca^{2+} (8 mM and 1 mM, respectively) to block neurally evoked muscle contractions. Measurements were made 5 minutes before and 10 minutes after treatment with methyl mercury. At least 100 EPPs were analyzed for each preparation. The star indicates a value less than control ($p < 0.05$). (Reprinted, by permission, from Atchison and Narahashi 1982, p. 43.)

(Atchison and Narahashi 1982; Atchison et al. 1986; Traxinger and Atchison 1987a,1987b). A lower concentration (20 μM) of MeHg caused block of the EPP after approximately 40 minutes (Atchison and Narahashi 1982; Traxinger and Atchison 1987b).

In all cases reported, the decline in EPP amplitude was progressive with time, proceeding to complete block. Thus, block of the EPP does not attain a steady state short of complete block. For this reason, a strict concentration-dependence does not occur. There appears to be a lower threshold concentration below which block of evoked release does not occur (Atchison and Narahashi 1982), but this may simply reflect that the latent period to produce block at these concentrations was longer than the period over which the measurements were made and the effect was missed. Thus, it is not possible to state unequivocally that there is a threshold concentration of mercury needed to block evoked transmitter release.

Some investigators reported a transient increase in EPP amplitude in the presence of mercury preceding the block of the EPP. The onset of this increase in EPP amplitude occurred after 10 to 20 minutes (Manalis and Cooper 1975; Juang 1976b; Binah et al. 1978; Cooper and Manalis 1983) and lasted from 10 to 35 minutes. For example, at the frog neuromuscular junction, Manalis and Cooper (1975) reported that inorganic mercury (1–10 μM) first increased EPP amplitude 50 times the control values before subsequently depressing it. Juang (1976b) reported a similar phenomenon with 10 μM methyl mercury, but did not observe any such effect with 10 μM HgCl$_2$. Atchison and Narahashi (1982) observed a slight though statistically nonsignificant stimulatory effect of 4 μM methyl mercury on the EPP at the rat motor end-plate, but no stimulation at higher concentrations of methyl mercury (20 and 100 μM). More recently, Traxinger and Atchison (1987a) reported slight, transient, and statistically nonsignificant increases in EPP amplitude with a concentration of 100 μM MeHg in experiments using the "cut fiber" preparation. Similar effects of methyl mercury have been observed on transmission at autonomic ganglia and in the central nervous system. Methyl mercury (5 μM) increased the amplitude of the postsynaptic compound action potential recorded from the rabbit superior cervical ganglion slightly, while 10–20 μM inhibited the action potential (Alkadhi and Taha 1982). At 100 μM, methyl mercury reduced the amplitude of the postsynaptic potential recorded extracellularly from isolated olfactory cortical slices of guinea pig brain (Kuroda, Atchison, and Narahashi, unpublished observation). It may be that transmission block occurs too rapidly at these higher concentrations to permit a marked stimulation of evoked release to be observed.

Presynaptic effects of methyl mercury on nerve-evoked transmitter release should be observed as effects on mean quantal content (m), the number of transmitter quanta released by a nerve volley. Measurements of m by a number of different investigators (Juang 1976a; Binah et al. 1978; Atchison and Narahashi 1982) indicated that the effects of methyl mercury and HgCl$_2$ on mean EPP amplitude paralleled those on mean quantal content, indicating that a predominant component of mercurial-induced block of synaptic transmission could be attributed to presynaptic effects. Further analysis of neurotransmitter release statistical parameters (McLachlan 1978) indicated that the depression of m produced by methyl mercury was due primarily to depression of the immediately available store of neurotransmitter (n) (Atchison and Narahashi 1982) (Figure 11.4). The probability of transmitter release (p) was actually increased by methyl mercury (Atchison and Narahashi 1982).

Block of evoked transmitter release by mercurials appears to be independent of external Ca^{2+} concentration. Increasing the bath concentration of Ca^{2+} from 2 mM to 4 or 8 mM did not prolong the time of the EPP to block, nor did it decrease the degree of block produced by methyl mercury (Atchi-

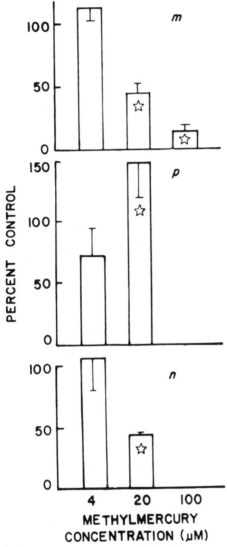

Figure 11.4. Effects of methyl mercury on statistical parameters of neurotransmitter release at the rat neuromuscular junction. Determinations of quantal content (*m*), probability of release (*p*), and immediately available store (*n*) were made during a 5-minute period 10 minutes before (control) and 15 minutes after administration of methyl mercury (4, 20, or 100 μM). Quantal content was determined by the method of failures. Each value is the mean percent (± SEM of pretreatment control). The star represents a value that is statistically different from control ($p <$ 0.05). (Reprinted, by permission, from Atchison and Narahashi 1982, p. 45.)

son et al. 1986; Traxinger and Atchison 1987*a*). Moreover, once the EPP was blocked completely, washing the preparation for 30–45 minutes with a higher extracellular $[Ca^{2+}]$ could not reverse the block, nor could washing with 4-aminopyridine (50 or 100 μM, $n = 5$), which increases Ca^{2+} influx during the action potential (Atchison and Traxinger 1986). When transmitter release was supported by Ca^{2+} (2 mM), increasing either the stimulus intensity or duration at the time that the EPP was first blocked caused a temporary restoration of transmission (12 out of 13 experiments) (Atchison and Traxinger 1986). However, with continued application of MeHg, transmission was again blocked even at the higher intensities and longer durations of stimulation. When Sr^{2+} was substituted for Ca^{2+} to support evoked release, block of the EPP again occurred at 8–10 minutes (Traxinger and Atchison 1987*a*). When Sr^{2+} was substituted for Ca^{2+} on an equimolar basis, reversal was obtained less often (3 out of 6 experiments) with increased intensity or duration of stimulation (Atchison and Traxinger 1986; Traxinger and Atchison 1987*b*). However, in preparations treated with 4 mM Sr^{2+}, recovery was produced in 100 percent (3 of 3 experiments) of the preparations by increasing stimulus intensity or duration. In three experiments, Ca^{2+}-containing liposomes were used to bypass the membrane Ca^{2+} channel (Atchison, unpublished observation). When transmission was blocked with MeHg, direct intracellular application of Ca^{2+} could not reverse the MeHg-induced block. Similarly, mercury-induced release of catecholamines from the bovine adrenal was not affected by increasing Ca^{2+} concentration in the perfusion medium (Hart and Borowitz 1974).

One potential mechanism by which the MeHg-induced block of transmitter release may occur is suppression of voltage-dependent entry of Ca^{2+} into the nerve terminal following the action potential. Because of their extremely small size, motor nerve terminals cannot be impaled with microelectrodes. Thus, intracellular recordings of Ca^{2+} currents cannot be undertaken, nor can Ca^{2+}-selective electrodes be used to measure increases in $[Ca^{2+}]_i$. One way around this problem is to use synaptosomes and measure $^{45}Ca^{2+}$ uptake during depolarization. Nachshen (1984) reported that inorganic, divalent mercury ($HgCl_2$) suppressed the uptake of ^{45}Ca during K^+-induced depolarization or following predepolarization in rat brain synaptosomes. The effect of MeHg (10–500 μM) on total ^{45}Ca uptake in K^+-depolarized ($[K^+] = 41$ mM) synaptosomes was measured, and compared to that obtained in the presence of $HgCl_2$ (10–500 μM) or controls (Atchison et al. 1986). Inorganic mercury produced a concentration-dependent suppression of depolarization-induced ^{45}Ca uptake. Peak inhibition occurred at 200 μM $HgCl_2$, which suppressed ^{45}Ca uptake to approximately 5 percent of premercury control values. These results corroborate those obtained previously by Nachshen (1984). MeHg also decreased total ^{45}Ca uptake, although the maximal inhibition produced (70 percent at 200 μM) was less than that produced by $HgCl_2$.

The effect of MeHg was more apparent following 10 seconds of incubation in synaptosomes predepolarized for 10 seconds with 41 mM K^+ prior to MeHg and ^{45}Ca addition to inactivate the "fast" Ca^{2+} channel than following a 1-second incubation. A significant decrease in ^{45}Ca uptake occurred at 200 and 500 μM MeHg following the 10-second incubation. ^{45}Ca uptake following a 1-second incubation was also depressed by MeHg; this effect occurred at lower concentrations of MeHg (20–50 μM), although the maximal percent block was not as high as that produced during 10 seconds of depolarization. Ca uptake during 10 seconds is thought to represent flux through slow, non-inactivating Ca channels while uptake during 1 second is thought to be due to a rapid, inactivating Ca channel (Nachshen and Blaustein 1980). It appears that MeHg is more efficacious as a blocker at the slow channel, but more potent at the fast channel. The total uptake of ^{45}Ca as a function of extracellular Ca in the absence of MeHg saturated at approximately 0.5 mM $= [Ca]_o$. When 200 μM MeHg was present, ^{45}Ca uptake also saturated at 0.5 mM Ca^{2+}, although the total uptake was only 35–40 percent of that in the absence of MeHg. Thus, MeHg appears to behave as a noncompetitive, irreversible inhibitor to Ca entry through both a slow noninactivating and a rapid inactivating membrane Ca channel. These results are consistent with the apparently irreversible block of Ca-dependent, nerve-evoked transmitter release induced by MeHg at the vertebrate neuromuscular junction.

Effects on Spontaneous Neurotransmitter Release

The effects of mercurials on spontaneous transmitter release are biphasic with continued exposure. The time course for this effect differs from that observed for effects on evoked release. The initial effect observed is a dramatic increase in the resting release of neurotransmitter, observed as an increase in MEPP or MEPSP frequency. Values of MEPP frequency have been increased by mercurials from control values of 0.3–3.0 per second to frequencies of 10–100 per second in the frog, rat, and mouse (Barrett et al. 1974; Juang 1976*b;* Atchison and Narahashi 1982; Miyamoto 1983; Atchison et al. 1984), usually following a latency of 2–40 minutes, depending on the concentration of mercury employed. Binah et al. (1978) and Cooper and Manalis (1983) reported that $HgCl_2$ increased MEPP frequency immediately upon exposure, but this has not been reported by others. The latent period can be cut dramatically by depolarizing the preparation using elevated extracellular K^+ (15–20 mM) (Miyamoto 1983; Atchison 1984). The increase in spontaneous release does not appear to be concentration-dependent—similar frequencies are produced by concentrations from 10 to 100 μM. Reports vary as to whether $HgCl_2$ is more or less potent than methyl mercury; Miyamoto (1983) reported that $HgCl_2$ increased MEPP frequency at a threshold concentration of 3 μM, compared with 100 μM for methyl mercury, while Binah et al. (1978) reported that $HgCl_2$ was more potent than the organomercurial mersalyl. On the other hand, Juang (1976a, 1976b) showed that $HgCl_2$ and methyl mercury at 10 μM were approximately equi-effective in increasing MEPP frequency at the frog end-plate, but $HgCl_2$ was less effective than methyl mercury in stimulating transmitter release at the isolated guinea pig ganglion. Increased spontaneous release of ACh was also seen when mercury was given systemically, as opposed to by bath application. Juang and Yonemura (1975) found that MEPSP frequency was increased significantly in ganglia removed from guinea pigs between 30 minutes and 5 days after intraperitoneal injection of 1mg MeHg.

The Ca^{2+} dependence of the effects of MeHg on spontaneous release has also been investigated. Spontaneous release of transmitter differs from nerve-evoked release in certain minor respects, such as the response of the process to changes in membrane potential, but there are many fundamental similarities in terms of the underlying mechanisms, the dependence on Ca^{2+}, and so forth. Moreover, spontaneous release does not require the presence of a nerve action potential to cause release, and thus spontaneous release is a very useful tool for studying the release process when the possibility of block of the presynaptic action potential exists because it bypasses that step. (Block of the presynaptic action potential would certainly cause block of the EPP, which depends on the presence of a nerve impulse.) The goal was to determine whether MeHg-induced stimulation of spontaneous release of acetylcholine was independent of extracellular Ca^{2+} concentration and whether MeHg increased spontaneous ACh release by intracellular mechanisms. Increasing bath Ca^{2+} concentration from 1 to 2 or 4 mM decreased the latent period required by 100 μM MeHg to increase spontaneous ACh release as measured by miniature end-plate potential (MEPP) frequency from 48 to 34 to 22 min, respectively (Atchison 1986). Further increasing bath Ca^{2+} to 8 mM actually increased the latent period back to 49 minutes, an effect that could be explained by screening of or binding to negative surface charges on the terminal external membrane by Ca^{2+}. Increasing $[Ca^{2+}]_o$ had no consistent effect on the magnitude of the MeHg-induced increase in MEPP frequency, while in controls, MEPP frequency increased monotonically as $[Ca^{2+}]_o$ was increased (Figure 11.5). Depolarization of the preparation with elevated extracellular K^+ (15 mM) shortened the latent period for increased MEPP frequency from approximately 30 minutes to 1–5 minutes and also shortened the time required for MeHg to cause complete cessation of MEPPs (Figure 11.6). In experiments conducted in K^+-depolarized preparations to which no Ca^{2+} was added, MeHg increased MEPP frequency, although not as much as in solutions containing Ca^{2+}. Similarly, under conditions of Ca^{2+} deprivation (pretreatment with 10 mM EGTA and Ca^{2+}-free solutions), MeHg still increased MEPP frequency.

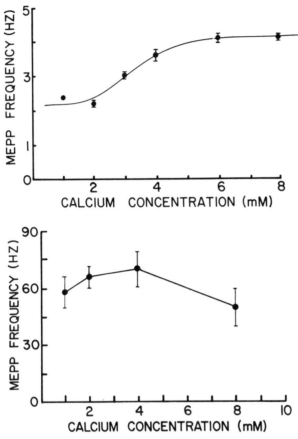

Figure 11.5. Effects of increasing $[Ca^{2+}]_o$ on MEPP frequency in the absence (*top*) and presence (*bottom*) of methyl mercury. MEPPs were recorded during a 5-minute interval in the absence and presence of MeHg at the time of peak increase in MEPP frequency using the $[Ca^{2+}]_o$ indicated. Each preparation was exposed to a single $[Ca^{2+}]_o$. Each value is the mean ($\pm$ SEM) of at least five preparations. (After Atchison 1986a.)

Ca^{2+} is not the only ion that can support the release of neurotransmitter. Sr^{2+} and Ba^{2+} also support the release of ACh at the neuromuscular junction, although their efficacy and the effects they have on the release process differ from those of Ca^{2+} (Silinsky 1981; Dodge et al. 1969). Since MeHg induces an increase in Ca-dependent spontaneous release of ACh, Ba^{2+} or Sr^{2+} was substituted for Ca^{2+} to support MeHg-induced release of ACh in hopes of determining whether the cationic selectivity of the ACh release process was altered by MeHg. In these studies, Ca^{2+} was replaced in the bath solution by either Sr^{2+} or Ba^{2+} in concentrations that produced a control MEPP fre-

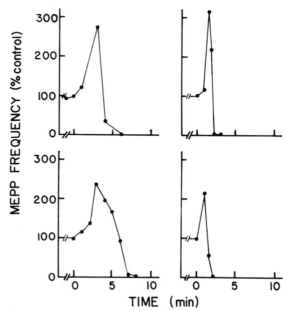

Figure 11.6. Time course of effects of methyl mercury on MEPP frequency in four rat hemidiaphragm preparations exposed to high $[K^+]_0$. Preparations were pretreated with physiological saline containing 20 mM KCl to induce chemical depolarization for 35 to 45 minutes prior to exposure to MeHg, which commenced at time "zero." MEPPs were recorded continuously from the same cell before and during application of MeHg. Note that the MeHg-induced increase and decrease in MEPP frequency are complete by 10 minutes in each case. (After Atchison 1986*a*).

quency that was equi-effective with Ca^{2+}. When preparations were subsequently challenged with 100 μM MeHg, peak MEPP frequencies in Sr^{2+} (2 mM), Ba^{2+} (2mM), and Ca^{2+} (2 mM) were 34.1 $\pm$ 6 Hz, 33.7 $\pm$ 6 Hz, and 35 $\pm$ 3 Hz, respectively ($n = 5$–6). Thus, Sr^{2+} and Ba^{2+} were equally active in supporting MeHg-evoked spontaneous release. That is, MeHg's effect on the transmitter release process is *not* Ca^{2+}-specific (Traxinger and Atchison 1987*a*).

Brief, repetitive stimulation produces a progressive increase in MEPP frequency which decays gradually with multiple components back to control levels after stimulation (Liley and North 1953; Miledi and Thies 1971; Erulkar and Rahamimoff 1978; Zengel and Magleby 1981). The term "asynchronous evoked release" is used to describe the evoked increases in MEPP frequency (Silinsky 1985). The extracellular divalent cation potency sequence for evoked asynchronous release in the frog is $Ba^{2+} > Sr^{2+} > Ca^{2+}$ (Silinsky and Mellow 1981). Clearance of the cations by nerve terminal organelles or membrane processes is generally thought to be responsible for the decay of MEPP frequency following stimulation (Magleby and Zengel

1982; Silinsky 1985) although other Ca^{2+}-activated factors may be involved (Zengel and Magleby 1982). MEPPs and EPPs were evoked at 1-minute intervals by repetitive stimulation of the phrenic nerve during a 4-minute control period in 2 mM Ca^{2+}, 2 mM Sr^{2+}, or 0.5 mM Ba^{2+} and subsequently in the cation, plus 100 μM MeHg. MeHg did not alter the rate constants for either the fast or the slow component of MEPP frequency decay in Sr^{2+} or Ba^{2+} solutions. However, the fractional increase in MEPP frequency ($F_{m(t)}$) was greater with MeHg during both the fast and slow phases of MEPP frequency of decay in Sr^{2+} and Ba^{2+} solutions. In Ca^{2+} solutions, $F_{m(t)}$ was elevated in MeHg during the entire 60-second period after stimulation. Asynchronous evoked release was also blocked by MeHg; the mean latency to block was significantly longer (12.0 $\pm$ 0.8 min) than the mean latency to block (8.4 $\pm$ 0.5 min) of synchronous evoked release. These results suggest that the MeHg-induced effect on spontaneous release of ACh appears to be due to MeHg-induced release of divalent cation from bound intracellular stores as opposed to block of cation uptake into intraterminal buffering systems (Traxinger and Atchison 1987a).

The relative independence of the MeHg-evoked increase in spontaneous and potassium-evoked ACh release from extracellular Ca^{2+} implies that MeHg acts to release some *intracellular* source of Ca^{2+}. One major component of the intracellular Ca^{2+} storage pool is the mitochondrion. Perhaps MeHg causes nerve terminal mitochondria to discharge Ca^{2+}. If this is the case, it might be possible to antagonize or block this effect of MeHg by altering normal mitochondrial function. To test this the interaction of MeHg with several mitochondrial inhibitors on the spontaneous release of ACh was studied (Levesque and Atchison 1987). The agents tested were dicoumarol, 2,4-dinitrophenol, valinomycin, and ruthenium red. The first two uncouple oxidative phosphorylation in the mitochondrion. Valinomycin is a K^+ ionophore that first hyperpolarizes the terminal before uncoupling oxidative phosphorylation, while ruthenium red is a specific inhibitor of the mitochondrial Ca^{2+} transport system. All these chemicals produced a transient increase in ACh release when administered alone. In each case we tested the interaction of the inhibitor with MeHg by first applying the mitochondrial inhibitor, and then, when its effect had subsided, applying MeHg. MeHg was able to evoke a large increase in MEPP frequency within 10 minutes when given in conjunction with the uncouplers. Similarly, the potassium ionophore valinomycin, which alters mitochondrial function, could not prevent the increased discharge of quantal ACh in response to MeHg. However, it was not possible to observe an increase in MEPP frequency with MeHg when given to ruthenium-red-poisoned preparations. Thus, ruthenium red can antagonize the action of MeHg. This effect was not due to transmitter depletion by ruthenium red, because 2 mM La^{3+} evoked a massive discharge of ACh in ruthenium-red-poisoned preparations. Thus, blocking the mitochondrial Ca^{2+} uniporter appears to block the effectiveness of MeHg, but simply suppressing mitochondrial function does not prevent the action of MeHg on spontaneous release.

With continued bath application of mercury salts, spontaneous transmitter release declines until eventually no further release can be recorded. The time course for stimulation and subsequent block of spontaneous release is concentration-dependent. Block of spontaneous release by methyl mercury is not due to depletion of vesicular neurotransmitter stores, because treatment of the preparation at the time that MEPPs disappeared with lanthanum chloride ($LaCl_3$), which is a profound stimulator of spontaneous release (Heuser and Miledi 1971), was able to induce high frequencies of MEPPs (Atchison et al. 1984; Atchison 1986). Moreover, since normal appearing MEPPs were evoked by La^{3+}, and since ACh depolarizations were normal at the time that spontaneous release ceased (Atchison and Narahashi 1982), diminished postsynaptic sensitivity to ACh does not seem to account for the block of spontaneous release. An unexpected finding was that when MEPP frequency was reduced to zero by MeHg, washing with elevated K^+ solutions containing no MeHg caused a return of MEPPs. Washing with 1 or 2 mM d-penicillamine, but not 0.4 mM, was also able to restore spontaneous release in MeHg-poisoned preparations in which MEPPs had disappeared (Atchison 1986). These results suggest (1) that the latent period preceding the MeHg-induced increase in spontaneous quantal secretion is related to accumulation by the cell of either MeHg or free intracellular Ca^{2+}; (2) that extracellular Ca^{2+} contributes to but is not required for the MeHg-induced increase in quantal release; (3) that the late suppression of quantal secretion is due to direct effects of MeHg on the release process; and (4) that under some conditions the block of spontaneous release of ACh by MeHg can be relieved.

The effects of mercurials on spontaneous release of transmitter are not limited to ACh alone; other neurotransmitters are affected similarly. For example, catecholamine release from the bovine adrenal medulla and from the guinea pig vas deferens was also increased by inorganic and organic mercurials (Borowitz 1974; Hart and Borowitz 1974; Nakazato et al. 1979), while a subsequent decrease in spontaneous catecholamine secretion from the adrenal medulla was also reported for inorganic mercury (Borowitz 1974). Serotonin (5-hydroxytryptamine) was released from rabbit platelets by methyl mercury (Tuomisto and Komulainen 1983). Thus, the effects of mercurials on transmitter release appear to be due to a more generalized action.

The increased MEPP frequency associated with mercurials is not prevented by blocking either the axon membrane Na^+ channels with tetrodotoxin (Atchison and Narahashi 1982; Miyamoto 1983) or by blocking membrane Ca^{2+} channels with high concentrations of Mg^{2+} (Atchison and

Narahashi 1982) or Co^{2+} (Miyamoto 1983). Simultaneous block of *both* Na^+ and Ca^{2+} channels prevents the increase in MEPP frequency associated with $HgCl_2$, but not that associated with methyl mercury (Miyamoto 1983). The implication is that inorganic mercuric ions can enter the nerve terminal through both Na^+ and Ca^{2+} channels. On the other hand, methyl mercury may enter the cell not only through the channels but also directly through the membrane, because of its increased lipophilicity.

More recent studies (Atchison 1985; 1986*b*) indicate that the latent period could be shortened by use of ionophores for Ca^{2+} (A23187, 25 μM) but not Na^+ (monensin, 100 μM). In the presence of 100 μM MeHg alone, the peak increase in MEPP frequency occurred 40 $\pm$ 5 minutes ($n = 8$) after application of MeHg. Pretreatment with A23187 (25 μM) shortened this latent period to 25 $\pm$ 1 minutes ($n = 6$). When extracellular Ca^{2+} was removed, A23187 still shortened the latent period for MeHg's effect to 27 $\pm$ 5 minutes ($n = 6$). A Ca^{2+} channel agonist (Bay K-8644, 750 nM) also shortened the delay preceding the MeHg-elicited surge in spontaneous release of ACh (Atchison 1986*b*). The effect of Bay K-8644 was more pronounced in MeHg-containing Ca^{2+}-free solutions. Monensin (20–100 μM), an ionophore with greater affinity for monovalent cations than divalent cations, did not decrease the latent period for MeHg to increase MEPP frequency ($n = 6$). Veratridine (10 μM), an Na^+ channel opener, shortened significantly the latent period in bath solutions containing Ca^{2+} (2 mM) and in Ca^{2+}-deficient solutions. The results with A23187 and Bay K-8644 suggest that MeHg can utilize a path similar to that of Ca to enter the nerve terminal. The results with veratridine indicate some complex interaction between Na and Ca with MeHg within the nerve terminal. Replacement of the Na^+ in the bath with a nonpermeant cation, methylamine, did not prevent the MeHg-induced increase in MEPP frequency, although it did prolong the time to peak somewhat and reduced the peak MEPP frequency (Atchison 1986). Thus, extracellular Na is not required for the MeHg-induced increase in spontaneous release of ACh.

Postsynaptic Actions

The blocking effects of mercurials on stimulus-evoked release of ACh at the neuromuscular junction could be due either to presynaptic effects or to postsynaptic effects, the EPP being the final net result of both processes. Measurements of mean MEPP amplitude taken at the time of depressed EPP amplitude have indicated in general no significant effect of mercurials (Atchison and Narahashi 1982; Miyamoto 1983; Atchison et al. 1984). Juang (1976*b*) noted a slight decrease in mean MEPP amplitude with 40 μM $HgCl_2$ and a slight increase with 40 μM MeHg, but the magnitude of these changes was small. Since postsynaptic processes responsible for both the MEPP and the EPP are identical (i.e., receptor-agonist binding, receptor activation, ionic channel opening with resulting postsynaptic conductance changes; see

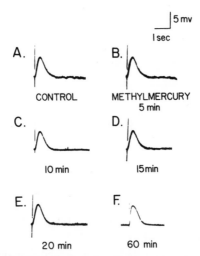

Figure 11.7. End-plate depolarizations produced by iontophoretic application of acetylcholine before and after methyl mercury (100 μM). The records were all taken from one end-plate, except for the 60-minute record, which was taken from a different end-plate in the same preparation. (Reprinted, by permission, from Atchison and Narahashi 1982, p. 45.)

Hubbard et al. 1969; Katz 1969), a lack of effect of mercury on MEPP amplitude suggests that there is no significant postsynaptic blocking effect of mercurials at the time the EPP is blocked. This, coupled with the measurements of statistical release parameters, implies that the block of synaptic transmission is primarily presynaptic.

It is still possible, however, that postsynaptic sensitivity to ACh is diminished by inorganic mercury or by methyl mercury, particularly with prolonged exposure, when MEPPs are no longer present. This hypothesis has been tested by iontophoretic application of exogenous ACh onto the motor end-plate of mercurial-poisoned preparations (Manalis and Cooper 1975; Atchison and Narahashi 1982). End-plate depolarizations due to ACh are not decreased in amplitude by concentrations of mercurials as high as 100 μM or for periods of exposure for up to 60 minutes, by which time MEPPs are no longer observed (Figure 11.7). Thus, at the motor end-plate, mercurials appear to produce few postsynaptic effects.

In contrast to this, other experiments have indicated that mercurials *do* affect the postsynaptic membrane. For example, iontophoretic application of the organomercurial *p*-chloromercuribenzoate depolarized the postsynaptic membrane of the electroplax in a manner similar to ACh and carbachol (del Castillo et al. 1972). On the other hand, exposure of N1E-115 neuroblastoma cells to methyl mercury *decreased* both the fast nicotinic and slow muscarinic responses to iontophoretic application of ACh (Figure 11.8) (Quandt et al. 1982). However, depolarizing action produced in response to dopamine was not decreased by methyl mercury (Figure 11.9), indicating that nonspecific postsynaptic effects such as membrane depolarization were not responsible for the actions of methyl mercury. These studies agree with a number of biochemical studies that indicate that methyl mercury decreases the binding of cholinergic agonists to nicotinic (Shamoo et al. 1976; Eldefrawi et al. 1975; 1977) and muscarinic (Bondy and Agrawal 1980; Eldefrawi et al. 1977; Von Burg et al. 1980) receptors. Indeed, this apparent lack of effect of

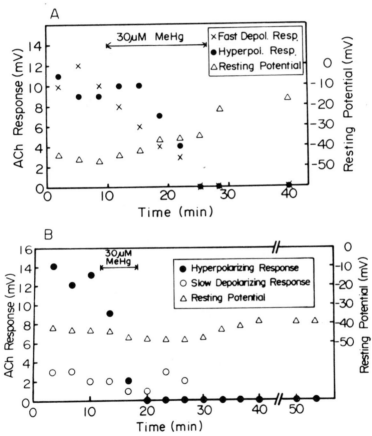

Figure 11.8. The effects of 30 μM MeHg on the resting membrane potential, and the potential responses induced by iontophoretic application of acetylcholine. (A) The effects on a cell producing the fast depolarizing (nicotinic) response and the hyperpolarizing (muscarinic) response. Both responses were decreased by methyl mercury with small membrane depolarizations. (B) The effects on another cell producing the hyperpolarizing response and the slow depolarizing (muscarinic) response. Both the responses were decreased with negligible changes in the resting membrane potential. The effects of methyl mercury are irreversible after prolonged washing. Temperature 33° C. (Reprinted, by permission, from Quandt et al. 1982, p. 214.)

mercurials on the postsynaptic membrane of the neuromuscular junction is puzzling, given the well-known affinity of inorganic and organic mercurials for sulfhydryl groups. The ACh receptor is known to contain sulfhydryl groups, modification of which leads to decreased affinity of the receptor to cholinergic agonists (Karlin and Bartels 1966). Presumably, methyl mercury should interact with the sulfhydryl groups to modify the ACh receptor and decrease the postsynaptic response to ACh. Perhaps the action of mercurials on the end-plate postsynaptic membrane is slow to develop, and thus was missed because of the high margin of transmission safety that exists at the motor end-plate.

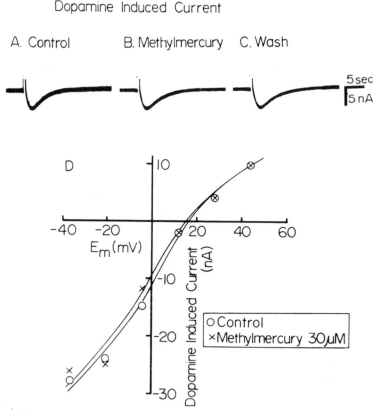

Figure 11.9. Absence of an effect of methyl mercury on dopamine-induced current in the voltage-clamped neuroblastoma cell. (A) Current induced by iontophoretic application of dopamine at the holding membrane potential of −30 mV. (B) As in A, but 10 minutes after application of 30 μM MeHg. (C) After washing with drug-free solution. (D) Current-voltage relationship of dopamine-induced current before and after application of 30 μM MeHg. Temperature 33 °C. (Reprinted, by permission, from Quandt et al. 1982, p. 217.)

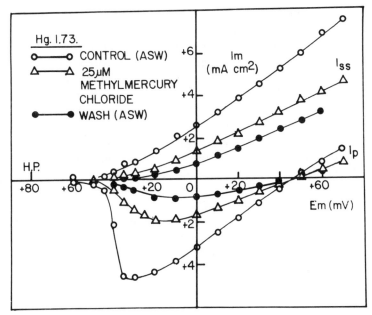

Figure 11.10. Current-voltage (I-V) relationships for peak sodium current (I_p) and steady-state potassium current (I_{ss}) before and during a 15-minute application of 25 μM methyl mercury chloride and after washing with normal artificial sea water (ASW) for 90 minutes. H. P. is the holding potential. (Reprinted, by permission, from Shrivastav et al. 1976, p. 1078.)

Effects on Nerve and Muscle Membrane

In addition to affecting synaptic transmission, mercurials also directly affect conduction of nerve impulses by effects on axon membranes. Impulse conduction has been shown to be impaired by methyl mercury in the preganglionic axon of the superior cervical ganglion of the rabbit (Taha and Alkadhi 1982) by acute administration and in dorsal root axons of rats by both acute and subchronic exposure (Somjen et al. 1973) and blocked completely by acute administration in the squid giant axon (Shrivastav et al. 1976).

The effects of mercurials on the underlying cationic conductances are observed in both sodium and potassium currents. Suppression of sodium currents by methyl mercury (20–60 μM) has been reported for the squid axon (Shrivastav et al. 1976) (Figure 11.10), lobster axon (Pennock and Goldman 1972), and mouse N1E-115 neuroblastoma cell (Quandt et al. 1982). Steady-state potassium currents appear to be affected equally well as the peak sodium currents at 20 μM MeHg in the neuroblastoma cell, but increasing the concentration of methyl mercury to 100 μM, produced no further block of potassium currents, while sodium currents were reduced substantially (Figure 11.11).

Despite the block of action-potential conduction, resting membrane potential is often not affected appreciably by mercurials. For example, Quandt et al. (1982) found that 20–40 μM MeHg produced only a 4–5 mV depolarization, yet reduced the action potential amplitude by 50–80 percent of control (Figure 11.12). Depolarization of resting membrane potential was observed with concentrations of organic and inorganic mercury of 500 μM and 1 mM, respectively, in the squid giant axon (Huneeus-Cox et al. 1966; Shrivastav et al. 1976), 250 μM in frog sciatic nerve (del Castillo and Hufschmidt 1951), 100 μM in barnacle muscle fibers (Hift and Schultz 1976), 26–370 μM in crab muscle (Marco et al. 1979), and 400 μM in frog skeletal muscle fibers (Juang 1976*b*) (Figure 11.13). On the other hand, Miyamoto (1983) reported that both HgCl$_2$ and methyl mercury depolarized the postsynaptic membrane of skeletal muscle, while Barrett et al. (1974) reported that methyl mercury depolarized the resting potential in the frog by 10–50 mV. Thus, the effect of mercurials on resting membrane potential remains unresolved. The cause of the block of nerve action potential conduction appears to be inhibition of

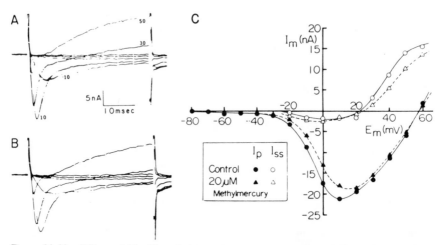

Figure 11.11. Effects of 20 μM methyl mercury on components of voltage-dependent ionic current. A neuroblastoma cell was voltage clamped and perfused internally and externally using the suction pipette method. The membrane potential was held at −40 mV. A 1-second prepulse to −80 mV was then given prior to step depolarizations to the test potentials. Temperature 12° C. (A) Representative superimposed traces of membrane current in response to selected depolarizations to the levels indicated were recorded from a cell in normal saline solution. Inward current is downward. Time-independent leakage currents were subtracted electronically. Early inward currents are due to current flow through the Na channel. Later outward currents are due primarily to current through the K channel. (B) Currents recorded from the same cell as in A following a 3-minute exposure to external saline solution containing 20 μM MeHg. (C) Current-voltage relationship for the early peak currents (I$_p$) and steady-state currents (I$_{ss}$) at the end of the 40 msec test depolarization obtained in normal saline solution (*circles*) or solution containing methyl mercury (*triangles*). (Reprinted, by permission, from Quandt et al. 1982, p. 210.)

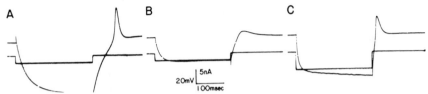

Figure 11.12. Effects of methyl mercury on the action potential. The top trace represents the time course of membrane potential recorded from a neuroblastoma cell, upward excursions being depolarizations. The lower trace gives the current through the recording microelectrode, downward deflections being inward current. (A) An "anode break" action potential is elicited following the termination of hyperpolarizing current. The resting potential was -40 mV. (B) Six minutes following a change of the external perfusate from normal saline solution to one containing 40 μM MeHg, the membrane depolarized by 4 mV. The membrane potential change during the application of current was reduced, indicating a decrease in input resistance. The action potential is markedly depressed. (C) The current through the microelectrode was then increased to bring the change in membrane potential toward the previous value, resulting in a partial recovery of the anode break action potential. Temperature 22° C. (Reprinted, by permission, from Quandt et al. 1982, p. 209.)

sodium activation mechanisms, since methyl mercury was more efficacious at inhibition of peak sodium currents than of steady-state potassium currents (Quandt et al. 1982). In every case tested, the effects of mercurials on ionic conductances could not be reversed by washing with mercury-free solutions.

Postulated Mechanisms

In summary, the effects of mercurials on synaptic transmission observed consistently are (1) depression of synchronous nerve-evoked transmitter release, (2) a biphasic increase and decrease of asynchronous spontaneous

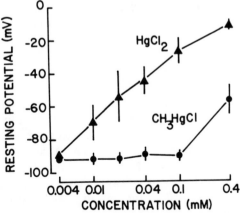

Figure 11.13. Resting membrane potentials of muscle fibers after 30-minute exposure to methyl mercury or $HgCl_2$ vs. millimolar concentrations of the compounds. Each symbol and vertical bar indicates the mean $\pm$ SD of resting potentials from 20–45 fibers in two to three muscles. (Reprinted, by permission, from Juang 1976*b*, p. 341.)

release, and (3) no effect on postsynaptic sensitivity to the transmitter. The most parsimonious explanation for these results invokes both extracellular and intracellular actions of mercury.

It is speculated that extracellular actions of mercury are responsible for the block of nerve-evoked transmitter release, but this effect could be due to intracellular actions, extracellular actions, or both. Like other polyvalent cations, mercury has been shown to impair influx of Ca^{2+} into isolated nerve terminals through voltage-dependent ionic channels (Nachshen 1983). In addition, increasing extracellular Ca^{2+} has been shown to interrupt briefly the progressive depression of the postsynaptic compound action potential at the superior cervical ganglion of the guinea pig (Alkadhi and Taha 1982). Conceivably, mercury can compete with Ca^{2+} for entry into the nerve terminal. This could explain the depressant action of mercury on nerve-evoked release as evidenced by its depression of the EPP and EPSP. At present, however, there is no direct evidence that mercurials block voltage-dependent Ca^{2+} conductances, so this possibility remains untested.

Analysis of statistical parameters associated with neurotransmitter release indicates that the action of methyl mercury on nerve-evoked release is attributable in part to effects within the cell. This can be inferred from the decrease in the parameter n, the immediately available transmitter store. It has been hypothesized that this parameter reflects some physical entity within the nerve terminal on which Ca^{2+} acts to cause release of the transmitter; examples include active release sites and filled vesicles in apposition to the plasmalemma (McLachlan 1978). The depressant action of methyl mercury on n could then reflect such actions as inhibiting vesicle mobilization, screening of membrane/vesicle interaction sites, inappropriate positioning of vesicles with respect to the membrane, and a decrease in vesicle number or other as yet undefined actions within the cell (Blioch et al. 1968).

Increases in the probability of release, p, by methyl mercury appear to be inconsistent with the notion that mercury impedes Ca^{2+} entry into the terminal. The parameter p is thought to reflect ionized Ca^{2+} concentration within the nerve terminal (McLachlan 1978), and thus an increase in p would predict that methyl mercury increased cytoplasmic Ca^{2+} concentration, an effect that again could be attributed to either extracellular or intracellular actions. The inconsistency can be resolved by assuming that the effect of methyl mercury to increase p is due to *intracellular* actions. This seems more likely than an extracellular effect, since inorganic mercury has been shown to block $^{45}Ca^{2+}$ influx into rat brain synaptosomes (Nachshen 1983). The paradoxical increase in p and decrease in n (both variables depend on intracellular Ca^{2+} concentration) can be explained in turn by hypothesizing that mercurials increase the intracellular Ca^{2+} concentration yet in some way impair the ability of Ca^{2+} to enable the vesicle to interact with the cell membrane. It should be noted that there is presently no direct evidence supporting or refuting this hypothesis.

Effects of mercurials on spontaneous neurotransmitter release are thought to be due to intracellular effects. The evidence on which this hypothesis is based is indirect. One of these clues is that the effects of mercurials on spontaneous release follow a much slower time course than those on evoked release, with a latent period that depends on the concentration of mercury employed. This latent period is presumed to be related to the entry of the mercurial into the cell and accumulation at its target site. This is supported by the observation that depolarizing the cell with elevated extracellular K^+ shortens the latency and speeds up the entire time course dramatically (Miyamoto 1983; Atchison 1985; 1986). This effect is assumed to be due to increased entry of the mercurial through voltage-dependent membrane ionic channels (Ca^{2+} and perhaps Na^+) following K^+-induced depolarization (Atchison 1985; 1987). Once inside the cell, mercurials may increase spontaneous transmitter release by a number of mechanisms, including increasing intracellular free Ca^{2+} or screening of fixed negative surface charges on the internal membrane. Increased intracellular Ca^{2+} by mercurials is supported by the observation that the probability of release, p, is increased by methyl mercury (Atchison and Narahashi 1982), as well as by the observation that MeHg can increase MEPP frequency in preparations exposed to Ca-free solutions or in preparations that were depleted of Ca (Atchison 1986a). Increased free Ca^{2+} within the nerve terminal will cause MEPP or MEPSP frequency to increase (Hubbard et al. 1968; Matthews and Wickelgren 1977). A variety of other chemicals that increase MEPP frequency dramatically, such as warfarin, tetraphenylboron, and ruthenium red, are proposed to do so as a result of increasing Ca^{2+} by a variety of different mechanisms (Glagoleva et al. 1970; Rahamimoff and Alnaes 1973; Alnaes and Rahamimoff 1975; Marshall and Parsons 1975). Regulation of intracellular Ca^{2+} in the nerve terminal is complex; it involves buffering systems in mitochondria, microsomes, and perhaps synaptic vesicles; resting, voltage-independent Ca^{2+} flux; voltage-dependent Ca^{2+} influx; and an exchange system that ultimately extrudes excess free Ca^{2+} (Blaustein 1974; Blaustein et al. 1978a, 1978b, 1980a, 1980b; Rahamimoff et al. 1978; McGraw et al. 1980). It is not certain which, if any, of these nerve terminal processes are affected by mercurials, but it is known that inorganic and organic mercurials can inhibit Ca^{2+} uptake into isolated mitochondria (Binah et al. 1978). More recent indirect evidence (Levesque and Atchison 1987) indicates that MeHg may interact with mitochondria to cause release of Ca from bound stores. Ruthenium red, which blocks Ca uptake and release from the Ca uniporter in the mitochondrial membrane, blocks the effect of MeHg to stimulate MEPP frequency.

The effects of mercurials on evoked release and spontaneous release are consistent with the hypothesis that mercurials act to depolarize the presynaptic nerve terminal. Depolarization would lead to both a decrease of evoked release and an increase of spontaneous neurotransmitter release. If the depolarization were severe enough, it could lead ultimately to block of axonal conduction, which would cause failure of synaptic transmission. As indicated above, mercurials depolarize both isolated nerve and muscle preparations. While the data regarding depolarizing effects of mercurials at the end-plate membrane are conflicting, these data do not necessarily reflect the effects of mercury on the nerve terminal membrane. Indeed, there are two reasons that it is highly likely that mercurials could depolarize the nerve terminal without affecting the resting potential of the muscle end-plate membrane. First, the prejunctional nerve terminal has a much greater surface-to-volume ratio than the skeletal muscle fiber, so the terminal would be more sensitive to changes in the internal ionic concentrations. Second, skeletal muscle fibers, unlike nerves, have a large chloride conductance (Hodgkin and Horowitz 1959), which protects the muscle cell from minor alterations in cationic conductance. Thus, small changes in Na^+, K^+, or Ca^{2+} conductance might not be observed as a change in resting potential in the myofiber. Results obtained in the presence of tetrodotoxin, a specific blocker of the axon Na^+ channel (Narahashi 1974), indicate that mercurial-induced depolarization, if it occurs, does not simply entail block of Na^+ channels (Atchison and Narahashi 1982; Miyamoto 1983). However, other possibilities, such as inhibition of nerve ionic exchange systems or increased leakage current, still remain. Both possibilities have been demonstrated to occur with methyl mercury (Su and Okita 1975; Shrivastav et al. 1976; Holmes and Okita 1979).

In conclusion, acute exposure to both inorganic and organic mercury salts affects neuronal function. Conduction of impulses by the axon, and chemical transmission at synapses—the two fundamental processes involved in information flow within the nervous system—are both affected. The effects appear to be exerted at both extracellular membrane sites and intracellular sites. The precise mechanisms remain to be elucidated. The relationship that these effects of acute and subchronic exposure to mercurials have, if any, to the pattern of neurotoxicity observed following chronic human exposure also remains to be seen.

Acknowledgments

The research for this chapter was supported by NIH grant ES03299 and by a grant from the Michigan State University Agricultural Experiment Station (Experiment Station Manuscript 12115).

References

Alkadhi, K. A., and Taha, M. N. (1982). Antagonism by calcium of the inhibitory effect of methylmercury on sympathetic ganglia. *Arch Toxicol* 51:175–181.

Alnaes, E., and Rahamimoff, R. (1975). On the role of mitochondria in transmitter release from motor nerve terminals. *J Physiol* (Lond) 248:285–306.

Atchison, W. D. (1984). Neuromuscular effects of methylmercury on transmitter release. *Proceedings of the Ninth International Congress of Pharmacology, July 29–August 4, 1984,* London 2029P.

———(1985). Effects of calcium and sodium ionophores on the methylmercury-induced increase in spontaneous release of ACh. *Pharmacologist* (abstr.) 27:159.

———(1986). Extracellular calcium-dependent and -independent effects of methylmercury on spontaneous and potassium-evoked release of acetylcholine at the neuromuscular junction. *J Pharmacol Exp Ther* 237:672–680.

———(1987). The effects of activation of sodium and calcium entry on spontaneous release of acetylcholine induced by methylmercury. *J Pharmacol Exp Ther* 241(1) (in press).

Atchison, W. D.; Clark, A. W.; and Narahashi, T. (1984). Presynaptic effects of methylmercury at the mammalian neuromuscular junction. In *Cellular and Molecular Neurotoxicology,* edited by T. Narahashi, pp. 23–43. New York: Raven Press.

Atchison, W. D.; Joshi, U.; and Thornburg, J. E. (1986). Irreversible suppression of calcium entry into nerve terminals by methylmercury. *J Pharmacol Exp Ther* 238:618–624.

Atchison, W. D., and Narahashi, T. (1982). Methylmercury-induced depression of neuromuscular transmission in the rat. *Neurotoxicol* 3(3):37–50.

Atchison, W. D., and Traxinger, D. L. (1986). Reversal attempts for methylmercury-induced block of nerve-evoked release of acetylcholine. *Toxicol Lett* 31(Suppl):144.

Baker, P. F.; Hodgkin, A. L.; and Ridgeway, E. B. (1971). Depolarization and calcium entry in squid giant axons. *J Physiol* (Lond) 218:709–755.

Bakir, F.; Damluji, S.; Amin-Zaki, L.; Murtadha, M.; Khalidi, A.; Al-Rawi, N. Y.; Tikriti, S.; Dhahir, H. L.; Clarkson, T. W.; Smith, J. C.; and Doherty, R. A. (1973). Methylmercury poisoning in Iraq. *Science* 181:230–240.

Balnave, R. J., and Gage, P. W. (1973). The inhibitory action of manganese on transmitter release at the neuromuscular junction of the toad. *Br J Pharmacol* 47:339–352.

Barrett, J.; Botz, D.; and Chang, D. B. (1974). Block of neuromuscular transmission by methyl mercury. In *Behavioral Toxicology: Early Detection of Occupational Hazards,* edited by C. Xintaras, B. L. Johnson, and I. deGroot. Washington, D.C.: Department of Health, Education, and Welfare, vol. 5, pp. 277–287.

Binah, O.; Meiri, U.; and Rahamimoff, H. (1978). The effects of $HgCl_2$ and mersalyl on mechanisms regulating intracellular calcium and transmitter release. *Eur J Pharmacol* 51:453–457.

Blaustein, M. P. (1974). The interrelationship between sodium and calcium fluxes across cell membranes. *Rev Physiol Biochem Pharmacol* 70:34–82.

Blaustein, M. P.; McGraw, C. F.; Somlyo, A. V.; and Schweitzer, E. S. (1980a). How is the cytoplasmic calcium concentration controlled in nerve terminals? *J Physiol* (Paris) 76:459–470.

Blaustein, M. P.; Ratzlaff, R. W.; and Kendrick, N. K. (1978a). The regulation of intracellular calcium in presynaptic nerve terminals. *Ann NY Acad Sci* 307:195–211.

Blaustein, M. P.; Ratzlaff, R. W.; and Schweitzer, E. S. (1978b). Calcium buffering in presynaptic nerve terminals, II: Kinetic properties of the nonmitochondrial Ca sequestration mechanism. *J Gen Physiol* 72:43–67.

———(1980b). Control of intracellular calcium in presynaptic nerve terminals. *Fed Proc* 39:2790-2795.

Blioch, Z. L.; Glagoleva, I. M.; Liberman, E. A.; and Nenashev, V. A. (1968). A study of the mechanism of quantal transmitter release at a chemical synapse. *J Physiol* (Lond) 199:11-35.

Bondy, S. C., and Agrawal, A. K. (1980). The inhibition of cerebral high affinity receptor sites by lead and mercury compounds. *Arch Toxicol* 46:249-256.

Borowitz, J. L. (1974). Mechanism of adrenal catecholamine release by divalent mercury. *Toxicol Appl Pharmacol* 28:82-87.

Branisteanu, D. D., and Volle, R. L. (1975). Modification by lithium of transmitter release at the neuromuscular junction of the frog. *J Pharmacol Exp Ther* 194:362-372.

Cooper, G. P., and Manalis, R. S. (1983). Influence of heavy metals on synaptic transmission: A review. *Neurotoxicol* 4(4):69-84.

del Castillo, J.; Bartels, E.; and Sobrino, J. A. (1972). Microelectrophoretic application of cholinergic compounds, protein oxidizing agents, and mercurials to the chemically excitable membrane of the electroplax. *Proc Natl Acad Sci USA* 69:2081-2085.

del Castillo, J., and Engbaek, L. (1954). The nature of the neuromuscular block produced by magnesium. *J Physiol* (Lond) 124:370-384.

del Castillo, J., and Hufschmidt, H. J. (1951). Reversible poisoning of nerve fibres by heavy metal ions. *Nature* (Lond) 167:146-147.

Dodge, F. A.; Miledi, R.; and Rahamimoff, R. (1969). Strontium and quantal release of transmitter at the neuromuscular junction. *J Physiol* (Lond) 200:267-283.

Eldefrawi, M. E.; and Eldefrawi, A. T. (1977). Acetylcholine receptors. In *Receptors and Recognition,* vol. 4, series A, edited by P. Cuatrecasas and M. F. Greaves, pp. 197-258. London: Chapman and Hall.

Eldefrawi, M. E.; Eldefrawi, A. T.; and Shamoo, A. E. (1975). Molecular and functional properties of the acetylcholine receptor. *Ann NY Acad Sci* 264:183-202.

Erulkar, S. D., and Rahamimoff, R. (1978). The role of calcium ions in tetanic and posttetanic increase in miniature end-plate potential frequency. *J Physiol* (Lond) 278:501-511.

Fehling, C.; Abdulla, M.; Brun, A.; Dictor, M.; Schutz, A.; and Skerfving, S. (1975). Methylmercury poisoning in the rat: A combined neurological, chemical, and histopathological study. *Toxicol Appl Pharmacol* 33:27-37.

Glagoleva, I. M.; Liberman, E. A.; and Khashad, Z. (1970). Effect of uncouplers of oxidative phosphorylation on output of acetylcholine from nerve endings. *Biofizika* 15:76-83.

Hart, D. T., and Borowitz, J. L. (1974). Adrenal catecholamine release by divalent mercury and cadmium. *Arch Int Pharmacodyn* 209:94-99.

Heuser, J., and Miledi, R. (1971). Effect of lanthanum ions on function and structure of frog neuromuscular junctions. *Proc R Soc Biol* 179:247-260.

Hift, H., and Schultz, R. (1976). Methylmercury induced injury of single barnacle muscle fibres. *Environ Res* 11:367-385.

Hodgkin, A. L., and Horowitz, P. (1959). The influence of potassium and chloride ions on the membrane potential of single muscle fibres. *J Physiol* (Lond) 148:127–160.

Holmes, L. S., and Okita, G. T. (1979). The role of Na,K-ATPase in methylmercury induced teratogenesis. *Fed Proc* 38:680.

Hubbard, J. I.; Jones, S. F.; and Landau, E. M. (1968). On the mechanism by which calcium and magnesium affect the spontaneous release of transmitter from mammalian motor nerve terminals. *J Physiol* (Lond) 194:355–380.

Hubbard, J. I.; Llinas, R.; and Quastel, D. M. J. (1969). *Electrophysiological Analysis of Synaptic Transmission.* Baltimore: Williams and Wilkins.

Huneeus-Cox, F.; Fernandez, H. L.; and Smith, B. H. (1966). Effects of redox and sulfhydryl reagents on the bioelectric properties of the giant axon of the squid. *Biophys J* 6:675–689.

Juang, M. S. (1976a). Depression of frog muscle contraction by methylmercury chloride and mercuric chloride. *Toxicol Appl Pharmacol* 35:183–185.

———(1976b). An electrophysiological study of the action of methylmercuric chloride and mercuric chloride on the sciatic nerve-sartorius muscle preparation of the frog. *Toxicol Appl Pharmacol* 37:339–348.

Juang, M. S., and Yonemura, K. (1975). Increased spontaneous transmitter release from presynaptic nerve terminal by methyl mercuric chloride. *Nature* (Lond) 256:211–213.

Kajimoto, N., and Kirpekar, S. M. (1972). Effect of manganese and lanthanum on spontaneous release of acetylcholine at frog motor nerve terminals. *Nature, New Biol* 235:29–30.

Karlin, A., and Bartels, E. (1966). Effects of blocking sulfhydryl groups and of reducing disulfide bonds on the acetylcholine-activated permeability system of the electroplax. *Biochim Biophys Acta* 126:525–535.

Katz, B. (1962). The transmission of impulses from nerve to muscle and the subcellular unit of synaptic action. *Proc R Soc Biol* 155:455–477.

———(1969). *The Release of Neural Transmitter Substances.* Springfield, Ill.: Charles C Thomas.

Keynes, G. (1969). The history of myasthenia gravis. In *Myasthenia Gravis*, edited by R. Green, pp.1–13. London: Heineman Medical Books.

Kostial, K., and Landeka, M. (1975). The action of mercury ions on the release of acetylcholine from presynaptic nerve endings. *Experientia* 31:834–835.

Le Quesne, P. M.; Damluji, S. F.; and Rustam, H. (1974). Electrophysiological studies of peripheral nerves in patients with organic mercury poisoning. *J Neurol Neurosurg Psychiatry* 37:333–339.

Levesque, P. C., and Atchison, W. D. (1987). Interactions of mitochondrial inhibitors with methylmercury on spontaneous quantal release of acetylcholine. *Toxicol Appl Pharmacol* 87:315–324.

Liley, A. W., and North, K. A. K. (1953). An electrical investigation of effects of repetitive stimulation on mammalian neuromuscular junction. *J Neurophysiol* 16:509–527.

Magleby, K. L., and Zengel, J. E. (1982). A quantitative description of stimulation-induced changes in transmitter release at the frog neuromuscular junction. *J Gen Physiol* 80:613–638.

Manalis, R. S., and Cooper, G. P. (1975). Evoked transmitter release increased by inorganic mercury at the frog neuromuscular junction. *Nature* (Lond) 257:690–691.

Marco, L. A.; Isaacson, L.; and Torri, J. C. (1979). Effects of mercuric chloride on the resting membrane potentials of blue crab (*Callinectes sapidus*) muscle fibers. *Toxicol* 12:41–46.

Marshall, I. G., and Parsons, R. L. (1975). The effects of tetraphenylboron on spontaneous transmitter release at the frog neuromuscular junction. *Br J Pharmacol* 54:333–338.

Matthews, G., and Wickelgren, W. (1977). Effects of guanidine on transmitter release and neuronal excitability. *J Physiol* (Lond) 266:69–89.

McGraw, C. M.; Somlyo, A. V.; and Blaustein, M. P. (1980). Probing for calcium at presynaptic nerve endings. *Fed Proc* 39:2796–2802.

McLachlan, E. M. (1978). The statistics of transmitter release at a chemical synapse. In *International Review of Neurophysiology,* vol. 3, no. 17, edited by R. Porter, pp. 49–177. Baltimore: University Park Press.

Miledi, R., and Thies, R. (1971). Tetanic and post-tetanic rise in frequency of miniature end-plate potentials in low calcium solutions. *J Physiol* (Lond) 212:245–257.

Miyamoto, M. D. (1983). Hg^{2+} causes neurotoxicity at an intracellular site following entry through Na and Ca channels. *Brain Res* 267:375–379.

Nachshen, D. A. (1983). Block of calcium channels in synaptosomes by polyvalent cations. *Biophys J* 41:292a(Abstr.).

——(1984). Selectivity of the Ca binding site in synaptosome Ca channels: Inhibition of Ca influx by multivalent metal cations. *J Gen Physiol* 83:941–967.

Nachshen, D. A., and Blaustein, M. P. (1980). Some properties of potassium-stimulated calcium influx in presynaptic nerve endings. *J Gen Physiol* 76:709–728.

Nakazato, Y.; Asano, T.; and Ohta, A. (1979). The in vitro effect of mercury compounds on noradrenaline output from guinea pig vas deferens. *Toxicol Appl Pharmacol* 48:171–177.

Narahashi, T. (1974). Chemicals as tools in the study of excitable membranes. *Physiol. Rev.* 54:813–889.

Pennock, B. E., and Goldman, D. E. (1972). The action of lead and mercury on lobster axon. *Fed Proc* 31:219.

Quandt, F. N.; Kato, E.; and Narahashi, T. (1982). Effects of methylmercury on electrical responses of neuroblastoma cells. *Neurotoxicol* 3:205–220.

Rahamimoff, R., and Alnaes, E. (1973). Inhibitory action of ruthenium red on neuromuscular transmission. *Proc Natl Acad Sci* 70:3613–3616.

Rahamimoff, R.; Erulkar, S. D.; Lev-Tov, A.; and Meiri, H. (1978). Intracellular and extracellular calcium ions in transmitter release at the neuromuscular synapse. *Ann NY Acad Sci* 307:583–598.

Rustam, H., and Hamadi, T. (1974). Methyl mercury poisoning in Iraq: A neurological study. *Brain* 97:499–510.

Rustam, H.; Von Burg, R.; Amin-Zaki, L.; and El Hassani, S. (1975). Evidence for a neuromuscular disorder in methylmercury poisoning. *Arch Environ Health* 30:190–195.

Shamoo, A. E.; MacLennan, D. H.; and Eldefrawi, M. E. (1976). Differential effects of mercurial compounds on excitable tissue. *Chem Biol Interact* 12:41–52.

Shrivastav, B.; Brodwick, M. S.; and Narahashi, T. (1976). Methylmercury: Effects on electrical properties of squid axon membranes. *Life Sci* 18:1077–1082.

Silinsky, E. M. (1981). On the calcium receptor that mediates depolarization-secretion coupling at cholinergic motor nerve terminals. *Br J Pharmacol* 73:413–429.

———(1985). The biophysical pharmacology of calcium-dependent acetylcholine secretion. *Pharmacol Rev* 37:81–132.

Silinsky, E. M., and Mellow, A. M. (1981). The relationship between strontium and other divalent cations in the process of transmitter release from cholinergic nerve endings. In *Handbook of Stable Strontium,* edited by S. Skoryna, pp. 263–285. New York: Plenum Press.

Somjen, G. G.; Herman, S. P.; and Klein, R. (1973). Electrophysiology of methylmercury poisoning. *J Pharmacol Exp Ther* 186:579–592.

Su, M., and Okita, G. T. (1975). Studies of CNS teratogenesis induced by methylmercury. *Fed Proc* 34:810.

Taha, M. N., and Alkadhi, K. H. (1982). Effects of methylmercuric chloride on sympathetic preganglionic nerves. *Arch Toxicol* 50:142–147.

Traxinger, D. L., and Atchison, W. D. (1987*a*). Comparative effects of divalent cations on the methylmercury-induced alterations of acetylcholine release. *J Pharmacol Exp Ther* 240:451–459.

———(1987*b*). Reversal of methylmercury-induced block of nerve-evoked release of acetylcholine at the neuromuscular junction. *Toxicol. Appl. Pharmacol.* (accepted).

Tuomisto, J., and Komulainen, H. (1983). Release and inhibition of uptake of 5-hydroxytryptamine in blood platelets in vitro by copper and methylmercury. *Acta Pharm Toxicol* 52:292–297.

Von Burg, R., and Landry, T. (1975). Methylmercury induced neuromuscular dysfunction in the rat. *Neurosci Lett* 1:169–172.

———(1976). Methylmercury and the skeletal muscle receptor. *J Pharm Pharmacol* 28:548–551.

Von Burg, R.; Northington, F. K.; and Shamoo, A. (1980). Methylmercury inhibition of rat brain muscarinic receptors. *Toxicol Appl Pharmacol* 53:285–292.

Von Burg, R., and Rustam, H. (1974). Electrophysiological investigations of methylmercury intoxication in humans: Evaluation of peripheral nerve by conduction velocity and electromyography. *Electroencephalogr Clin Neurophysiol* 37:381–392.

Weakly, J. N. (1973). The action of cobalt ions on neuromuscular transmission in the frog. *J Physiol* (Lond) 234:597–612.

Zengel, J. E., and Magleby, K. L. (1981). Changes in miniature endplate potential frequency during repetitive nerve stimulation in the presence of Ca^{2+}, Ba^{2+}, and Sr^{2+} at the frog neuromuscular junction. *J Gen Physiol* 77:503–529.

———(1982). Augmentation and facilitation of transmitter release: A quantitative description at the frog neuromuscular junction. *J Gen Physiol* 80:583–611.

T W E L V E

Tissue Culture: A Useful Model for Studying the Mechanism of Methyl Mercury Toxicity on Nerve Tissue

Kedar N. Prasad

Heavy metals are known to cause neurological disorders in humans and in animals. In addition, other inorganic and organic pollutants in the environment may have the potential to induce neurological disorders. The molecular mechanisms leading to neurological abnormalities following exposure to neurotoxic substances are difficult to study in the central nervous system in vivo because of heterogeneous cell populations and other complexities associated with in vivo systems. A tissue culture model using clonal lines may be useful in studying the cellular and molecular mechanisms of neurotoxicity produced by heavy metals and other agents. Our results show that monolayer cultures of mouse neuroblastoma (NB) and rat glioma (C-6) cells may be very sensitive experimental models to investigate the cellular and molecular mechanisms of heavy-metal-induced damage of nerve tissues, even though these cells are of tumor origin. We have emphasized particularly the effects of methyl mercuric chloride.

The Use of Various Model Systems

The effect of mercury on nerve tissue has been investigated using several methods and model systems. These include the turnover of mercury (Friberg et al. 1972), histopathology of the brain (Berlin and Ulberg 1963; Berthoud et al. 1976; Chang and Hartmann 1972*a*; Takeuchi 1968), ultrastructural changes (Chang and Hartmann 1972*a*, 1972*b;* Chang et al. 1977, Eto and Takeuchi 1977), localization of mercury in brain cells (Garman et al. 1975; Miyakawa et al. 1970; Takeuchi 1968; Vallee and Ulner 1972), neurotransmitter uptake, release (Bondy et al. 1979; Landeka and Kostial 1975; MacKay and Iversen 1972), and contents (Hrdina et al. 1976; Spuhler and Prasad 1980; Taylor and DiStefano 1976), biotransformation of mercury (Friberg et al. 1972; Syversen 1974), cellular distribution of mercury (Berlin and Ulberg 1963; Berthoud et al. 1976; Chang and Hartmann 1972*b;* Cassano et al. 1969; Garman et al. 1975), changes in enzyme activity (Braubaker et al. 1973; Neathery and Miller 1973; Vallee and Ulner 1972), nucleic acid and protein synthesis (Braubaker et al. 1973; Chang et al. 1972; Cheung et al. 1977; Neathery and Miller 1973), binding with protein complexes

(Braubaker et al. 1973; Vallee and Ulner 1972), respiration (Cheung and Verity 1979; Fox et al. 1975), and electrophysiological studies of peripheral nerves (Bondy et al. 1979; Hrdina et al. 1976; Mannalis and Cooper 1975; Le Quesne et al. 1974; Shrivastav et al. 1976). The experimental models used in the above studies have been either brain tissues obtained after chronic administration of mercury to the animal, or brain homogenates and brain slices from the normal animal. In the latter models, exogenous concentrations of mercury compounds were added immediately before assaying cellular functions. These studies have provided useful information with respect to certain aspects of mercury-induced neurotoxicity, but many aspects of the molecular mechanisms of damage remain unknown. This may result in part from the complexity of whole organisms or brain slices on which the studies were performed. The concentrations of mercury compounds used in most studies were very high.

Monolayer cultures of neuroblastoma and glioma cells may be simpler models for studying the effects of heavy metals on nerve tissues. Although mouse NB cells and rat glioma (C-6) cells are of tumor origin, they do have several features of nerve and glial cells, respectively (Augusti-Tocco and Sato 1969; Benda et al. 1968; Coyle and Schwarcz 1976; De Vellis et al. 1970; Haftke and Seeds 1976; Pfeiffer et al. 1977; Prasad 1975). Many responses of NB cells and normal embryonic nerve tissue are similar. For example, like NB cell cultures (Prasad 1975), cultures of dorsal root ganglia from chick embryos (Roisen et al. 1972), mouse sensory ganglia (Haas et al. 1972), and mouse cerebrum (Shapiro 1973) show morphological differentiation after treatment with cAMP-stimulating agents. As in NB cells (Prasad 1975), dibutyryl cAMP increases the activity of tyrosine hydoxylase in sympathetic ganglia culture (MacKay and Iversen 1972) and the activity of dopamine β-hydroxylase in superior cervical ganglia (Kean and McLean 1972). The sensitivity of adenylate cyclase to norepinephrine (Schmidt and Robison 1970), the level of cAMP (Butcher and Sutherland 1962; Ebadi et al. 1971), and the activity of cAMP phosphodiesterase (Weiss et al. 1971) increase during differentiation of normal nervous tissue. A similar observation has been made in NB cell cultures (Prasad 1975). Many responses of glioma cells and normal glial cells are similar. For example, like rat brain primary cultures, glioma cells release a factor into the medium that induces process formation in the NB cell line (Monard et al. 1975). The agonists of β-receptors increase the intracellular level of cAMP in both glioma and normal glial cells (Perkins et al. 1975). Dibutyryl cAMP produces morphological differentiation in both glioma and normal embryonic glial cells (MacIntyre et al. 1972; Vernadakis and Nidess 1976).

The clones of NB (NBP_2 and $NBA_{2(1)}$) and glioma (C-6) cells have been well defined with respect to their morphology and biochemical properties. In addition, monolayer cultures of NB and C-6 cells provide an adequate amount of sample material for biochemical analysis of cellular functions. Therefore, we have extensively utilized these clones of nervous tissue to investigate the mechanisms of heavy metals.

The Relative Sensitivity of Glioma and Neuroblastoma Cells to Neurotoxic Substances

We found (Prasad et al. 1979*b*) that C-6 cells were more sensitive than NB cells to methyl mercuric chloride (CH_3HgCl) for the criterion of growth inhibition (resulting from cell death and inhibition of cell division) (Figure 12.1). Although a much higher concentration of mercuric chloride ($HgCl_2$) was required to produce effects similar to those produced by CH_3HgCl, it produced no differential effect on C-6 and NB cells. Tri-*n*-butyl lead acetate

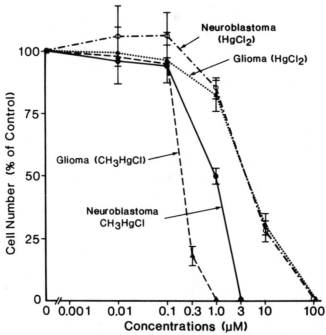

Figure 12.1. Sensitivity of NB and C-6 (glioma) cells to CH_3HgCl. Cells (NB, 50,000; C-6, 100,000) were plated in Falcon plastic dishes (60 mm); mercury compounds were added 24 hours after plating. Drug and medium were changed every day for the NB cells, and 1 and 3 days after treatment for the C-6 cells. The number of cells was counted 3 days after treatment for the NB cells, and 4 days after treatment for the C-6 cells. The number of NB cells in control culture 3 days after treatment was $218 \pm 29 \times 10^4$, and the number of C-6 cells in control culture 4 days after treatment was $80 \pm 12 \times 10^4$. The number of cells in treated culture was expressed as percentage of control. Each value represents an average of at least six samples. The bar at each point is the standard deviation. The vertical bars of the points not shown in the figure were too small to be shown on the graph.

was much more toxic than CH_3HgCl, but it did not produce a differential effect (Prasad 1982). Acrylamide, which is known to cause peripheral neuropathy (Brewer-Auld and Bedwell 1967; Fullerton and Barnes 1966), did not cause a differential effect on glioma and NB cells (Prasad 1982).

To understand the reasons for the differential sensitivity of C-6 and NB cells, the uptake, subcellular distribution, and biological half-life of $CH_3^{203}HgCl$ in these cells were studied (Ramanujam et al. 1979). Most of the radioactivity (about 70 percent of homogenate radioactivity) was associated with the cytosol and particulate fractions of NB and C-6 cells (Ramanujam et al. 1979). This is consistent with an earlier observation on brain cortical slices in which most of the mercury was present in the cytosol and microsomal fractions (Wuerthele et al. 1978). The purified chromatin fractions of C-6 and NB contained 1.9 percent and 3.4 percent of their homogenate radioactivities. Chang (1977) showed that the nuclear fraction of animal brain contained only a very small proportion of the administered organic mercury. Methyl mercuric chloride has been reported to bind primarily with the nuclear membrane, and only a very small amount was found within the nucleus (Berlin and Ulberg 1963; Cassano et al. 1979; Chang 1977; Ostlund 1969).

We have shown (Ramanujam et al. 1979) that only about 50–60 percent of the cytosol radioactivity was protein-bound in both C-6 and NB cells. However, the protein-bound radioactivity in C-6 cells was higher than that in NB cells. The total homogenates, lipoproteins, and cytosol of glioma cells also accumulated more $CH_3^{203}HgCl$ than the corresponding fractions of NB cells. Thus, the greater sensitivity of C-6 cells to CH_3HgCl may result in part from the fact that they accumulate more CH_3HgCl than NB cells. The specific radioactivity of the lipoprotein fraction of C-6 cells was particularly high, compared with that of NB cells. This would indicate that the binding affinity of CH_3HgCl for lipoproteins is greater in C-6 cells than in NB cells. The reasons for a higher uptake of radioactive CH_3HgCl in C-6 cells, compared with NB cells, are unknown. However, a similar observation has been made in brain tissues of humans who died of CH_3HgCl toxicity. It was observed (Oyaki et al. 1966; Takeuchi 1972) that most of the mercury was located in the glial cells of the brain. Thus, cell-culture models resemble the human brain with respect to accumulation of mercury in glia and neurons. However, this is in contrast to studies in rats, in which neurons accumulated more radioactive CH_3HgCl than glial cells (Chang and Hartmann 1972b; Somjen et al. 1973). The reasons for the discrepancy in cellular accumulation of CH_3HgCl in the cell-culture model and human brain, on the one hand, and in rat brain, on the other, are unknown, but the following possibilities can be mentioned: (1) species differences, (2) difference in experimental conditions, and (3) time interval between injection of methyl mercury compounds and assay of radioactivity. The last factor was found to be very important in the cell-culture model. When the uptake and subcellular distribution of radioactive CH_3HgCl were assayed 5 hours after incubation (time required for the uptake value to reach plateau was 4–6 hours of incubation in the presence of radioactive CH_3HgCl), C-6 cells accumulated more radioactivity than NB cells. However, if the cells were incubated in the presence of radioactive methyl mercuric chloride for only 15 minutes, the reverse was true (Prasad and Nobles 1978). Hence, the study must be performed at the time the cellular uptake of CH_3HgCl reaches equilibrium.

The binding of radioactive methyl mercuric chloride with various subcellular fractions may involve some uncertainties. For example, it is not known whether all the radioactivity of various fractions was incorporated during the incubation of intact cells, or whether portions of or all of the radioactivity could be attributed to redistribution of CH_3HgCl among the subcellular fractions during homogenization and subsequent fractionation. Indeed, such a possibility has been suggested by Yoshino et al. (1966). The instability of CH_3HgCl-protein complexes in solution makes it exceedingly difficult to derive conclusive information on the binding and subcellular distribution of $CH_3{}^{203}HgCl$. However, these data do provide some estimation of the relative distribution of CH_3HgCl in the subcellular fractions of these two cell types.

The biological half-life of CH_3HgCl in C-6 and NB cells was 4.1 hours and 7.2 hours, respectively. However, the biological half-life of CH_3HgCl in the mouse is 7 days, in the cat, 20 days, and in the human, 70 days (Weiss 1977). Since the biological half-life of CH_3HgCl in C-6 cells is shorter than that in NB cells, the greater sensitivity of C-6 cells is not the result of slower turnover of CH_3HgCl. It is possible that the total accumulation of CH_3HgCl in cells is more important than the turnover for the expression of growth-inhibitory effects of CH_3HgCl. This may in part be because the process responsible for the growth-inhibitory effects is initiated as soon as mercury compounds enter the cells and the binding activity is completed. The turnover of CH_3HgCl may be more important for the expression of chronic effects than for the expression of acute effects. Another reason for the greater sensitivity of C-6 cells to methyl mercuric chloride is that these cells release a factor(s) into the medium that enhances the effect of CH_3HgCl on C-6 cells (Prasad and Ramanujam 1980).

Methyl mercuric chloride produced a differential effect on another parameter. When CH_3HgCl was present continuously, only cytotoxic effects were observed in both cell types. If the NB cells were exposed to 1–2 μM CH_3HgCl for 1 or 2 days, however, and then examined 2 days after the removal of the mercury compound, a marked increase in morphological differentiation was observed, in addition to cell death (Prasad et al. 1979b). The increase in morphological differentiation in CH_3HgCl-treated NB cells is associated with a 10-fold increase in tyrosine hydroxylase activity (Prasad 1982). No morphological changes were observed in C-6 cells under similar experimental conditions. C-6 cells exhibited a greater degree of degenerative change in the area of lesser cell density (Prasad et al. 1979*b*). The reason for the CH_3HgCl-induced morphological differentiation in NB cells is unknown. One possibility can be mentioned. Mercury binds with a variety of molecules, including proteins and nucleic acids (Vallee and Ulner 1972). We speculate (Prasad et al. 1979*b*) that in NB cells there is a factor (or factors) that prevents the expression of morphological differentiation; organic mercury binds with this factor and makes it inactive, which then allows the expression of differentiated phenotypes in many of the surviving cells.

Nakada and Imura (1980) report that mercuric chloride enhanced DNA synthesis of mouse C-6 and mouse NB cells at the concentration of 1–10 μM, although CH_3HgCl at the same concentration showed no effect. In our studies (Prasad et al. 1979*b*), a 50 percent reduction in the cell number was achieved by 0.1 μM CH_3HgCl in rat C-6 cells, 1 μM in NB cells (NBP$_2$), and 1.64 μM in mouse fibroblasts (L-cells). A concentration of about 5 μM $HgCl_2$ inhibited the growth of both mouse NB and rat C-6 cells by 50 percent. Thus, our cell lines appear to be more sensitive to mercury compounds than those used by other investigators (Prasad et al. 1979*b*). This may in part be because the clones and growth media used were different. Koerker (1980) shows that methyl mercuric hydroxide at a concentration of 1 μM caused cytotoxicity in mouse NB cells in culture, which was reversible after removal of the mercury compounds. Recovery from the cytotoxic effects of methyl mercuric hydroxide was reduced in the presence of 3 μM of cycloheximide, an inhibitor of protein synthesis (Koerker 1980).

Modification of the Effect of Mercury Compounds

The Effect of cAMP-Stimulating Agents on Methyl Mercuric Chloride

Study of the modification of the effect of mercury compounds is important for several reasons. Such studies may increase our understanding of the mechanisms of the effect of these heavy metals on nervous tissue. The modifying agents may reduce the acute and chronic deleterious effects of mercury compounds on nervous tissue. We have succeeded in identifying some new modifying agents that are present naturally in the body and therefore may have an important role in modulating the extent of damage produced by methyl mercuric chloride. The effects of some of these compounds are discussed below.

Prostaglandin E_1 (PGE$_1$), a stimulator of adenylate cyclase activity, and RO20-1724, an inhibitor of cyclic nucleotide phosphodiesterase activity, are known to induce morphological differentiation in NB cell culture by increasing the intracellular level of cAMP (Prasad 1975). Methyl mercuric chloride reduced (Prasad et al. 1979*c*), PGE$_1$, and 4-(3-butoxy-4-methoxybenzyl)-2-

imidazolidinone (RO20-1724) induced morphological differentiation in NB cell culture. Methyl mercuric chloride depolymerizes the neurotubules (Abe et al. 1975), which is considered essential for the expression of a differentiated phenotype in NB cells (Prasad 1975). PGE_1 induced morphological changes in C-6 cells, but RO20-1724 did not. Methyl mercuric chloride did not reduce the extent of PGE_1-induced morphological differentiation in C-6 cells. This suggests either that the expression of cytoplasmic processes in C-6 and NB cells is in part differently regulated, or that the cellular concentration of CH_3HgCl in C-6 cells is not enough to depolymerize the microtubules.

PGE_1 by itself inhibited the growth of C-6 and NB cells in a dose-dependent fashion, but the C-6 cells were more sensitive to PGE_1 than the NB cells (Prasad et al. 1979c). Methyl mercuric chloride enhanced the PGE_1-induced growth inhibition in C-6 cells, and this effect was particularly marked at a concentration of 1 μg/ml (Figure 12.2). CH_3HgCl also increased the PGE_1-

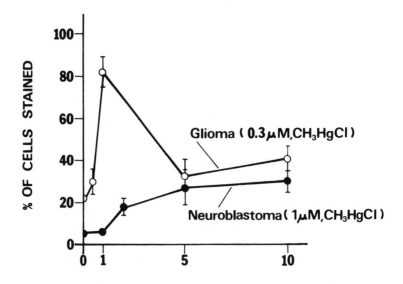

PROSTAGLANDIN E₁ CONCENTRATIONS (µg/ml)

Figure 12.2. Effect of PGE_1 on NB and C-6 cells. C-6 (100,000) and NB (50,000) cells were plated in Lux culture dishes (60 mm). CH_3HgCl was added immediately after addition of various concentrations of PGE_1. All drugs were added 24 hours after plating. Drug and medium were changed in NB cells 2 days after treatment, but not changed in C-6 cells. The number of viable cells per dish was determined 3 days after treatment. The mean value of cell number in culture treated with a given concentration of PGE_1 was considered 100 percent, and the inhibition of growth in culture treated with CH_3HgCl and PGE_1 was calculated as cell number in culture treated with the same concentration of PGE_1. Each value represents an average of 8–9 samples. The bar at each point is one standard deviation. The bars not shown in the figure were equal to sizes of symbols. (Reprinted, by permission, from Prasad et al. 1979c.)

induced growth inhibition in NB cells (Prasad et al. 1979*c*), but this effect became independent of PGE_1 concentrations after a concentration of 2 μg/ml (Figure 12.2). The reasons for a greater degree of growth inhibition and cell death in CH_3HgCl-treated C-6 cells in the presence of a lower concentration of PGE_1 (1 μg/ml) is unknown. The fact that PGE_1 at high concentrations (5–10 μg/ml) causes a marked increase in morphological differentiation of C-6 cells, whereas at a lower concentration (1 μg/ml) it did not, suggests that the growth-inhibitory effect of CH_3HgCl is reduced during PGE_1-induced morphological differentiation of C-6 cells. This phenomenon is not observed in NB cells. PGE_1 caused a sustained increase in the intracellular level of cAMP in NB cells, but it caused only a transient increase in C-6 cells. Therefore, the enhanced effect of CH_3HgCl on NB cells in the presence of PGE_1 may in part be related to elevation of the cellular cAMP level, whereas this may not be the case in C-6 cells. Among various prostaglandins, PGE_1, PGE_2, and $PGE_{2\alpha}$ at a lower concentration (1 μg/ml) did not inhibit the growth of NB and C-6 cells in culture, but PGE_1 and PGE_2 dramatically enhanced the growth-inhibitory effect of CH_3HgCl, whereas $PGE_{2\alpha}$ failed to modify the effect of CH_3HgCl (see Table 12.1). PGE_2 (1 μg/ml) inhibited the growth of C-6 cells in culture by 28 percent of control, but in combination with CH_3HgCl, it produced an additive effect (see Table 12.1).

RO20-1724, an inhibitor of cyclic nucleotide phosphodiesterase activity, by itself inhibited the growth of C-6 and NB cells in a dose-dependent fashion (Prasad et al. 1979*c*). However, the C-6 cells were less sensitive than the NB

Table 12.1   Modification by prostaglandins of CH_3HgCl effect in glioma (C-6) cells in culture

Treatment	Cell No. (% of Untreated Control ± SD)
Ethyl alcohol + CH_3HgCl (0.2 μM)	43.0 ± 12.0
PGE_1 (1 μg/ml)	101.0 ± 8.0
PGE_1 + CH_3HgCl	2.3 ± 0.5
PGE_2 (1 μg/ml)	109.0 ± 8.0
PGE_2 + CH_3HgCl	4.2 ± 1.9
PGA_2 (1 μg/ml)	72.0 ± 10.0
PGA_2 + CH_3HgCl	22.0 ± 8.0
PGF_2^α (1 μg/ml)	117.0 ± 14.0
PGF_2^α + CH_3HgCl	42.0 ± 9.0

Source: Reprinted, by permission, from Prasad 1982.
Note: Cells (10^5) were plated in Lux culture dishes (60 mm); prostaglandin (PG) and CH_3HgCl were added 24 hours after plating. Since PGs are soluble in 50 percent ethyl alcohol, an equivalent amount of solvent was also added as a control. No medium or drug was changed for a period of 3 days. The number of trypan blue-stained cells was counted among the attached cell population, and the total number of cells was counted in a Coulter Counter 3 days after treatment. The number of viable cells per dish was determined by subtracting the number of stained cells from the total number. The average value of cell number in untreated controls was considered 100 percent. Each value represents an average of at least 6 samples.

cells at a lower concentration, although at a high concentration (200 μg/ml) both cell types exhibited similar sensitivity to this drug (Prasad et al. 1979c). In the presence of RO20-1724, methyl mercuric chloride produced a contrasting effect on C-6 and NB cells in culture. RO20-1724 completely protected C-6 cells against CH_3HgCl-induced toxicity. A concentration of 100 μg/ml of RO20-1724 provided complete protection against the cytotoxic effect of 0.3 μM CH_3HgCl (Figure 12.3). Methyl mercuric chloride slightly enhanced the growth-inhibitory effect of RO20-1724 on NB cells. The reasons for the protective effect of RO20-1724 against the cytotoxic effect of CH_3HgCl on C-6 cells are unknown. However, this is not unique to RO20-1724, since similar results are obtained in the presence of other inhibitors of cyclic nucleotide phosphodiesterase, such as papaverine and isobutylaxanthine (Prasad et al. 1979c). The protective effect of inhibitors of cyclic nucleotide phosphodiesterase against the cytotoxic effect of CH_3HgCl on C-6 cells is not

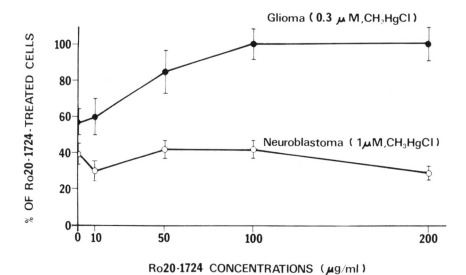

Figure 12.3.   Effect of RO20-1724 on C-6 cells in presence of CH_3HgCl. C-6 (100,000) and NB (50,000) cells were plated in Lux culture dishes (60 mm). CH_3HgCl was added immediately after addition of various concentrations of 4-(3-butoxy-4-methoxybenzyl)-2-imidazolidinone (RO20-1724). All drugs were added 24 hours after plating. Drug and medium were changed in NB cells 2 days after treatment, but they were not changed in C-6 cells. The number of viable cells per dish was determined 3 days after treatment. The mean value of cell number in culture treated with a given concentration of RO20-1724 was considered 100 percent, and the inhibition of growth in culture treated with CH_3HgCl and RO20-1724 was calculated as percentage of cell number in culture treated with the same concentration of RO20-1724. Each value represents an average of 8–9 samples. The bar at each point is one standard deviation. The bars not shown in the figure were equal to sizes of symbols. (Reprinted, by permission, from Prasad and Ramanujam 1980.)

associated with a sustained increase in cellular cAMP. It is suggested (Prasad et al. 1979c) that both CH_3HgCl and phosphodiesterase inhibitors may compete for the same sites that are responsible for CH_3HgCl-induced growth inhibition in C-6 cells, and that inhibitors of phosphodiesterase may have a higher affinity for binding with these sites than does CH_3HgCl. This is not true in NB cells, in which CH_3HgCl enhances the growth-inhibitory effect of inhibitors of cyclic nucleotide phosphodiesterase.

The Effect of Vitamin E on CH3HgCl-Induced Toxicity

Vitamin E (D1-alpha-tocopheryl acetate) at a concentration of as little as 10^{-5} IU/ml provided significant protection against the growth-inhibitory effect of CH_3HgCl on C-6 cells (Figure 12.4), whereas it did not modify the effect of CH_3HgCl on NB cells (Prasad and Ramanujam 1980). The CH_3HgCl (0.4 μM) treated (3 days) C-6 culture contained 95 percent trypan blue-stained cells, whereas the control culture contained less than 1 percent. The C-6 cells treated with 0.4 μM CH_3HgCl and 10^{-2}–10^{-4} IU/ml vitamin E

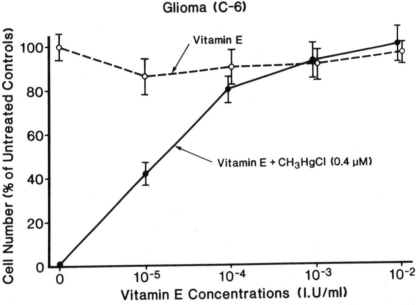

Glioma (C-6)

Figure 12.4. Effects of vitamin E on CH_3HgCl-induced toxicity. C-6 cells (10^5) were plated in Lux culture dishes (60 mm); vitamin E and CH_3HgCl were added 24 hours later. No drug or medium was changed during a 3-day period. The number of viable cells per dish was determined 3 days after treatment. The number of cells in untreated control cultures was considered 100 percent, and the cell number in treated cultures was expressed as percentage of untreated control. Each value represents an average of 9 samples. The bar at each point is one standard deviation. (Reprinted, by permission, from Prasad and Ramanujam 1980.)

showed less than 1 percent trypan blue-stained cells. The protective effect of vitamin E against CH_3HgCl-induced toxicity of C-6 cells may not be entirely the result of its antioxidant property, because sodium *L*-ascorbate, sodium *D*-ascorbate, or glutathione did not alter the effect of CH_3HgCl on C-6 cells (Prasad and Ramanujam 1980). The mechanism of protection against CH_3HgCl-induced toxicity of C-6 cells by vitamin E is unknown.

Vitamin E also protects quails, rats, and golden hamsters against neurotoxicity in vivo produced by methyl mercury (Chang et al. 1978; Kasuya 1975; Weiss et al. 1971). It is unknown whether vitamin E protects glial cells, neurons, or both in vivo against CH_3HgCl-induced neurotoxicity. The response of C-6 cell culture in the presence of vitamin E and CH_3HgCl is similar to that observed in vivo; therefore, the information obtained on cell-culture models could be useful in explaining the mechanism of damage in vivo. Vitamin E at a concentration of 0.01 IU/ml failed to protect C-6 or NB cells against the toxicity of tri-*n*-butyl lead acetate and inorganic mercury ($HgCl_2$). Therefore, vitamin E-induced protection is rather specific for CH_3HgCl.

Enhancement of the Effect of CH_3HgCl by Vitamin C

Sodium *L*-ascorbate (vitamin C) at nonlethal concentrations markedly potentiated the growth-inhibitory effect of methyl mercuric chloride on NB cells (Figure 12.5), whereas it did not modify the effect of CH_3HgCl on C-6 cells (Prasad and Ramanujam 1980). The effect of ascorbate was most pronounced at a CH_3HgCl concentration of 1 μM. Sodium *D*-ascorbate was equally effective in potentiating the effect of CH_3HgCl on NB cells, but glutathione did not produce such an effect (Prasad and Ramanujam 1980). It is unknown whether vitamin C would enhance the effect of CH_3HgCl on neurons in vivo.

Enhancement of the Effect of CH_3HgCl by Glioma Factor(s)

We have shown (Prasad and Ramanujam 1980) that the cytotoxic effect of CH_3HgCl on cells was much greater in cultures in which the medium was not changed during a 3-day experimental period than those in which the medium was changed daily. The number of cells in control cultures was similar, irrespective of any change of growth medium. This suggests that C-6 cells released a "factor(s)" into the medium that does not affect the growth rate of control cells. However, this "factor" increased the effect of CH_3HgCl on C-6 and NB cells (see Table 12.2).

The responses of NB cells to methyl mercuric chloride were similar irrespective of change of growth medium during the experiment (Prasad and Ramanujam 1980), indicating that NB cells do not produce any factor that increases the cytotoxicity of CH_3HgCl. The hybrid cells (NB x glioma, NCB-20 supplied by Dr. Marshall Nirenberg of the National Institutes of

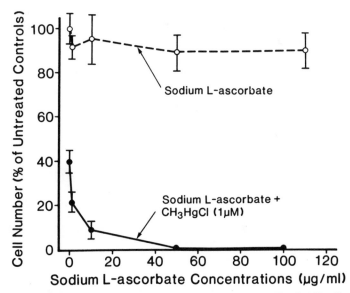

Figure 12.5. Effect of vitamin C on CH_3HgCl growth inhibiting effect in NB cells. NB cells (5×10^4) were plated in Lux culture dishes (60 mm); sodium *L*-ascorbate and CH_3HgCl were added 24 hours later. Drug and medium were changed daily, and the number of viable cells per dish was determined 3 days after treatment. The number of cells in untreated control cultures was considered 100 percent, and the cell number in treated cultures was expressed as percentage of untreated control. Each value represents an average of 9 samples. The bar at each point is one standard deviation. The bars not shown in the figure were equal to sizes of symbols. (Reprinted, by permission, from Prasad and Ramanujam 1980.)

Table 12.2   Effect of glioma "factor(s)" in CH_3HgCl-induced growth inhibition in NB and glioma (C-6) cells in culture

	Cell No. (% of Untreated Control ± SD)	
Treatment "Glioma Factor(s)" (Growth Medium)	$NBA_{2(I)}$	*Glioma (C-6)*
0:5, CH_3HgCl	46 ± 4 (1.0 μM)	88.0 ± 7.0 (0.3 μM)
3:1, Control	75 ± 3	80.0 ± 3.0
3:1, CH_3HgCl	9 ± 2	0.5 ± 0.2
1:1, Control	80 ± 7	85.0 ± 6.0
1:1, CH_3HgCl	31 ± 4	22.0 ± 4.0

Source: Reprinted, by permission, from Prasad and Ramanujam 1980.
NB (50,000) and C-6 (10^5) cells were plated in Lux culture dishes (60 mm).
Glioma-conditioned medium containing glioma "factor(s)" and CH_3HgCl were added 24 hours after plating. The glioma-conditioned medium, regular growth medium, and CH_3HgCl were changed daily in glioma cells, but in NB cells they were changed 2 days after treatment. The number of viable cells per dish was determined 3 days after treatment. Each value represents an average of 6 samples.

Health) also release a "factor(s)" into the medium that enhances the growth-inhibitory effect of CH_3HgCl on mouse NB cells in culture. This shows that the gene responsible for producing this "factor" in glioma cells is dominant, since the trait continues to be produced in hybrid cells.

It is unknown whether normal glial cells produce a similar factor. If they do, we suggest that one of the molecular mechanisms of the effect of CH_3HgCl on nerve tissue may be mediated by a glial factor (or factors) that affects glial cells as well as certain kinds of neurons.

Enhancement of the Effect of CH₃HgCl by Glutamate

Methyl mercuric chloride (1 μM), mercuric chloride (2 μM), manganese chloride (5 μM), cadmium chloride (5 μM), cupric sulfate (10 μM), cobalt

Table 12.3   Modification by metals of glutamate effect on NB cells (P_2 clone) in culture

Treatment	Cell No. per Dish (% of Control Culture ± SD)
Na-glutamate (3.9 mM)	56±4*
CH_3HgCl (1 μM)	59±6
Na-glutamate + CH_3HgCl	14±3*
$HgCl_2$ (2 μM)	59±5
Na-glutamate + $HgCl_2$	21±3*
$MnCl_2$ (5 μM)	55±6
Na-glutamate + $MnCl_2$	10±3*
Organic Pb (0.5 μM)	51±5
Na-glutamate + organic Pb	31±5†
$CdCl_2$ (5 μM)	28±2
Na-glutamate + $CdCl_2$	15±3†
$CuSO_4$ (10 μM)	69±4
Na-glutamate + $CuSO_4$	32±4†
$CoCl_2$ (50 μM)	70±5
Na-glutamate + $CoCl_2$	28±3*
$Fe_2(SO_4)_3$ (50 μM)	85±6
Na-glutamate + $Fe_2(SO_4)_3$	34±3*
LiCl (50 μM)	98±5
Na-glutamate + $LiCl_2$	54±2‡

Source: Reprinted, by permission, from Prasad and Ramanujam 1980.
*Synergistic effect.
†Additive effect.
‡No effect.
Note: NB cells (50,000) were plated in Lux culture dishes (60 mm); glutamate and metals were added 24 hours after plating. Medium and agents were changed 2 days after treatment, and the number of cells per dish was determined 3 days after treatment. Each value represents an average of 6–8 samples. To test whether glutamate had any effect in combination with metal compounds in enhancing the growth inhibition of cells, the mean percentage of untreated control cultures for the glutamate plus metal-compound-treated cultures was compared with that of metal-treated or glutamate-treated cultures by the use of two independent sample t-tests at $p = 0.01$. If there was a significant effect of glutamate in combination with a metal compound, an additional test was performed to establish whether the combination of glutamate with a metal compound produced an additive or synergistic effect.

chloride (50 μM), and ferric sulfate (50 μM) by themselves inhibit the growth of NB cells to varying degrees, ranging from 15 to 49 percent (Table 12.3). The number of trypan blue-stained cells varied 3–5 percent. The combination of methyl mercuric chloride with glutamate produced a synergistic effect on growth inhibition of NB cells in culture (Prasad et al. 1980). The extent to which the effect of the combined treatment was modified depended on the concentrations of glutamate (Figure 12.6) and CH$_3$HgCl. The number of trypan blue-stained cells in culture treated with glutamate and CH$_3$HgCl was about 8 percent. The high concentration of CH$_3$HgCl (2 μM) caused 100

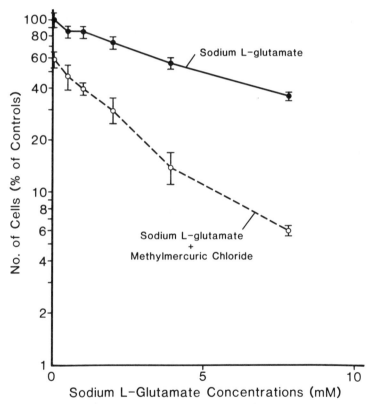

Figure 12.6. Modification of glutamate effect on NB cells (P2 clone) in culture by organic mercury. NB cells of clone NPB$_2$ were plated (50,000/dish) in Lux culture dishes (60 mm). Sodium *L*-glutamate or sodium *L*-glutamate plus CH$_3$HgCl (1 μM) was added 24 hours after plating. Drug and medium were changed 2 days after plating, and the number of viable cells per dish was determined 3 days after treatment. The mean value of the cell number in control cultures was considered 100 percent, and the number of cells in treated culture was expressed as percentage of cell number in control cultures. Each value represents the mean of 6 samples. The vertical line at each point is one standard deviation. (Reprinted, by permission, from Prasad and Ramanujam 1980.)

percent lethality; therefore, a concentration of CH_3HgCl higher than 1 μM was not used in this study. The combination of glutamate with inorganic mercury (Table 12.3) or with manganese chloride (Figure 12.7) also produced a synergistic effect on growth inhibition of NB cells in culture. The number of trypan blue-stained cells in the culture treated with mercuric chloride and glutamate was about 17 percent, whereas in cultures treated with manganese chloride and glutamate it was about 5 percent. Manganese chloride at a concentration of 20 μM was lethal to NB cells in culture. The combination of glutamate (3.9 μM) with $CoCl_2$ and $Fe_2(SO_4)_3$ also produced

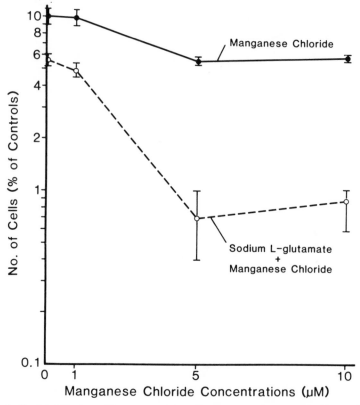

Figure 12.7. Modification of glutamate effect on NB cells (P2 clone) in culture by manganese chloride. NB cells of clone NPB_2 were plated (50,000/dish) in Lux culture dishes (60 mm). Manganese chloride or manganese chloride plus sodium *L*-glutamate (3.9 mM) was added 24 hours after plating. Drug and medium were changed 2 days after treatment, and the number of viable cells per dish was determined 3 days after treatment. The mean value of the cell number in control cultures was considered 100 percent, and the number of cells in treated culture was expressed as percentage of cell number in control cultures. Each value represents the mean of 6–9 samples. The vertical line at each point is one standard deviation. (Reprinted, by permission, from Prasad and Ramanujam 1980.)

a synergistic effect on growth inhibition. Other metals, such as lead tributyl acetate, cadmium, and copper, in combination with glutamate, produced an additive effect on growth inhibition of NB cells in culture. CH_3HgCl (1 μM) and $MnCl_2$ (5 μM) failed to modify the effect of D-glutamate (3.9 mM), L-aspartate (4.0 mM), or α-ketoglutarate (3.3 mM). The combination of carbachol (4.0 mM), an analog of acetylcholine (an excitatory neurotransmitter), with CH_3HgCl (1 μM) inhibited the growth of NB cells to an extent that is produced by CH_3HgCl alone (Prasad et al. 1980).

Certain metal compounds dramatically modify the effect of glutamate on NB cells in culture. The extent of modification depends on the particular metal compound. It should be pointed out that organic mercury produces neurological disorders that are referred to as Minamata disease (Takeuchi 1968), manganese produces neurological syndromes similar to those of Parkinsonism (Chandra et al. 1974; Committee on Biological Effects of Atmospheric Pollution 1973), and glutamate and/or kainate produces morphological and biochemical changes in the brain similar to those observed in Huntington's disease (Coyle et al. 1978; Coyle and Schwarcz 1976; Goli and Hong 1977; Kanazawa et al. 1977; McGeer and McGeer 1976). The fact that the combination of glutamate with mercury or manganese compounds produces a synergistic effect on growth inhibition of NB cells suggests that the interaction of this excitatory neurotransmitter with mercury and manganese compounds may influence the time of onset and the extent of the neurological syndromes produced by these agents. The mechanism of the modification of the effects of glutamate by mercury and manganese is unknown. It is interesting to note that organic lead, which produces neurological disorders (Hernberg 1980), does not potentiate the effect of glutamate on NB cells in culture. Neuroblastoma cells contain specific receptors for glutamic acid, but not for kainic acid (see Table 12.4). Therefore, it is possible that receptors for glutamic acid may be involved in the synergistic effect of CH_3HgCl and glutamic acid.

Table 12.4 Binding of [^{3}H]-glutamic acid with 50,000 $\times$ g pellet of mouse neuroblastoma cells (NBP$_2$)

Treatment	Bound [^{3}H]-Glutamic Acid (pM/mg protein $\pm$ SD)
No glutamate	5.10$\pm$0.30
1 mM glutamate	—
1 mM kainate	6.00$\pm$0.30
No glutamate, 1 mM CaCl$_2$	7.80$\pm$0.20
No glutamate, 4° C	0.24$\pm$0.08
No glutamate (after storage at -20° C for 20 hr)	1.20$\pm$0.04

Note: Bound [^{3}H]-glutamic acid = total binding $-$ binding in presence of 1mM glutamate or kainate. Reaction mixture (250 μl) contained Tris-HCl, 20 mM, pH 7.4; protein, 67–133 μg; [^{3}H]-glutamic acid, 11.9 nM. Incubations were done at 30° C until specified otherwise.

The Effect of CH₃HgCl on the cAMP System

The intracellular level of cAMP increased by about twofold in CH$_3$HgCl-treated C-6 and NB cells in culture (Prasad et al. 1979c). Therefore, we suggest that one of the biochemical lesions of CH$_3$HgCl-induced neurotoxicity may be an abnormal metabolism of cAMP in nerve tissue (Prasad et al. 1979c). It is unknown whether the increase in the cAMP level after treatment with CH$_3$HgCl is the result of stimulation of adenylate cyclase activity or of inhibition of cAMP phosphodiesterase activity.

The Effect of CH₃HgCl on the Sensitivity of Adenylate Cyclase to Neurotransmitters

PGE$_1$ significantly increased the intracellular level of cAMP in both C-6 and NB cells 10 minutes after treatment. However, this effect was markedly reduced ($p = 0.058$) in chronically treated (0.1 μM) C-6 cells, but not in chronically treated (0.1 and 0.2 μM) NB cells (see Table 12.5). Chronic CH$_3$HgCl treatment at 0.05 μM in C-6 cells also reduced the PGE$_1$ response, but to a lesser extent than did treatment at 0.1 μM (Prasad 1975). The addition of an equivalent volume of ethanol did not affect the level of cAMP in control or chronically treated cells. The response of PGE$_1$-sensitive adenylate cyclase did not change in either C-6 or NB cells after acute treatment with CH$_3$HgCl.

Table 12.5   Effect of methyl mercuric chloride (CH$_3$HgCl) on prostaglandin E$_1$ sensitive adenylate cyclases in glioma and neuroblastoma cells in culture

Treatment	Cyclic AMP Level (pM/mg protein $\pm$ SD)	
	Glioma (C-6)	Neuroblastoma (P₂)
Control	21$\pm$2	20$\pm$3
PGE$_1$ (10 μg/ml)	53$\pm$6	36$\pm$5
CH$_3$HgCl, 0.1 μM, acute treatment	30$\pm$3	22$\pm$5
PGE$_1$ + CH$_3$HgCl, acute treatment	51$\pm$7	36$\pm$4
CH$_3$HgCl, 0.1 μM, chronic treatment	20$\pm$5	20$\pm$4
PGE$_1$ + CH$_3$HgCl, chronic treatment	29$\pm$4	36$\pm$5

Note: Plating densities: for NB cells, 0.5×10^5 in control, PGE$_1$, and 0.1 μM CH$_3$HgCl groups, and 1×10^5 in the 0.2 μM CH$_3$HgCl group; for C-6 cells, 1×10^5 in control, PGE$_1$, and 0.05 μM CH$_3$HgCl groups, and 2×10^5 in the 0.1 μM CH$_3$HgCl group. Cells were treated with CH$_3$HgCl either immediately after plating (chronically treated cells) or 1 day after plating (acutely treated cells). After 5 days in culture, fresh growth medium and CH$_3$HgCl were changed 30 minutes before the addition of PGE$_1$. The cells were incubated in the presence of PGE$_1$ for 10 minutes and then harvested for cAMP assay. Each value is the mean of 8 samples $\pm$ SEM. The values of cAMP levels in control and prostaglandin E$_1$ (PGE$_1$)-treated C-6 and NB cells were different at $p = 0.001$. The values of cAMP levels in control C-6 cells after treatment with PGE$_1$ and in chronically treated C-6 cells after treatment with PGE$_1$ were different at $p = 0.058$ (Spuhler and Prasad 1980).

Dopamine (10 μM) and norepinephrine (10 μM) in the presence of RO20-1724 (a cyclic nucleotide phosphodiesterase inhibitor) increased the intracellular level of cAMP about twice as much as did RO20-1724 alone. RO20-1724 by itself increased cellular cAMP by about threefold to fourfold. The responses of dopamine- and norepinephrine-sensitive adenylate cyclases in NB cells (NBA$_{2(1)}$) (Abe et al. 1975) did not change after acute treatment with 0.5 μM CH$_3$HgCl (Somjen et al. 1973). Norepinephrine (10 μM) by itself increased the intracellular level of cAMP in C-6 cells by about eightfold to tenfold, and this effect remained unaltered in acutely and chronically treated C-6 cells (Spuhler and Prasad 1980).

The reasons for a decreased response of PGE$_1$-sensitive adenylate cyclase in chronically treated C-6 cells are unknown. The following possibilities can be mentioned. (1) Chronic treatment of C-6 cells with CH$_3$HgCl causes an increase in cAMP phosphodiesterase activity, which becomes the limiting factor in the accumulation of cAMP after the treatment of cells with PGE$_1$. (2) The number of PGE$_1$ receptors is decreased after chronic treatment with CH$_3$HgCl. (3) A modification of the plasma cell membrane results in a lessened affinity of PGE$_1$ to cyclase receptors. The present data cannot be extrapolated to an in vivo condition. However, one can raise the question of whether one of the biochemical lesions of CH$_3$HgCl-induced damage to nerve tissue might not be a reduction in the sensitivity of adenylate cyclase to PGE$_1$ in glial cells.

Methyl mercury blocks muscarinic receptors in the rat brain (Burg et al. 1980). It is interesting to note that the ability of CH$_3$HgCl to block quinuclidinyl benzilate (QNB, a high-affinity antagonist of muscarinic receptors) binding to muscarinic receptors was 100 times less than that of HgCl$_2$. It is known that CH$_3$HgCl undergoes biotransformation to divalent mercury in mammals. The amount of HgCl$_2$ in the brain after single or multiple doses of CH$_3$HgCl is usually less than 4 percent (Norseth and Clarkson 1970).

The Effect of CH$_3$HgCl on the Uptake of Neurotransmitters

Treatment of NB cells with 1 μM CH$_3$HgCl reduced the accumulation of choline in NB cells (Prasad et al. 1979a). The concentration of CH$_3$HgCl required to inhibit high-affinity choline uptake in NB cells (Prasad et al. 1979a) was one-tenth that required for its inhibition in adult mouse brain homogenates (Bondy et al. 1979). The reduced uptake of choline may in part account for a decreased level of acetylcholine in the cortical area of the rat brain (Hrdina et al. 1976). The energy-dependent uptake of dopamine and GABA was not shown in NB cells (Prasad et al. 1979a) but was demonstrable in adult mouse brain homogenates (Bondy et al. 1979), perhaps partly because this clone of NB is of a cholinergic type, with relatively undifferentiated cells. Treatment of NB and C-6 cells with low concentrations of CH$_3$HgCl produced a contrasting effect on the accumulation of glycine and glutamate. The energy-dependent accumulation of radioactive glycine or glutamate increased in NB cells after treatment with CH_3HgCl (1 μM), whereas it decreased in CH_3HgCl-treated C-6 cells.

These data show that low concentrations of 0.3–1.0 μM CH_3HgCl produce disturbances in the high-affinity uptake of certain putative neurotransmitters in nerve tissues in vitro. These results emphasize that one must be cautious in interpreting data that measure the level of neurotransmitters in the total brain tissue, because changes in the levels of certain putative neurotransmitters could be in the opposite direction, depending on the cell type.

The Effect of CH_3HgCl on the Growth Rate, Morphology, and Effect of cAMP After Chronic Treatment

The morphology and doubling time (24–35 hours for C-6 cells, 18–20 hours for NB cells) of chronically treated C-6 cells (0.05 μM and 0.1 μM) and NB cells (0.1 μM and 0.2 μM) were similar to those of untreated cultures (Ramanujam and Prasad 1979). We are not selecting any specific type of cell during chronic treatment, since the concentrations of CH_3HgCl used in this study neither caused cytotoxicity nor affected the growth rate. PGE_1 produced 85 percent morphological differentiation in C-6 cells that were not treated with CH_3HgCl. A similar effect of PGE_1 was observed in chronically treated C-6 cells. In NB cultures that were not treated with CH_3HgCl PGE_1 and RO20-1724 caused 45 percent and 75 percent morphological differentiation, respectively. A similar effect of cAMP-stimulating agents was observed in chronically treated NB cultures (Ramanujam and Prasad 1979).

The Effect of CH_3HgCl on Gene Expression

Changes in the Relative Amounts of Proteins

There were dramatic increases and decreases in the intensities of specific proteins of the cytosol (see Figure 12.8), particulate (Figure 12.9), and crude nuclear fractions (Figure 12.10) of acutely (0.1 μM CH_3HgCl) and chronically (0.05 μM CH_3HgCl) treated C-6 cells. The qualitative changes in the relative amounts of proteins and their phosphorylation levels are summarized in Tables 12.6 and 12.7. Marked alterations in the amounts of proteins were seen in glioma cells chronically treated with as little as 0.05 μM (12.5 ng/ml) CH_3HgCl. In addition, there were marked differences in the relative amounts of proteins between acutely and chronically treated C-6 cells. The staining intensities of most bands (all bands of nuclear fraction, and half the bands of cytosol and particulate fractions) in acutely treated C-6 cells were similar to those found in the untreated cells. However, the intensities of all bands presented in Tables 12.7 and 12.8 show marked alterations in the chronically (0.1 μM) treated C-6 cells. There were mostly quantitative differences be-

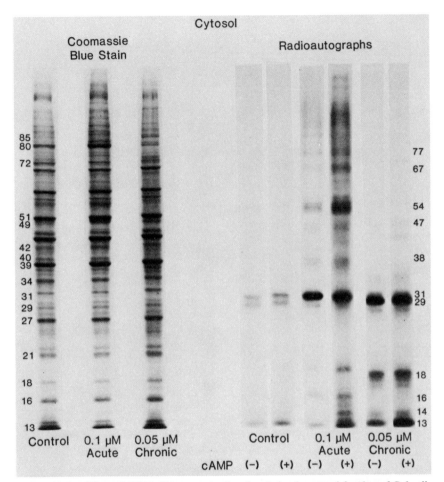

Cytosol

Coomassie
Blue Stain

Radioautographs

85
80
72

51
49

42
40
39

34
31
29
27

21

18

16

13

Control   0.1 µM   0.05 µM
           Acute   Chronic

77
67

54
47

38

31
29

18

16
14
13

Control   0.1 µM   0.05 µM
                Acute   Chronic

cAMP (−) (+)   (−) (+)   (−) (+)

Figure 12.8.   Effect of CH₃HgCl on protein phosphorylation in cytosol fraction of C-6 cells, as shown by results of polyacrylamide gel electrophoresis. The approximate molecular weights of proteins are expressed as multiples of 1,000 (K). The observed change in the phosphorylation of protein species represents a steady-state situation and is the sum of phosphorylation and dephosphorylation reactions. (Reprinted, by permission, from Ramanujam and Prasad 1979.)

tween concentrations of 0.05 µM and 0.1 µM CH₃HgCl in chronically treated C-6 cells. The degrees of change were greater in cells treated with higher concentrations of CH₃HgCl.

In contrast to the chronically treated C-6 cells, NB cells did not show any significant change (Ramanujam and Prasad 1980) in the amounts of proteins in the cytosol (Figure 12.11), particulate (Figure 12.12), and crude nuclear fractions (Figure 12.13) after chronic treatment with CH₃HgCl (0.1 µM and 0.2 µM).

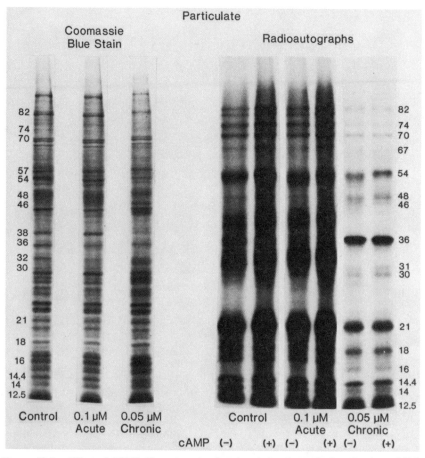

Figure 12.9. Effect of CH₃HgCl on protein phosphorylation in particulate fraction of C-6 cells, as shown by results of polyacrylamide gel electrophoresis. See legend of Figure 12.8 for additional information. (Reprinted, by permission, from Ramanujam and Prasad 1979.)

Changes in Levels of Protein Phosphorylations

Because the phosphorylation of brain proteins has been implicated in regulation of the expression of neuronal functions it was important to investigate whether CH₃HgCl alters the phosphorylation of cellular proteins. The phosphorylation levels of proteins of untreated C-6 cells and NB cells were highest in the particulate (Figures 12.9 and 12.12) and lowest in the cytosol fractions (Figures 12.8 and 12.11). The phosphorylation levels of most proteins in the particulate and cytosol fractions were cAMP-dependent in C-6 cells (Tables 12.6 and 12.7), whereas only one band (NB, MW 12.6 K) or two (glioma, MW 13.2 and 32 K) were cAMP-dependent in the crude nuclear

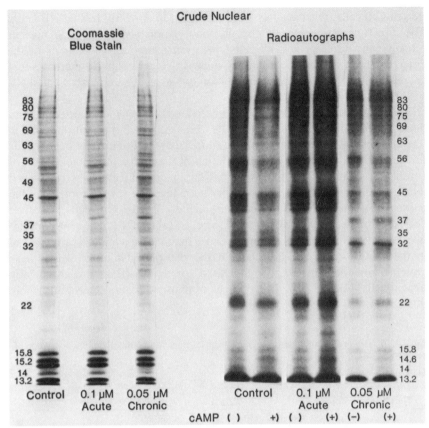

Figure 12.10. Effect of CH₃HgCl on protein phosphorylation in crude nuclear fraction of C-6 cells, as shown by results of polyacrylamide gel electrophoresis. See legend of Figure 12.8 for additional information. (Reprinted, by permission, from Ramanujam and Prasad 1979.)

fraction. Note that the use of confluent cells in these experiments may account in part for a low phosphorylation level in the cystosol. However, the overall phosphorylation levels of cytosol proteins in NB cells were greater than those of C-6 cells; the reverse was true for particulate and nuclear fractions (Ramanujam and Prasad 1980).

Chronic treatment of glioma and NB cells produced marked alterations (increases and decreases) in net phosphorylation profiles of specific proteins (Ramanujam and Prasad 1979, 1980). Increases and decreases in the levels of phosphorylation were observed in the cytosol fractions of NB and C-6 cells. However, the direction of the changes in the phosphorylation levels of the particulates of C-6 cells was opposite that of NB cells. For example, the phosphorylation levels of the particulate fraction decreased in chronically treated C-6 cells, whereas they were increased in similarly treated NB cells. The direction of changes in the phosphorylation levels of crude nuclear proteins was different in both cell types. For example, the proteins of the crude nuclear fraction of chronically treated C-6 cells showed increases and decreases in the levels of phosphorylation, whereas in chronically treated NB cells they showed only decreases.

The phosphorylation levels of acutely treated C-6 cells were different from those of chronically treated C-6 cells. For example, the phosphorylation levels of several proteins were increased in the cytosol of acutely treated cells (Table 12.6), whereas the phosphorylation of these proteins in the cytosol of chronically treated C-6 cells either showed no significant change or showed increases and decreases. The phosphorylation levels of several proteins of the particulate remained unchanged in the acutely treated C-6 cells, but they decreased in the chronically treated C-6 cells (Table 12.7). The phosphorylation levels of crude nuclear proteins either remained unchanged or increased in the acutely treated C-6 cells, but the phosphorylation levels of these proteins remained unchanged, increased, or decreased in the chronically treated cells (Table 12.8). The changes in phosphorylation levels of acutely treated NB cells have not been studied.

Table 12.6 Effect of methyl mercuric chloride on changes in amounts and phosphorylation of cytosol proteins of glioma cells

Molecular Weight (× 1,000)	Control	Acute 0.1 μM	Chronic 0.1 μM	0.05 μM
Coomassie Blue Stained Protein Bands				
85.0	Detectable	Unchanged	+	Unchanged
80.0	Detectable	+	−	−
49.0	Detectable	+	+	+
39.4	Detectable	Unchanged	−	−
Net Phosphorylation Profiles				
77.0*	Undetectable	+	Unchanged	Unchanged
54.0*	Undetectable	+	Unchanged	Unchanged
47.0*	Undetectable	+	Unchanged	Unchanged
30.0*	Detectable	+	−	+
18.0*	Undetectable	+	Unchanged	+
16.0*	Undetectable	+	Unchanged	Unchanged
13.0*	Detectable	+	+	+

*Refers to cAMP-dependent phosphorylation.

Note: From radioautographs, changes in the relative quantities and levels of phosphorylation of specific proteins in the acutely and chronically treated C-6 cells are presented as increased (+), decreased (−), or unchanged with respect to the corresponding proteins in the untreated cells. The observed change in the level of phosphorylation of a protein species represents a steady-state situation and is the sum of phosphorylation and dephosphorylation reactions (Ramanujam and Prasad 1979).

The levels of phosphorylation of specific proteins appear to be very sensitive to CH_3HgCl in both C-6 and NB cells. The reasons for the high sensitivity of phosphorylation reactions to CH_3HgCl are unknown, as is the biological significance of these changes. However, it is interesting to note that extensive modifications of gene expression are observed in cells that do not show any significant alteration in morphology, doubling time, and the effect of cyclic AMP-stimulating agents on morphological differentiation. It should be emphasized that alterations of gene expression in chronically treated cells have been studied using cells of the confluent phase of growth. If similar changes are observed in the chronically treated cells of the exponential phase of growth, one can suggest that cells need very little phosphorylation activity for maintaining growth rate, morphology, and certain biological responses. The mechanism of CH_3HgCl-induced changes in gene expression is unknown. However, it is pertinent to point out that 2–3 percent of added radioactive CH_3HgCl binds to the chromatin fraction of C-6 and NB cells (Ramanujam et al. 1979), and this amount may be enough to alter gene expression in the same cells. The alterations in gene expression in chronically

Table 12.7 Effect of methyl mercuric chloride on changes in amounts and phosphorylation of proteins of particulate fraction of glioma cells

Molecular Weight ($\times$ 1,000)	Control	Acute 0.1 μM	Chronic 0.1 μM	0.05 μM
Coommassie Blue Stained Protein Bands				
58.0	Detectable	−	−	−
46.0	Detectable	Unchanged	+	+
38.0	Detectable	Unchanged	−	−
32.0	Detectable	−	+	+
14.0	Detectable	+	+	+
12.5	Detectable	Unchanged	+	+
Net Phosphorylation Profiles				
83.0*	Detectable	Unchanged	−	−
74.0*	Detectable	Unchanged	−	−
70.0*	Detectable	Unchanged	−	−
54.0*	Detectable	Unchanged	−	−
36.0*	Detectable	Unchanged	−	−
21.0*	Detectable	Unchanged	−	−
14.0*	Detectable	Unchanged	−	−

*Refers to cAMP-dependent phosphorylation.
Note: From radioautographs, changes in the relative quantities and levels of phosphorylation of specific proteins in the acutely and chronically treated C-6 cells are presented as increased (+), decreased (−), or unchanged with respect to the corresponding proteins in the untreated cells. The observed change in the level of phosphorylation of a protein species represents a steady-state situation and is the sum of phosphorylation and dephosphorylation reactions (Ramanujam and Prasad 1979).

treated cells may also in part result from the effect of CH_3HgCl at the translational level. In fact, treatment of rats with methyl mercuric chloride has been reported to cause disorganization of the ribosomal structures in spinal ganglion neurons (Carmichael and Cavanagh 1976).

Conclusion

Our results show that glioma cells are more sensitive to methyl mercuric chloride than NB cells. Several agents, such as PGE_1, inhibitors of cyclic nucleotide phosphodiesterase, vitamin E, vitamin C, glioma factors, and glutamic acid, modify the effect of CH_3HgCl markedly. However, the extent of modification depends on the cell type and the particular modifying agents.

Our results show that cAMP-dependent and -independent phosphorylations of specific proteins are very sensitive to CH_3HgCl in both C-6 and NB cells. In addition, PGE_1-linked adenylate cyclase of C-6 cells is also very sensitive to the chronic effects of CH_3HgCl. Therefore, these biological

Table 12.8 Effect of methyl mercuric chloride on changes in amounts of phosphorylation of crude nuclear proteins of glioma cells

Molecular Weight (× 1,000)	Control	Acute 0.1 μM	Chronic 0.1 μM	0.05 μM
Coommassie Blue Stained Protein Bands				
59.0	Detectable	Unchanged	+	+
49.0	Detectable	Unchanged	+	+
32.0	Detectable	Unchanged	+	+
22.0	Undetectable	Unchanged	+	+
18.0	Undetectable	Unchanged	−	−
14.0	Detectable	Unchanged	−	−
Net Phosphorylation Profiles				
75.0	Detectable	+	Unchanged	Unchanged
56.0	Detectable	+	Unchanged	Unchanged
49.0	Undetectable	Unchanged	+	Unchanged
40.0–45.0	Detectable	+	−	−
37.0*	Undetectable	Unchanged	−	−
32.0–35.0	Detectable	+	−	−
22.0	Detectable	+	−	−
13.2*	Detectable	Unchanged	−	−

*Refers to cAMP-dependent phosphorylation.

Note: From radioautographs, changes in the relative quantities and levels of phosphorylation of specific proteins in the acutely and chronically treated C-6 cells are presented as increased (+), decreased (−), or unchanged with respect to the corresponding proteins in the untreated cells. The observed change in the level of phosphorylation of a protein species represents a steady-state situation and is the sum of phosphorylation and dephosphorylation reactions (Ramanujam and Prasad 1979).

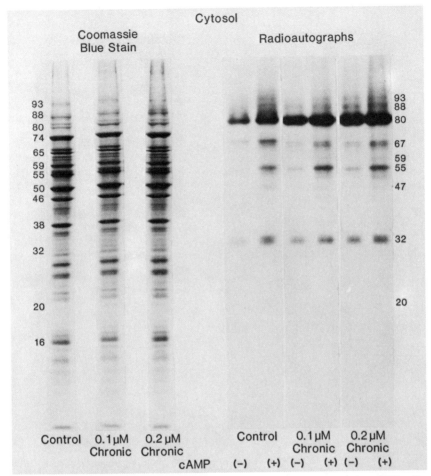

Figure 12.11. Effect of CH₃HgCl on protein phosphorylation in cytosol fraction of NB cells, as shown by results of polyacrylamide gel electrophoresis. See legend of Figure 12.8 for additional information. (Reprinted, by permission, from Ramanujam and Prasad 1979.)

systems can be used to evaluate the effects of other environmental pollutants that are known to possess or have potential to exhibit neurotoxic effects. It is now well established that the phosphorylation of neuronal proteins is an important biological event associated with a variety of neuronal functions. If CH₃HgCl produces a similar change in the phosphorylation levels of neuronal proteins of the central nervous system in vivo, one can suggest that changes in cAMP-dependent and -independent protein phosphorylation may be one of the important biochemical lesions, which could, in part, account for the expression of abnormal neurological symptoms, including alterations

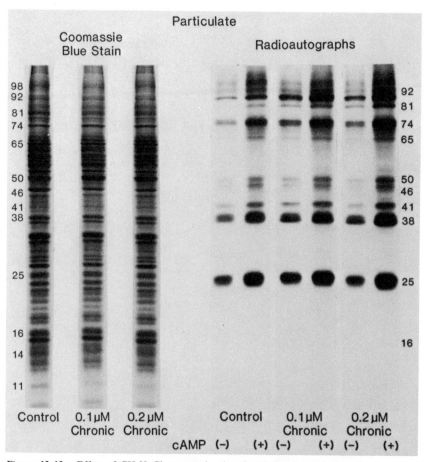

Figure 12.12. Effect of CH₃HgCl on protein phosphorylation in particulate fraction of NB cells, as shown by results of polyacrylamide gel electrophoresis. See legend of Figure 12.8 for additional information. (Reprinted, by permission, from Ramanujam and Prasad 1979.)

in behavior. The present study shows that the combination of glutamate with mercury or manganese compounds produced a synergistic effect on growth inhibition (as the result of cell death and inhibition of cell division). If such interactions are also observed in the central nervous system in vivo, the time of onset and extent of neurological disorders induced by mercury and manganese may be influenced by the availability of glutamate. Our data show that monolayer cultures of neuroblastoma and glioma cells may be useful in identifying the sensitive biological parameters that are affected by heavy metals. In addition, the tissue-culture model may also be useful in studying the modification of effects of heavy metals by endogenous and exogenous agents.

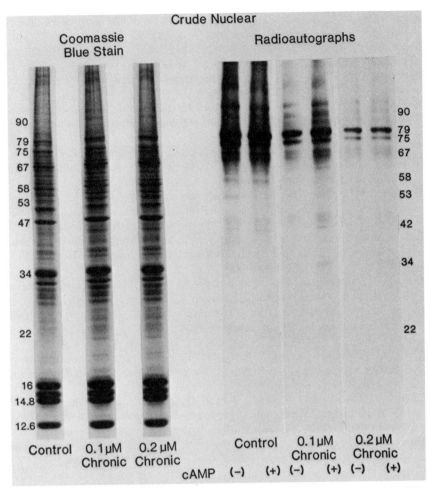

Figure 12.13. Effect of CH₃HgCl on protein phosphorylation in crude nuclear fraction of NB cells as shown by results of polyacrylamide gel electrophoresis. See legend of Figure 12.8 for additional information. (Reprinted, by permission, from Ramanujam and Prasad 1979.)

Acknowledgments

This work was supported by NIH Grant 1 RO1 ES NS 01576 and by the Hereditary Disease Foundation. We thank Marianne Gaschler for her technical assistance.

References

Abe, T.; Haga, T.; and Kurokawa, M. (1975). Blockage of axoplasmic transport and depolymerization of reassembled microtubules by methylmercury. *Brain Res* 86:504–508.

Augusti-Tocco, G., and Sato, G. (1969). Establishment of functional clonal lines of neurons from mouse neuroblastoma. *Proc Natl Acad Sci USA* 64:311–315.

Benda, P.; Lightbody, J.; Sato, G.; Levine, L.; and Sweet, W. (1968). Differentiated rat glial cell strain in tissue culture. *Science* 161:370–371.

Berlin, M., and Ulberg, S. (1963). Accumulation and retention of mercury in the mouse. *Arch Environ Health* 6:589–616.

Berthoud, H. R.; Garman, R. H.; and Weiss, B. (1976). Food intake, body weight, and brain histopathology in mice following chronic methylmercury treatment. *Toxicol Appl Pharmacol* 36:19–30.

Bondy, S. C.; Harrington, M. E.; Anderson, C. L.; and Prasad, K. N. (1979). The effect of low concentrations of organic lead compound on the transport and release of putative neurotransmitters. *Toxicol Lett* 3:35–41.

Braubaker, P. E.; Klein, R.; Herman, S. P.; Lucier, G. W.; Alexander, L. T.; and Long, M. D. (1973). DNA, RNA, and protein synthesis in brain, liver, and kidney of asymptomatic methylmercury treated rats. *Exp Mol Pathol* 18:263–280.

Brewer-Auld, R., and Bedwell, S. F. (1967). Peripheral neuropathy with sympathetic overactivity from industrial contact with acrylamide. *Can Med Assoc J* 96:652–654.

Burg, R. V.; Northington, F. K.; and Shamoo, A. (1980). Methylmercury inhibition of rat brain muscarinic receptors. *Toxicol Appl Pharmacol* 53:285–292.

Butcher, R. W., and Sutherland, E. (1962). Adenosine 3′,5′-phosphate in biological materials: Purification and properties of cyclic 3′,5′-phosphate in human urine. *J Biol Chem* 237:1244–1255.

Carmichael, N., and Cavanagh, J. B. (1976). Autoradiographic localization of *H*-uridine in spinal ganglion neurones of the rat and the effects of methylmercury poisoning. *Acta Neuropathol* 34:137–148.

Cassano, G. B.; Viola, P. L.; Ghetti, B.; and Amaducci, L. (1969). The distribution of inhaled mercury vapors in brains of rats and mice. *J Neuropathol Exp Neurol* 28:308–320.

Chandra, S. V.; Seth, P. K.; and Mankeshwar, J. K. (1974). Manganese poisoning: Clinical and biochemical observations. *Environ Res* 7:374–380.

Chang, L. W. (1977). Neurotoxic effect of mercury: A review. *Environ Res* 14:329–373.

Chang, L. W.; Gilbert, M.; and Sprecher, T. (1978). Modification of methylmercury toxicity by vitamin E. *Environ Res* 17:356–366.

Chang, L. W., and Hartmann, H. A. (1972a). Ultrastructural studies of the nervous system after mercury intoxication, II: Pathological changes in nerve fibers. *Acta Neuropathol* 20:316–334.

——— (1972b). Electron microscopic histochemical study on the localization and distribution of mercury in the nervous system after mercury intoxication. *Exp Neurol* 35:122–137.

Chang, L. W.; Martin, A. H.; and Hartmann, H. A. (1972). Quantitative autoradiographic study on the RNA synthesis in the neurons after mercury intoxication. *Exp Neurol* 37:62–67.

Chang, L. W.; Reuhl, K. R.; and Spyker, J. M. (1977). Ultrastructural study of the latent effects of methylmercury on the nervous system after prenatal exposure. *Environ Res* 13:171–185.

Cheung, M., and Verity, M. A. (1979). Mechanisms of methylmercury inhibition of synaptosome protein synthesis. *Trans Am Soc Neurochem* 10:62a.

Cheung, M.; Verity, M.; Brown, W. J.; and Czer, G. (1977). Methylmercury inhibition of synaptosome and brain slice protein synthesis: In vivo and in vitro studies. *J Neurochem* 29:673–679.

Committee on Biological Effects of Atmospheric Pollution (1973). *Reviews on Manganese.* Washington, D.C.: National Academy of Sciences.

Coyle, J. T.; Molliver, M. E.; and Kuhar, M. J. (1978). In situ injection of kainic acid: A new method for selectively lesioning neuronal cell bodies while sparing axon passage. *J Comp Neurol* 180:301–323.

Coyle, J. T., and Schwarcz, R. (1976). Lesions of striatal neurons with kainic acid provide a model for Huntington's chorea. *Nature* 263:244–246.

DeVellis, J.; Inglish, D.; and Galey, F. (1970). Effects of cortisol and epinephrine on glial cells in culture. In *Cellular Aspects of Growth and Differentiation in Nervous Tissue,* edited by D. Pease, pp. 23–32. Los Angeles: University of California Press.

Ebadi, M. S.; Weiss, B.; and Costa, E. (1971). Distribution of cyclic adenosine monophosphate in rat brain. *Arch Neurol* 24:353–357.

Eto, K., and Takeuchi, T. (1977). Pathological changes of human nerves in Minamata disease (methylmercury poisoning): Light and electron microscopic studies. *Virchow's Arch* 23:109–128.

Fox, J. H.; Patel-Mandlik, K.; and Cohen, M. M. (1975). Comparative effects of organic and inorganic mercury on brain slice respiration and metabolism. *J Neurochem* 24:757–762.

Friberg, L.; Vostal, J.; and Nordberg, G. F. (1972). Inorganic mercury: Relation between exposure and effects. In *Mercury in the Environment,* edited by L. Friberg and J. Vostal, pp. 113–139. Cleveland: CRC Press.

Fullerton, P. M., and Barnes, J. M. (1966). Peripheral neuropathy in rats produced by acrylamide, *Br J Ind Med* 23:210–221.

Garman, R.; Weiss, B.; and Evans, H. L. (1975). Alkylmercurial encephalopathy in the monkey. *Acta Neuropathol* (Berlin) 32:61–74

Goli, K., and Hong, J. S. (1977). Interaction of dopamine, GABA, and substance P in striatonigral neuronal regulation. *Fed Proc* 36:394.

Haas, D. C.; Heir, D. A.; Arnason, B. G. W.; and Young, M. (1972). On a possible relationship of cyclic AMP to the mechanisms of action of nerve growth factor. *Proc Soc Exp Biol Med* 14:45–47.

Haftke, S. C., and Seeds, N. W. (1976). Neuroblastoma: The E. coli of neurobiology? *Life Sci* 16:1649–1657.

Hernberg, S. (1980). Biochemical and clinical effects and responses as indicated by blood concentration. In *Lead Toxicity,* edited by R. Singhal and J. Thomas, pp. 367–400. Baltimore: Urban and Schwarzenberg.

Hrdina, P. D.; Peters, D. A. V.; and Singhal, R. L. (1976). Effect of chronic exposure to cadmium, lead, and mercury on brain biogenic amines in the rat. *Res Commun Chem Pathol Pharmacol* 15:483–493.

Kanazawa, I.; Bird, E.; O'Connell, R.; and Powell, D. (1977). Evidence for a decrease in substance P: Contents of substantia nigra in Huntington's chorea. *Brain Res* 120:387–392.

Kasuya, M. (1975). The effect of vitamin E on the toxicity of alkyl mercurials on nervous tissue in culture. *Toxicol Appl Pharmacol* 32:347–354.

Kean, P., and McLean, W. G. (1972). Effect of dibutyryl cyclic AMP on levels of dopamine β-hydroxylase in isolated superior cervical ganglia. *Arch Pharmacol* 275:465–469.

Kobayashi, H.; Yuyama, A.; Matsusaka, N.; Takeno, K.; and Yanagiya, I. (1980). Effect of methylmercury on brain acetylcholine concentrations and turnover in mice. *Toxicol Appl Pharmacol* 54:1–8.

Koerker, R. L. (1980). The cytotoxicity of methylmercuric hydroxide and colchicine in cultured mouse neuroblastoma cells. *Toxicol Appl Pharmacol* 53:458–469.

Landeka, M., and Kostial, K. (1975). The action of mercury ions on the release of acetylcholine from presynaptic nerve endings. *Experientia* 31:834–835.

Le Quesne, P.M.; Damluji, S.F.; and Rustam, H. (1974). Electrophysiological studies of peripheral nerves in patients with organic mercury poisoning. *J Neurol Neurosurg Psychiatry* 37:333–339.

MacIntyre, E. H.; Wintersgill, C. J.; Perkins, J. P.; and Vatter, A. E. (1972). The response in culture of human tumor astrocytes and neuroblasts to N^6O^2-dibutyryl adenosine 3′,5′-monophosphoric acid. *J Cell Sci* 11:639–662.

MacKay, A. V., and Iversen, L. I. (1972). Increased tyrosine hydroxylase activity of sympathetic ganglia cultured in the presence of dibutyryl cyclic AMP. *Brain Res* 48:424–426.

Mannalis, R. S., and Cooper, G. P. (1975). Evoked transmitter release increased by inorganic mercury at frog neuromuscular junction. *Nature* 257:690–691.

McGeer, E. G., and McGeer, P. L. (1976). Duplications of biochemical changes of Huntington's chorea by intradermal injections of glutamic acid and kainic acid. *Nature* 263:517–519.

Miyakawa, T.; Deshimaru, M.; Sumiyoshi, S.; Teraoka, A.; Udo, N.; Hattori, E.; and Tatetsu, S. (1970). Experimental organic mercury poisoning: Pathological changes in peripheral nerves. *Acta Neuropathol* (Berl) 15:45–55.

Monard, D.; Stockel, K.; Goodman, R.; and Thoenen, H. (1975). Distinction between nerve growth factor and glial factor. *Nature* 258:444–445.

Nakada, S., and Imura, N. (1980). Stimulation of DNA synthesis and pyrimidine deoxyribonucleoside transport systems in mouse glioma and mouse neuroblastoma cells by inorganic mercury. *Toxicol Appl Pharmacol* 53:24–28.

Neathery, M. W., and Miller, W. J. (1973). Metabolism and toxicity of cadmium, mercury, and lead in animals: A review. *J Dairy Sci* 58:1767–1781.

Norseth, T., and Clarkson, T. W. (1970). Studies on the biotransformation of ^{203}Hg-labeled methylmercury chloride in rats. *Arch Environ Health* 21:717–727.

Ostlund, K. (1969). Studies on the metabolism of methylmercury and dimethylmercury in mice. *Acta Pharmacol Toxicol* 27(Suppl. 1):1–30.

Oyaki, Y.; Tanaka, M.; Kubo, H.; and Cichibu, H. (1966). Neuropathological studies on organomercury intoxication with special reference to distribution of mercury granules. *Prog Neurol Res* 10:744–750.

Perkins, J. P.; Moore, M. M.; Kalisker, A.; and Su, Y. F. (1975). Regulations of cyclic AMP content in normal and malignant brain cells. *Adv Cyclic Nucleotide Res* 5:641–660.

Pfeiffer, S. E.; Betschart, B.; Cook, J.; Mancini, P.; and Morris, R. (1977). Glia cell lines. In *Cell, Tissue, and Organ Cultures in Neurobiology,* edited by S. Fedoroff and I. Hertz, pp. 287–346. New York: Academic Press.

Prasad, K. N. (1975). Differentiation of neuroblastoma cells in culture. *Biol Rev* 50:129–165.

―――― (1982). Tissue culture model to study the mechanism of the effect of heavy metals on nerve tissue. In *Mechanism of Actions of Neurotoxic Substances,* edited by K. N. Prasad and A. Vernadakis, pp. 67–94. New York: Raven Press.

Prasad, K. N.; Harrington, M. E.; and Bondy, S. C. (1979*a*). Effects of methylmercuric chloride on high affinity uptake of certain putative neurotransmitters in neuroblastoma and glioma cell cultures. *Toxicol Lett* 4:373–377.

Prasad, K. N.; Nayak, M.; Edward-Prasad, J.; Cummings, S.; and Pattisapu, K. (1980). Modification of glutamate effects on neuroblastoma cells in culture by heavy metals. *Life Sci* 27:2251–2259.

Prasad, K. N., and Nobles, E. (1978). Glioma cells are more sensitive to methylmercury than neuroblastoma cells in culture. *Trans Am Soc Neurochem* 9:25a.

Prasad, K. N.; Nobles, E.; and Ramanujam, M. (1979*b*). Differential sensitivities of glioma cells and neuroblastoma cells to methylmercury toxicity in cultures. *Environ Res* 19:189–201.

Prasad, K. N.; Nobles, E.; and Spuhler, K. (1979*c*). Effect of methylmercuric chloride in the presence of cyclic AMP-stimulating agents on glioma and neuroblastoma cells in culture. *Environ Res* 19:321–338.

Prasad, K. N., and Ramanujam, S. (1980). Vitamin E and vitamin C alter the effect of methylmercuric chloride on neuroblastoma and glioma cells in culture. *Environ Res* 21:343–349.

Prasad, K. N.; Ramanujam, S.; and Gaudreau, D. (1979*d*). Vitamin E induces morphological differentiation and increases the effect of ionizing the radiation on neuroblastoma cells in culture. *Proc Soc Exp Biol Med* 161:570–573.

Ramanujam, M.; Bondy, S. C.; and Prasad, K. N. (1979). Binding of radioactive methylmercuric chloride in subcellular fractions of neuroblastoma and glioma cells in culture. *Toxicol Lett* 3:265–271.

Ramanujam, M., and Prasad, K. N. (1979). Alterations in gene expression after chronic treatment of glioma cells in culture with methylmercuric chloride. *Biochem Pharmacol* 28:2979–2984.

―――― (1980). Effect of methylmercuric chloride on gene expression in neuroblastoma and glioma cells after acute and chronic treatments. *Biochem Pharmacol* 29:539–552.

Roisen, F. J.; Murphy, R. A.; Pichichero, M. E.; and Braden, W. G. (1972). Cyclic adenosine monophosphate stimulation of axonal elongation. *Science* 175:73–74.

Schmidt, M. J., and Robison, C. A. (1970). Cyclic AMP, adenyl cyclase, and the effect of norepinephrine in the developing rat brain. *Fed Proc* 29:479a.

Schwarcz, R. C.; Bennett, J. P.; and Coyle, J. T. (1977). Loss of striatal serotonin synaptic receptor binding induced by kainic acid lesions: Correlation with Huntington's disease. *J Neurochem* 28:867–869.

Schwarcz, R. C., and Coyle, J. T. (1977). Neurochemical sequelae of kainate injections in corpus striatum and substantia nigra of rat. *Life Sci* 20:431–436.

Shapiro, D. L. (1973). Morphological and biochemical alterations in foetal rat brain cells cultured in the presence of monobutyryl cyclic AMP. *Nature* 241:203–204.

Shrivastav, B. B.; Brodwick, M. S.; and Narahashi, T. (1976). Methylmercury: Effects on electrical properties of squid axon membranes. *Life Sci* 18:1077–1082.

Somjen, G. G.; Herman, S. P.; Klein, R.; Brubaker, P. E.; Briner, W. H.; Goodrich, J. K.; Krigman, M. R.; and Haseman, J. K. (1973). The uptake of methylmercury (^{203}Hg) in different tissue related to its neurotoxic effects. *J Pharmacol Exp Ther* 187:602–611.

Spuhler, K., and Prasad, K. N. (1980). Inhibition by methylmercuric chloride of prostaglandin E_1-sensitive adenylate cyclase activity in glioma but not in neuroblastoma cells in culture. *Biochem Pharmacol* 29:201–203.

Syversen, T. L. M. (1974). Biotransformation of Hg-203 labelled methylmercuric chloride in rat brain measured by specific determination of Hg^{2+}. *Acta Pharmacol Toxicol* 35:277–283.

Takeuchi, T. (1968). Experiments with organic mercury, particularly with methylmercury compounds: Similarities between experimental poisoning and Minamata disease. In *Minamata Disease,* edited by M. Kutsuma, pp. 229–252. Tokyo: University of Tokyo Press.

———— (1972). Biological reactions and pathological changes in human beings and animals under conditions of organic mercury contamination. In *Environmental Mercury Contamination,* edited by R. Hartung and B. D. Dinman, pp. 247–289. Ann Arbor: Ann Arbor Science.

Taylor, L. L., and DiStefano, V. (1976). Effect of methylmercury on brain biogenic amines in developing rat pup. *Toxicol Appl Lett* 38:489–497.

Vallee, B. L., and Ulner, D. D. (1972). Biochemical effects of mercury, cadmium, and lead. *Ann Rev Biochem* 41:91–128.

Vernadakis, A., and Nidess, R. (1976). Biochemical characteristics of C-6 glia cells. *Neurochem Res* 1:385–402.

Weiss, B. (1977). The behavioral toxicology of metals. *Fed Proc* 37:22–27.

Weiss, B.; Shein, H. M.; and Snyder, R. (1971). Adenylate cyclase and phosphodiesterase activity of normal and SV_{40} virus transformed hamster astrocytes in cell culture. *Life Sci* 10:1253–1260.

Welsh, S. O., and Soares, J. H. Jr. (1976). The protective effect of vitamin E and selenium against methylmercury toxicity in the Japanese quail. *Nutr Rep Ing* 13:43–51.

Wuerthele, S. M.; Lovell, K. L.; Jones, M. Z.; and Moore, K. E. (1978). A histological study of kainic acid induced lesions in the rat brain. *Brain Res* 149:489–497.

Yoshino, Y.; Mozai, T.; and Nakao, K. (1966). Distribution of mercury in the brain and its subcellular units in experimental organic mercury poisonings. *J Neurochem* 13:397–406.

Contributors

Zoltan Annau, Ph.D., Department of Environmental Health Sciences, The Johns Hopkins University School of Hygiene and Public Health, Baltimore, Maryland

William D. Atchison, Ph.D., Department of Pharmacology and Toxicology, Neuroscience Program, and Center for Environmental Toxicology, Michigan State University, East Lansing, Michigan

Thomas M. Burbacher, Ph.D., Department of Pathology, University of Washington, Seattle, Washington

Louis W. Chang, Ph.D., Department of Pathology, University of Arkansas for Medical Sciences, Little Rock, Arkansas

Christine U. Eccles, Ph.D., Department of Pharmacology and Toxicology, School of Pharmacy, University of Maryland, Baltimore, Maryland

Hannu Komulainen, Department of Pharmacology and Toxicology, University of Kuopio, Department of Environmental Hygiene and Toxicology, National Public Health Institute, Kuopio, Finland

Laszlo Magos, M.C., F.R.C.Path., Medical Research Council, Toxicology Unit, Carshalton, Surrey, England

David O. Marsh, M.D., Department of Neurology and Division of Toxicology, University of Rochester School of Medicine and Dentistry, Rochester, New York

N. Karle Mottet, M.D., Department of Pathology, University of Washington, Seattle, Washington

Paul Mushak, Ph.D., Department of Pathology, University of North Carolina, Chapel Hill, North Carolina

Kedar N. Prasad, Ph.D., Department of Radiology, University of Colorado Health Sciences Center, Denver, Colorado

Adil E. Shamoo, Ph.D., Department of Biochemistry, University of Maryland School of Medicine, Baltimore, Maryland

Cheng-Mei Shaw, M.D., Department of Pathology, University of Washington, Seattle, Washington

Tore L. M. Syversen, Ph.D., Department of Pharmacology and Toxicology, University of Trondheim, Trondheim, Norway

David J. Thomas, Ph.D., Department of Pediatrics, The Johns Hopkins University School of Medicine, Baltimore, Maryland

Jouko Tuomisto, Ph.D., Department of Pharmacology and Toxicology, National Public Health Institute, Kuopio, Finland

Index

Absorption
 d-penicillamine, protective role of, 26
 gastrointestinal, 26–27
 in guinea pigs, 26
 in human skin, 26
 of methyl mercury dicyandiamide, 26
 percutaneous, 25–26
 in piglets, 26
 pulmonary, 25
 in rats, 26
Adenylate cyclase in C-6 and NB cells
 dopamine-sensitive, 237
 norepinephrine-sensitive, 237
 PGE-sensitive, 236
Analysis
 dimethyl mercury, 3
 gas-liquid chromatography, 3–7
 hair, 1–2, 9
 high-performance liquid chromatography,
  8
 methyl and inorganic mercury, 8–10
 sampling and sample handling, 1–2
 speciation, 1, 8–10
 Westöö method of, 6–7, 9

Behavioral effects
 active avoidance, 122–23
 apomorphine-induced stereotypy, 124
 conditioned suppression, 122
 continuous reinforcement, 123
 convulsive behavior, 122
 cross-fostering, effects of, on, 122
 d-amphetamine and motor activity, 124
 neonatal behavior, 124
 open field activity, 122
 passive avoidance, 122–23
 swimming behavior, 122
 time of treatment, role of, 125
 ultrasonic vocalization, 124–25
 water escape, 123
Biodegradation, 30–33

Biological half time
 and body burden, 34–35
 clearance, 34
 elimination constant, 34–36
 steady state, 35
Biotransformation, 19. *See also*
  Biodegradation
Body burden, 34–35
Brain distribution
 brain/blood concentration ratio, 30
 brain stem, 31
 caudate nucleus, 31
 cerebellum, 30–31
 cerebral cortex, 30–31
 corpus callosum, 31
 dentate nucleus, 31
 dorsal and ventral roots, 31
 human, 30
 hypothalamus, 31
 lateral geniculate nucleus, 31
 midbrain, 31
 sciatic nerve, 31
 species comparisons of, 30–31
 spinal cord, 31
 spinal ganglia, 31
 subcellular distribution, 55–56

Calcium and calcium antagonists, 14–15,
  197–99, 200–205
Calmodulin, 16
Calomel, and acrodynia, 17
cAMP-stimulating agents in tissue culture
 morphological differentiation induced by,
  225–27
 phosphodiesterase inhibitors, 227–29
 prostaglandins, 225–27
Catecholaminergic neurotransmission
 catechol-O-methyltransferase, 175–76
 cGMP, 179
 in development, 175–76
 DOPA decarboxylase, 175
 dopamine levels, 176

Catecholaminergic *(cont.)*
  dopamine receptors, 175
  dopamine uptake, 175
  noradrenaline levels, 176
  noradrenaline uptake, 175
  tyrosine hydroxylase, 175–76
Cholinergic transmission, 173–75. *See also*
    Synaptic transmission
  acetylcholine esterase, 173
  choline acetyltransferase, 173
  choline uptake, 173, 237
  muscarinic receptor binding in, 19–20,
    173, 207, 237
  neurophysiology of, 190–208
Cross-fostering, 122

Developing nervous system, 118–26
  cerebellum, 119
  glutamic acid decarboxylase, 125
  myelin formation in, 120
  periods of development in, 119
  proliferation, migration, and differentiation
    in, 119
  ultrastructural effects in, 119–20
Dimethyl mercury, 25
Distribution
  in blood, 27–28
  in brain, 30–31
  extravascular, 28–32
  fetal and placental, 32
  effects of glutathione on, 27–28
  in hair, pelt, or fur, 31–32
  in hemoglobin, 27–28
  in humans, 30
  in kidney, 27, 28–29
  in liver, 28
  organ/blood concentration ratios, 28–29
  in rats, 27–32
  red blood cell/plasma ratio, 27
  in sheep, 31
  in spleen, 28
d-penicillamine, 20, 25–27, 204
Dose-response relationships
  and blood levels, 45, 48–50
  and clearance half time, 50
  and concentration in fish, 48
  in hair levels, 45, 47–51
  in humans, 45–51
  in Iraq, 48–49
  in Minamata, 48
  of neurological effects, 45–47
  in Niigata, 48

Dose-response relationships *(cont.)*
  and paresthesia, 45–46, 49–50
  postnatal, 48–50
  prenatal, 50–51
  and protein synthesis, 161–63
  selenium, protective effect of, 51

Endoplasmic reticulum, 16
Excretion
  bile, 37
  enterohepatic circulation, 37
  feces, 36–37
  glutathione, 37
  hair or fur, 38
  kidney, 37
  lactation, 38
  ligandin, role of, 37
  in monkey, 37
  in pigs, 36
  polythiol resin, effect of, on, 37
  in rats, 36–37
  in urine, 36–37

Fetal accumulation, 115–16

GABAergic transmission, 181
  benzodiazepine receptor binding, 181
  glutamic acid decarboxylase, 125
Gas-liquid chromatography
  alkaline digestion, 7
  atomic absorption, 5–6
  atomic emission, 5–6
  column/column packing, 3–4
  complexing/extracting agents, 7
  detection system, 3–6
  electron capture, 5
  of fish samples, 7
  mass spectrometer, 5
  Westöö method of, 6–7
Gene expression in C-6 and NB cells, 238–44
Glutamate, 181, 232–35
  and clinical disease, 235
  and manganese chloride, 234–35
  and mercury toxicity, enhancement of,
    233–35
  in neuroblastoma, 232–35
  uptake, 238
Glutamic acid decarboxylase, 125

Heavy metals
  as calcium antagonists, 14–15, 197–99,
    200–205

Heavy metals *(cont.)*
  and calmodulin, 16
  and chelating agents, 13
  covalent bonds with, 13–14
  inorganic, 13–15
  interaction with cell components, 15–16
  and intracellular organelles, 16
  ionic bonds with, 13–14
  organic, 15
  physico-chemical characteristics of, 13–15
  and plasma membrane, 16
  and proteins, 13–15
  and skeletal muscle, 15
  and soluble proteins, 16
  and sulfhydryl groups, 16–18, 20
  target sites of, 13–18
High-performance liquid chromatography, 8

Manganese, 17–18, 234–35
  and calcium transport, 17–18
  and sulfhydryl groups, 17–18
  in tissue culture, 234–35
Membrane, functions and components of, 16
Mercury vapor, 24–25
Methoxyethyl mercury, 24
Methyl and inorganic mercury, analysis of,
  8–10
  atomic absorption, 9
  gas-liquid chromatography, 9–10
  inorganic, 9
  Magos method, 9
  neutron activation, 9
  Westöö method, 9
Minamata disease, 18
Mitochondria, 16
Muscarinic receptors, 19–20, 173, 207, 237
Muscle twitch, 190–92

Nerve and muscle membrane
  barnacle muscle fibers, 210
  frog sciatic nerve, 210
  frog skeletal muscle, 210
  neuroblastoma, 209
  sodium activation mechanisms in, 211
  squid axon, 210
Neurochemical effects, 172–84
  catecholaminergic transmission, 175–79
  cholinergic transmission, 173–75
  GABA and amino acids, 181
  and pharmacokinetics, 181

Neurochemical effects *(cont.)*
  possible mechanisms of, 183
  serotonergic transmission, 179–81
Neurological effects, 45–50
  abnormal reflexes, 46–47
  ataxia, 45
  chorea, 46
  dysarthria, 45
  impaired vision, 45
  Iraq, 46
  Minamata, 45–46
  paresthesia, 45–46
  postnatal, 45–46
  prenatal, 46–47
  sensory deficits, 45
Neuromuscular disorders, 18–19
Neuronal migration, 47, 93
Neuropathology, 47, 54–72
  after acute exposure, 87–88
  of blood-brain barrier, 54
  cerebellar, 59–60, 87
  of cerebral cortex, 47, 87–92
  after chronic low-dose exposure, 88–92
  in dentate nucleus, 87
  of dorsal root ganglia, 60–61
  and glia, 59, 87
  of granular neurons, 59, 90–91
  in humans, 47
  of lateral geniculate, 87
  and lysosomes, 61
  in monkeys, 86–92, 106–7
  of myelin sheath, 66, 87
  of Purkinje neurons, 60
  and rough endoplasmic reticulum, 60–61
  of sensory neurons, 60–61
Neurophysiology in clinical studies, 190
Neurotransmitter release, spontaneous
  Bay K-8644, 205
  and calcium, intracellular, 203–4
  calcium dependence of, 200–205
  calcium ionophores and, 205
  lanthanum chloride and, 204
  MEPP frequency, 199–205
  postulated mechanisms, 211, 213–14
  ruthenium red, 203

Oxidation, 24
Oxidation states, 17

Paresthesia, 45–46, 49–50
Pathology, non-neuronal, 73, 77–86, 92–99

Pathology *(cont.)*
  cerebrovascular lesions, 91
  colon, 84
  fatty accumulation in liver, 85
  gastrointestinal tract, 79–84
  gingivitis, stomatitis, 80
  heart, 86
  kidney, 77–79
  liver, 85
  Paneth cells, 80–84
  proximal convoluted tubules, 77–78
  relationship to blood levels, 75–77
Phenyl mercury, 24
Placental transfer, 115–16
Postsynaptic actions, 205–8
  ACh receptor sulfhydryl groups, 208
  at motor end-plate, 206
  in neuroblastoma, 206–7
  at receptors, 207
Prenatal effects in humans, 46–47
Prenatal exposure, 114–26
  behavioral consequences of, 121–25 (*see also* Behavioral effects)
  and cytochrome P450, 118
  early childhood exposure, compared with, 114–15
  electrophysiological consequences of, 120–21
  embryocidal effects after, 116–17
  fetal liver and kidney effects after, 118
  nervous system, 118–26 (*see also* Developing nervous system)
  neuropathology after, 114
  and strain differences, 117
  teratogenic effects after, 116–18
Prostaglandins, 225–27, 236
Protein phosphorylation in tissue culture, 240–44
  after acute treatment, 242
  after chronic treatment, 241–42
Protein synthesis, 131–64
  in adrenal glands, effects of corticosterone on, 143–44
  in brain slices, 145–46
  in cell-free systems, 152–56
  in central nervous system, 131–50
  after chronic exposure in isolated neurons, 148
  and dose-effect relationships, 161–63
  after exposure in adults, 139–44
  and food intake and cachectic effects, 140–42

Protein synthesis *(cont.)*
  in glioma cells, 151–52
  in HeLa S3 cells, 150–51
  after in vitro exposure, 145–59
  in leukemic cells, 150
  in neuronal cells, 146–50
  and peptide chain elongation, 138–39
  after pre- and perinatal exposure, 134–39
  regional specificity of mercury and, 136–37
  in synaptosomal preparations, 156–59

Receptor interactions, 19–20
Reproductive effects, 92–99. *See also* Prenatal effects
  abortion rate, 92
  birth weights, 98
  brain anomalies, 95
  cerebral cortical degeneration, 97
  cerebral palsy, 93, 97
  embryopathic effects, 93–99
  and microtubules, 99
  mitotic rate, 98
  neuronal migration and, 93, 98
  neurotoxicity during pregnancy, 96
  pregnancy outcome, 92–93
  seminiferous tubules, 93
  spermatogenesis, 93

Secd dressings, fungicides, 104
Selenium, 51
Sensory deficits, 104–11. *See also* Visual effects
  blood levels associated with, 106–7
  in dogs, 108–9
  dose schedules and, 107
  in guinea pigs, 109
  gustatory impairment, 105
  hearing impairment, 105, 109
  human symptoms, 45–46, 104–5, 108–10
  Hunter-Russell syndrome, 104–5
  in monkeys, 104–8
  neuronal loss associated with, 106
  in rats, 104, 108
  recovery of function, 107
  sensory nerve, electrophysiological changes in, 110
  startle stimuli, 109–10
  touch sensation, 106
  two-point discrimination, 104
  visual effects, 104–9
  visual field constriction, 105, 107

Sensory nerve electrophysiology, 110
Serotonergic transmission, 179–81
Synaptic transmission, 192–209
    autonomic ganglia, 196
    calcium, voltage-dependent entry, 198
    calcium concentration, external, 196
    end-plate potentials, 193–99
    mean quantal content, 196
    miniature end-plate potentials, 193–94,
        199–205
    postulated mechanisms of, 211–14
    probability of release, 196
    release of acetylcholine, nerve-evoked,
        193–99
    release of acetylcholine, spontaneous,
        199–207, 211–13

Tissue culture
    adenylate cyclase sensitivity to
        neurotransmitters, 236–37
    cAMP-stimulating agents in, 225–29
    effects of manganese in, 234–35
    effects of vitamin C in, 230
    effects of vitamin E in, 229–30

Tissue culture *(cont.)*
    embryonic nerve tissue, compared with,
        221
    gene expression in, 238–44
    glioma factors in growth medium of,
        230–32
    glutamate and enhanced toxicity in, 232–35
    model systems of, 220–22
    neurotransmitter uptake in, 237–38
    protein phosphorylation in, 240–44
    relative sensitivity to mercurials in, 222–25

Vapor pressure, 25
Visual effects, 104–9. *See also* Sensory
        deficits
    blood levels associated with, 106–7
    critical fusion intensity, 107
    recovery of function, 107
    spatial contrast sensitivity, 108
    visual discrimination, 105–6
    visual evoked potential, 108–9
    visual field constriction, 105, 107
    Wisconsin General Test, 106–7

The Toxicity of Methyl Mercury

Designed by Chris L. Smith
Composed by BG Composition, Inc., in Times Roman text and display
Printed by Thomson-Shore on 60-lb. Glatfelter Spring Forge White and
bound in GSB #12 and stamped in black